Textbook of
Ayurveda

Other Books by Vasant D. Lad

Ayurveda: The Science of Self-Healing. 1985

Secrets of the Pulse: The Ancient Art
of Ayurvedic Pulse Diagnosis. 1996, 2006, 2nd ed.

The Complete Book of Ayurvedic Home Remedies. 1998

Strands of Eternity: A Compilation of
Mystical Poetry and Discourses. 2004

Ayurvedic Perspectives on Selected Pathologies 2005, 2018, 3rd ed.

The Textbook of Ayurveda: A Complete Guide
to Clinical Assessment, Volume Two. 2006

Pranayama for Self-Healing. DVD, 2010

The Textbook of Ayurveda: General Principles of Management
and Treatment, Volume Three. 2012

Applied Marma Therapy Cards. 2013

The Yoga of Herbs: An Ayurvedic Guide to Herbal Medicine. 1986
by Vasant Lad and David Frawley

Ayurvedic Cooking for Self-Healing.
1994, 1997, 2nd ed. Hardcover, 2015
by Usha and Vasant Lad

Marma Points of Ayurveda: The Energy Pathways
for Healing Body, Mind and Consciousness
with a Comparison to Traditional Chinese Medicine.
2008, Paperback, 2016
by Vasant Lad and Anisha Durve

Ayuryoga: VPK Basics. 2014
by Vasant Lad and Maria Garre

Textbook of Ayurveda

Fundamental Principles
of Ayurveda
Volume One

by
Vasant D. Lad, M.A.Sc.

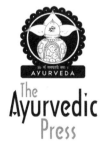

The
Ayurvedic
Press

Albuquerque, New Mexico

Copyright © **2002** by Vasant D. Lad

ALL RIGHTS RESERVED. First Edition 2002.
Printed in Malaysia.
21 20 19 18   6   7   8   9
This book is printed on acid-free paper.
ISBN-13: 978-1-883725-07-5

Cover design and illustration: Kevin Curry.
Illustrations by Shawn O'Connor. Illustrations in Chapters 4 and 8 by Carlos Luna. All art in this book is based on drawings by Vasant Lad.
Ganesha drawings in front pages by Vasant Lad.
Layout by Laura Humphreys.
Edited by Glen Crowther and Margaret Smith Peet.

Library of Congress Cataloging-in-Publication Data

Lad, Vasant, 1943-
    Textbook of Ayurveda / by Vasant Dattatray Lad.
        p. cm.
Includes bibliographical references and index.
        ISBN: 1-883725-07-0
    1. Medicine, Ayurvedic--History. 2. Medicine, Ayurvedic--Philosophy.
I. Title.
        R606 L33 2000
        615.5'3--dc21
                                                    00-009373

Published by **The Ayurvedic Press** • P.O. Box 23445 • Albuquerque, NM 87192-1445

For more information on Ayurveda, contact:
The Ayurvedic Institute
11311 Menaul Blvd. NE
Albuquerque, NM 87112
(505)291-9698 • Fax 505.294.7572 • www.ayurveda.com

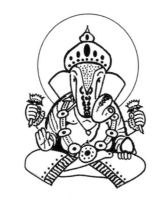

Dedication

|| श्रीः ||

This book is dedicated with all my heart to my loving wife, Usha, who has inspired and supported me in all walks of my life.

About the Cover

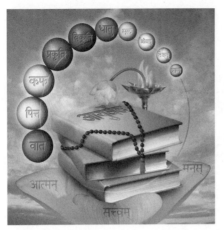

The image represented on the cover of this textbook originated in Dr. Lad's meditation. Out of the depth of his love for his students and for Āyurveda, he is sharing it as his vision of the order, beauty, and poetry of life.

The three books pictured here represent the three sages, Charaka, Sushruta, and Vāgbhata, who served as vehicles for the Āyur Vidya, and gave to the world the "Great Three" texts on Āyurveda. The ghee lamp signifies the flame of attention, intuition, and the dedicated study that unlocks the true meaning existing in the wealth of information presented in these three great texts. It is the light of inner knowledge and the light of life.

Illuminated by this light of truth, the ātma, one's Self, the manas, one's mind, and sattvam, the truth of existence, rest peacefully on the petals of the lotus. The lotus flower is the purity, sacredness, and simplicity that are characteristic of the devoted student's being. These qualities are the perfume of the life that is lived in harmony and cooperation with Nature.

The thread of wisdom that runs through and encircles the texts is the thread of true knowledge that remains unbroken and unchanged throughout the shifting ages and cultures. The timeless wisdom of Āyurveda joins the individual, manifested life with the eternal Cosmic Life. It also weaves itself through all the components of the individual body-mind: sattva, rajas, tamas; ojas, tejas, and prāna; the seven dhātus, and three doshas. The thread of Wisdom is the integrating factor that allows these components to function together in equilibrium, bringing harmony and peace to the body and mind.

The visions that come in the meditative mind convey the order and beauty of life in a way that cannot always be expressed in words. They express the poetry of life. The life that is lived in cooperation and harmony with Nature is itself poetry. Students are encouraged to meditate on this loving vision of Āyurveda and its role in the individual and Cosmic life.

Table of Contents

Foreword xv
Preface xix
About the Author xxi
The Use of Sanskrit xxiii

1 **Shad Darshan, The Six Philosophies of Life | 1**
Introduction 1
Sānkhya 5
    Purusha and Prakruti 5
    Mahad (Creative Intelligence) 6
    Ahamkāra 8
    Sattva, Rajas, Tamas 8
Nyāya and Vaisheshika 10
    The Four Pramāna–Sources of Valid Knowledge 11
    The Elements 12
    Soul (Ātman) 15
    Mind (Manas) 16
    Time (Kālā) 16
    Direction (Dig) 17
Mīmāmsa 18
Yoga 19
Vedānta 20
Buddhism 21

2 **Universal Attributes and Doshic Theory | 25**
The Five Elements and Their Attributes 25
The Five Elements and Tanmātrās 27
The Basic Attributes of Tridosha—Vāta, Pitta, Kapha 29
Attributes (Gunas) and Their Effects on Doshas 30
Prakruti: Your Unique Body Type 35
    Vikruti 36
    Characteristics of the Vāta Individual 39
    Characteristics of the Pitta Individual 39
    Characteristics of the Kapha Individual 40

3 **The Doshas and Their Subtypes | 45**
Vāta and Its Subtypes 45
    Prāna Vāyu 48
    Udāna Vāyu 50
    Samāna Vāyu 51
    Apāna Vāyu 52
    Vyāna Vāyu 53
Pitta and Its Subtypes 53
    Pāchaka Pitta 56

Rañjaka Pitta 57
Sādhaka Pitta 59
Ālochaka Pitta 63
Bhrājaka Pitta 64
Kapha and Its Subtypes 65
Kledaka Kapha 68
Avalambaka Kapha 70
Bodhaka Kapha 71
Tarpaka Kapha 74
Shleshaka Kapha 77
Summary 78

4   **Agni, The Digestive Fire | 81**
Agni, the Digestive Fire 81
Agni and the Five Elements 83
The Role of Agni in Digestion 84
Normal Functions of Agni 86
The Doshas and Agni 89
The Four Varieties of Agni 90
The 40 Main Types of Agni 92
The Subtypes of Agni 92
Summary 101

5   **Dhātus, The Seven Bodily Tissues | 103**
Introduction 103
Nutrition and Structure of the Dhātus 104
Dhātu By-products 106
Disorders of the Dhātus 106
Rasa Dhātu: the Plasma Tissue 107
By-products of Rasa Dhātu 109
Disorders of Rasa Dhātu 110
Fever 111
Decreased and Increased Rasa Dhātu 111
Rakta Dhātu: the Blood Tissue 113
Red Blood Cells 114
By-products of Rakta Dhātu 116
Disorders of Rakta Dhātu 117
The Health of the Blood Vessels 120
Māmsa Dhātu: the Muscle Tissue 122
Types of Muscles and Their Functions 124
By-products of Māmsa Dhātu 125
Disorders of Māmsa Dhātu 127
The Role of Māmsa Dhatu In Emotional Well Being 129
Meditation and Māmsa Dhātu 130
Meda Dhātu: the Fat Tissue 132
By-products of Meda Dhātu 134
Disorders of Meda Dhātu 135

Awareness and Meda 142
Asthi Dhātu: the Bone Tissue 144
  By-products of Asthi Dhātu 145
  Disorders of Asthi Dhātu 147
Majjā Dhātu: the Nerve Tissue and Bone Marrow 151
  Majjā and the Prenatal Development Stage 152
  The Functions of Majjā Dhātu 155
  By-products of Majjā Dhātu 161
  Dreams 161
  Disorders of Majjā Dhātu 162
Shukra and Ārtava Dhātus: Male and Female Reproductive Tissues 168
  By-products of Shukra and Ārtava Dhātus 169
Shukra Dhātu 169
Ārtava Dhātu 172
  Disorders of Shukra/Ārtava Dhātus 174
Conclusion 175

6   **Srotāmsi, The Bodily Channels and Systems | 177**
Introduction 177
Sroto Dushti 180
The Channels to Receive: Food, Prāna, Water 181
  Anna Vaha Srotas: The Channel of Food 181
  Prāna Vaha Srotas: The Respiratory Channel 183
  Ambu Vaha Srotas: The Channel for Water 184
The Channels to Nourish and Maintain the Body: The Dhātu Srotāmsi 185
  Rasa Vaha Srotas: The Channel for Plasma 185
  Rakta Vaha Srotas: The Channel for Blood 186
  Māmsa Vaha Srotas: The Channel for Muscle 186
  Meda Vaha Srotas: The Channel for Fat 186
  Asthi Vaha Srotas: The Channel for Bone 187
  Majjā Vaha Srotas: The Channel for the Nerves and Bone Marrow 188
  Shukra/Ārtava Vaha Srotas: The Channel for Reproductive Tissue 188
  Rajah Vaha Srotas: The Channel for Menstruation 189
  Stanya Vaha Srotas: The Channel for Lactation 189
Channels of Elimination: Feces, Urine, Sweat 189
  Purisha Vaha Srotas: The Channel for Feces 189
  Mūtra Vaha Srotas: The Channel for Urine 191
  Sveda Vaha Srotas: The Channel for Sweat 192
Mano Vaha Srotas: The Channel of the Mind 193
  States of Mind 193
  Manifestations of the Mind 194
  Chakras, Koshas, and the Mind 195
  Perception, Awareness, and the Mind 197
  Individual Mind and Universal Mind 198
  Mind in the Lower Three Chakras 200
  Heart Chakra: Bridge to Higher Consciousness 200
  The Mind and the Higher Three Chakras 201

States of Awareness 202
  The Universality of Mind 202
  Disorders of Mano Vaha Srotas 203
  Witnessing Awareness 204
Conclusion 205

7 **Ojas, Tejas, Prāna | 207**
Ojas 208
  Inferior and Superior Ojas 210
  Disorders of Ojas 213
  Causes of Disorders of Ojas 215
Tejas 216
  Qualities of Tejas 217
  Manifestations of Tejas 220
  Tejas and Karma 221
  Tejas and Kundalinī 223
Prāna 224
The Functional Integrity of Prāna, Tejas, and Ojas 228
Soma 229
Awareness 231

8 **Digestion and Nutrition | 235**
Rasa (Taste) 235
  How Taste Relates to the Elements 236
  Relation of Rasa to Tongue and Organs 237
Pharmacological and Psychological Actions of the Six Tastes 238
  Sweet 238
  Sour 240
  Salty 241
  Pungent 242
  Bitter 243
  Astringent 244
  Cravings 246
Vīrya (Potent Energy) 246
Vipāka (Post-Digestive Effect) 248
Prabhāva (Unique, Specific Action) 249
  Actions of Rasa, Vīrya, Vipāka, and Prabhāva 250
Digestion 251
  The Stages of Digestion 252
How to Eat a Balanced Diet 258
  Nutritional Disorders 259
Food Combining 260
The Three Laws of Nutrition 261
  Nutrition Begins at Conception 263
Cellular Metabolism (Pīlu Pāka) 265
  Pīlu Pāka and Pithara Pāka 266
  Desire 268

Thoughts, Feelings, and Emotions 270
Conclusion 273

9   **Conclusion | 275**
The Āyurvedic Definition of Health 275
The Doshas 276
The Interactions of the Doshas 277
Factors That Affect Our Health 278
Choosing a Balanced Lifestyle 279
Relationships, Emotions, and Meditation 279
Behavioral Medicine 280

Appendix | 283

Glossary | 295

Bibliography and Selected Readings | 311

Acknowledgements | 313

Index | 315

List of Tables

Shad Darshan: The Six Philosophies of Life 4

The Elements and Associated Types of Energy 14

The Senses and the Elements 27

The 20 Attributes and Their Relation ship to the Tridosha 31

The Attributes of the Vāta Individual 42

The Attributes of the Pitta Individual 43

The Attributes of the Kapha Individual 44

The Subtypes of Vāta 46

The Subtypes of Pitta 55

The Subtypes of Kapha 68

The Four Varieties of Agni 92

The Amino Acids and 20 Gunas 98

The Seven Dhātus 104

Signs and Symptoms of Rasa Disorders 110

Signs and Symptoms of Rakta Disorders 118

Blood Types Correlated to the Doshas 120

Signs and Symptoms of Māmsa Disorders 129

Signs and Symptoms of Meda Disorders 137

Signs and Symptoms of Asthi Disorders 149

Signs and Symptoms of Majjā Disorders 167

Signs and Symptoms of Shukra and Ārtava Disorders 174

Four Types of Sroto Dushti 180

The Chakras and the Koshas 196

Functions of Tejas 216

Five Elements and Foods 236

Taste and the Five Elements 237

Tastes and Their Related Organs 238

Effects of Tastes on the Doshas 245

Functions and Effects of Vīrya 247

Effects of Rasa and Vipāka on the Doshas 249

Digestion: Fields of Experience and Action 251

Examples of Attributes of Certain Foods 258

The Twenty Attributes (Gunas) and Their Effects on the Doshas 283

The Seven Bodily Tissues (Sapta Dhātu) 284

The 40 Main Types of Agni 285

Disorders of Ojas, Tejas, and Prāna 287
Srotāmsi, the Systems and Channels of the Body 288
Relationship of Sattva, Rajas, and Tamas to Foods and Behavior 290
Food Guidelines for Basic Constitutional Types 291

Foreword

आयुर्वेद

India is a land of magnificent diversity, a place where archaic structures, concepts and traditions rub shoulders with up-to-the-minute formations, where variety and extremity stride hand in hand. No country any less richly textured could have given birth, thousands of years ago, to Āyurveda, and no other country could have prompted the sometimes bewildering multiplicity of principles and practices that have sprouted from Āyurveda's roots.

New growth will inevitably burgeon from Āyurveda, and from its sister sciences such as Yoga, Jyotisha, and Vastu, each of which is an expression of the "living wisdom" that is a *vidya*. These vidyas are living beings, goddess manifestations of the totality of one aspect of the natural world. Āyurveda, for example, is the articulation in human terms of the *Ayur Vidya*, the "lore of life," the power of Nature that cures disease and promotes health. Doctors cannot themselves cure diseases; they can only act to assist Nature's healing efforts. All first-rate physicians serve as vehicles for the Ayur Vidya, but too often they perform this service unaware of the nature of the Ayur Vidya herself. Good Āyurvedic training fosters a profound personal relationship between the student and the Ayur Vidya, to enable the conscious descent of that vidya into the postulant.

The vidyas themselves are perennial, but their manifestations in our impermanent world are ever-changing. The ultimate, timeless version of a vidya is perpetually available to whoever can locate and tap into it; whoever can contact the muse that is the Ayur Vidya will find her guiding and inspiring their progress. Those who are unable to achieve the vidya herself can employ the more limited adaptations that human physicians have codified and elaborated for us. Taken together, the many elaborations of the Ayur Vidya represent the accumulated wisdom of how to effectively apply one aspect of nature's healing potential in a human context.

Living wisdom gains richness and fluency with each successful transfer from one proficient human vehicle to the next, developing its own life as it is exercised. For many centuries, the Ayur Vidya has offered the boon of Āyurveda to generations of Indian physicians, and to those from other lands (Tibet, China, Persia, Greece, Arabia) who have made the pilgrimage to India's temples of healing. Now, the good news of Āyurveda is finally making its way West.

Until recently the materialistic, mechanistic philosophical climate here in the West could not support the Ayur Vidya, but over the last half-century alternative ways of seeing the world have spread widely enough to permit Āyurveda to start naturalizing itself on Western soil. The first Ayur sprouts were weak and tentative, and many failed to thrive, but a few did take root and have flourished. One of the premier garden plots of Āyurvedic education in the USA is located in Albuquerque, New Mexico, at the Ayurvedic Institute. The Institute has strived since its inception to sow the seeds of the good news of Āyurveda into every available field, by means of lectures, books, and tapes. Early publications focused on Āyurveda's most basic tenets, and teaching materials have gradually gained in sophistication as students have become more familiar with Āyurvedic language.

With the publication of *The Textbook of Ayurveda*, Āyurvedic education enters a new era. This, the first course book of Āyurvedic medicine actually written for a Western audience, should facilitate the development of the first true Āyurvedic colleges in the Occident, institutions that one day will shelter generations of Ayur Vidya apprentices beneath their generous limbs. This book thus represents a new, exciting phase in the adaptation of the Ayur Vidya to once alien soil.

All such developments come via a vehicle, and in this case, the vehicle is Dr. Vasant D. Lad. I first met Dr. Lad in Pune, India in January of 1974, where he was already a favorite instructor at the Tilak Āyurveda College. Thanks in large part to his help and support I survived six years there, graduating finally with a degree in Āyurveda.

When in 1979 the opportunity arose for Dr. Lad to proceed to the USA on an Āyurvedic lecture tour, he was at first reluctant to embark for a foreign shore, leaving his home, his family, and his beloved India behind him. However, after he considered the possible good that could come from exposing Āyurveda to a broader audience, he reluctantly agreed to go. In India we think less of what privileges an individual is due, and more of the many debts that person has to pay. One of these debts is the *vidya rna*, the duty one has to strengthen and enhance one's vidya, and to spread its knowledge to those who are fit to receive it. When Dr. Lad reflected on the many blessings that the Ayur Vidya had already provided him—a livelihood, an ability to treat and cure, a respected position in the community, a fulfillment of his guru's wishes for him—he realized that it was incumbent on him to offer his own energies in return.

And so, off he went. Soon his family followed, and the Institute slowly took shape. Through all vicissitudes he trod forward, intent on his aim, and eventually his determination paid off, for the Ayurvedic Institute has become the leading American institution for Āyurvedic education.

This book is the culmination both of a lifetime of individual study and clinical practice of Āyurveda, and of a dedication of two decades of life force to the larger goal of extending the Ayur Vidya into realms that are for her new and exciting. It is yet another worthy offering that Dr. Lad makes at the altar of Ayur Vidya, and I salute it and him for the fruitful partnership that they have so long tended. May these pages benefit all sentient beings!

Robert E. Svoboda, Āyurvedāchārya
Albuquerque, December 2000

Preface

आयुर्वेद

For the last twenty years, I have traveled extensively teaching the various aspects of Āyurveda. The great three Āyurvedic texts—Charaka, Sushruta and Vāgbhata—Samhitās are quite authentic and contain several layers of meaning for the serious student. However, they are rather difficult for the beginner to follow and understand. I took an extract of these Three Greats and created a practical Ayurvedic Studies Program that I teach at The Ayurvedic Institute in Albuquerque, New Mexico.

I love my students. They are sincere, hardworking and study Āyurveda in both the Ayurvedic Studies Program and in the more advanced Gurukula Program. Over the years, the students have repeatedly requested a textbook for our classes. The entire curriculum is taught in an eight-month period and all of its material cannot be put together in a single volume. Hence, I have decided to write three volumes of a general textbook of Āyurveda covering the basic principles and philosophies of Āyurveda, the clinical assessment of health and disease, and the management of disease.

It gives me a great joy to write this preface for Volume I of the Textbook of Ayurveda. This book contains authentic teachings of the basic principles and philosophies of Āyurveda. I am quite sure that it will be a practical guide to all students of Āyurveda.

Love and light,

Dr. Vasant Lad
Albuquerque, New Mexico
March 2001

About the Author

आयुर्वेद

Ayurveda finds its home in the hearts of special beings whose dharma it is to preserve and maintain traditions of wisdom for the purpose of healing themselves and the world. Bridging the gap between the changing philosophies, sciences, and religions of the ages, it is passed down in the various cultures through these dedicated individuals. Dr. Lad's heart is one of the homes for that living flame, and his life and teachings are an expression of Ayurveda's true purpose in the world.

Dr. Lad brings a wealth of classroom and practical experience to the United States. He received the degree of Bachelor of Ayurvedic Medicine & Surgery (B.M.A.S.) from the University of Pune, in Pune, India in 1968 and a Master of Ayurvedic Science (M.A.Sc.) from Tilak Ayurved Mahavidyalaya in Pune, India in 1980. For 3 years he served as Medical Director of the Ayurveda Hospital in Pune, India. He also held the position of Professor of Clinical Medicine for seven years at the Pune University College of Ayurvedic Medicine, where he was an instructor for many years. Dr. Lad's academic and practical training includes the study of allopathic medicine (Western Medicine) and surgery as well as traditional Ayurveda. In 1979, he began traveling throughout the United States sharing his knowledge of Ayurveda. In 1981, he returned to New Mexico to teach Ayurveda. In 1984, he founded The Ayurvedic Institute and began as the director of the Institute.

Vasant Lad is respected throughout the world for his knowledge of Ayurveda. He is the author of 11 books on Ayurveda as well as hundreds of articles and other writings. Some of his titles include *Ayurveda, The Science of Self Healing,* and he is co-author of *The Yoga of Herbs* and *Ayurvedic Cooking for Self-Healing.* His book, *Secrets of the Pulse, The Ancient Art of Ayurvedic Pulse Diagnosis,* presents this fascinating subject for the first time. His work from Harmony Books, *The Complete Book of Ayurvedic Home Remedies,* is a compendium of classic Ayurvedic treatments for common and chronic ailments. This textbook is the first volume of a four volume set. The second volume was published in 2006 and the third in 2012. He is also the co-author of a book on marma therapy, *Marma Points of Ayurveda.* With over 500,000 copies of his books in print in the US, his work has been translated into more than 20 languages.

Dr. Lad presently is the Director of The Ayurvedic Institute in Albuquerque, New Mexico where he teaches the two levels of the Ayurvedic Studies Program and the more advanced Gurukula Program in India each year. Dr. Lad also travels throughout the world, consulting privately and giving seminars on Ayurveda, its history, theory, principles, and practical applications.

The Use of Sanskrit

आयुर्वेद

Knowledge of Āyurveda originates in the Sanskrit language. Sanskrit is a precise phonetic language that uses a set of written symbols not familiar to most Westerners. The phonetic representation of Sanskrit words using the English alphabet is called transliteration. We can transliterate Sanskrit to English characters, but not every sound translates directly. There are quite a few sounds that do not exist in the English language, requiring special characters to represent them accurately.

One example is वात ,which translates to vāta. The first 'a' in vāta is a 'long a', as in "father"; it is held for two beats. The second 'a' is a 'short a', as in "what." Another example is a sound somewhere between an 'i', a 'u' and an 'r' that occurs in the word प्रकृति. This word is transliterated as prakṛti. The 'ṛ' is pronounced as the 'ri' in the English spelling of the word Krishna. To make things even more complicated, among those who use Sanskrit the 'ṛ' is pronounced in northern India as the 'i' in "it" and in southern India as the 'u' sound in "root." Because of the regional variations in pronunciation, in this book both ru and ri are found in place of the technically correct 'ṛ'.

Another consideration is that the trailing 'a' in Sanskrit words is sometimes omitted because of the influence of the Hindi language. It is included in many of the words in this book. The trailing 'a' is also subject to grammatical changes depending on the letters that follow it and, for simplicity's sake, we generally ignore these rules. For example, the word *meda* (fat) can be transliterated as *medo, medas,* and meda depending on the word following it. Ordinarily, we use the most common form, meda, so that you, the reader, will have to learn only the one word. Of course, it would be wonderful if all our readers began the study of Sanskrit, inspired by the knowledge available in these ancient texts, but it is not our purpose here to teach that language.

In *The Textbook of Ayurveda*, we have chosen to use transliteration characters only for long vowels, denoted by an overscore or macron character, and for the 'nya' sound denoted by 'ñ'. The pronunciations of the vowels are:

> a as in about; ā as in father
> i as in ink; ī as in fee
> u as in put; ū as in food
> e as in pay; ai as in I
> o as in corn; au as in loud

In all of our texts, we have elected to italicize the first occurrence of the Ayurvedic terms used in the text,[1] since they are used repeatedly throughout the text.

Editor's Note

The editor would like to thank Glen Crowther for his attention to detail, his intelligence and patience, and his tireless efforts in editing this book. I would also like to thank Barbara Cook for her excellent work glossary as well as for her insightful suggestions on the text of the book. This book owes much to their scholarship and dedication to Āyurveda. Margaret Smith Peet brought her years of editorial experience and love of Āyurveda to this book; much of its flow and beauty is due to her gifts. Of course, we are all grateful to Dr. Lad for his profound knowledge of Āyurveda and his generosity in sharing it with his students.

Laura Humphreys
Editor

1. *The Chicago Manual of Style,* 15th ed. (Chicago: University of Chicago Press, 2003), 292.

1

Shad Darshan
The Six Philosophies of Life

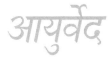

Introduction

Āyurveda is a system of healing that has its roots in ancient India. It is thought by many scholars to be the oldest healing system extant on our planet. *Āyuh* means life and *veda* means knowledge. The knowledge contained in Āyurveda deals with the nature, scope and purpose of life, and includes its metaphysical and physical aspects—health and disease, happiness and sorrow, pain and pleasure. Āyurveda defines life as the conjunction of body, mind and spirit found in Cosmic Consciousness and embracing all of Creation. Āyurveda states that the purpose of life is to know or realize the Creator, both within and without, and to express this Divinity in one's daily life. According to Āyurveda, every individual life is a microcosm of the Cosmos.

Āyurveda is a medical science and its purpose is to heal and to maintain the quality and longevity of life. It is an art of daily living that has evolved from practical, philosophical and spiritual illumination, rooted in the understanding of Creation. It offers a profound understanding of each person's unique body, mind, and consciousness, which is the foundation of health and happiness.

The principles of many natural healing systems now familiar in the West, such as herbal medicine and polarity therapy, have their roots in Āyurveda. Because of its broad scope, Āyurveda embraces all health care disciplines and weaves them into an integrated treatment plan for each individual. If a person needs surgery, surgical procedures are available. If a person needs psychological or spiritual counseling, or rejuvenation of the body, mind, and spirit, there are procedures for these as well. Āyurveda encompasses all these treatments and coordinates them appropriately. It is called a "living" science since it incorporates modern developments and techniques along with ancient wisdom. It is uniquely capable of suggesting a treatment regimen appropriate to each individual. Most other medical disciplines are too specialized to design a plan that includes elimination of the cause(s), treatment of the condition, rebuilding of the body and the continuing support of a rejuvenation program. In Āyurveda, all these elements are of paramount importance in the treatment process.

Āyurveda is quite old, with its roots going far back into Indian antiquity. It has been practiced continuously in India for thousands of years. In more recent times, the British introduced Western medicine to India, which they considered a superior form of medical treatment. Āyurveda was suppressed and its practice discouraged by government policies. Many Indians followed this movement to Western medicine and succumbed to the lure of quick fixes, shots, pills and drugs, thereby, like their western counterparts, avoiding personal responsibility for their own health. Today some Indians are returning to historical, native Āyurveda having realized that Western medicine tends simply to suppress symptoms and does not help to prevent problems from recurring. Although Western medicine is extremely helpful for acute conditions and trauma, it tends to overlook the importance of individual response to the stresses and conditions of life. There is no concept of specialization in Āyurveda, as there is in Western medicine. Āyurveda treats the whole person, not just the organ or system involved.

Every healing system has a basic foundation of philosophy. Āyurvedic philosophy is based on the Shad Darshan, the Six Philosophies of life, which developed from the ancient sages and scriptures of India. Many of these scriptures are known as Vedas, or bodies of knowledge. The Vedas are timeless; some say more than 10,000 years old. The four main Vedas—Rigveda, Yajurveda, Atharvaveda, and Sāmaveda—

are among the oldest bodies of recorded/written knowledge in human culture. There are also four secondary Vedas, called Upa-Vedas or subordinate Vedas, which developed from each of the main bodies of knowledge. "Āyur-Veda," translated as "The Science of Life," is an Upa-Veda. Although there is some debate, many scholars feel that Āyurveda is an Upa-Veda of the Atharvaveda. Others feel the origin was within the Rigveda.

The entire Vedic tradition is composed of highly spiritual wisdom and pure knowledge revealed through the hearts of enlightened *rishis* (seers). It is not a creation made by the mind of man but rather a revelation from the hearts of meditative sages. This ancient wisdom came from the caves and mountains of India where the rishis had ashrams and disciples. Students came to study with them, and the rishis imparted knowledge as they experienced it in a deep state of meditation. These early teachings were an oral tradition and, because there were no books, the students stored the knowledge in their minds and it became a part of them. As written music has no melody, so the written *mantra* has little energy. For that reason, the rishis believed that mantras should not be written down. They tried to impart this knowledge from one soul to another soul through the oral tradition.

The knowledge of Āyurveda has been passed down to us in *sūtras* or small phrases and the wisdom these sūtras contain is there to be unlocked by the inquiring mind. Much of the information in this book is based upon the truths contained in these sūtras, composed in the form of poetry during ancient times, more than 5,000 years ago. The words of a sūtra bring hidden knowledge to consciousness. However, the understanding of this knowledge and its hidden meaning need the guidance of a teacher.

The Sanskrit word sūtra means to suture with a thread. The small phrase of the sūtra is analogous to a thread passing through the eye of a needle. The eye of the needle is small but the trail of the thread leads to great hidden wisdom waiting for interpretation. A seed is a tree in minute form. A sūtra is analogous to the seed. The seed can have many meanings and can describe a variety of forms: a small sapling, a mature tree, flowers, fruits, acorns or nuts. It is clear that the seed embraces the totality. It is the microcosm within the macrocosm. The same is true of a sūtra.

The Charaka Samhitā, compiled approximately 400 C.E., is the oldest ancient Sanskrit Āyurvedic text still in existence and describes the five subdoshas of vāta. The Sushruta Samhitā text, compiled by the sage Nagarjuna, first described surgery, blood and the five pitta subdoshas. Vāgbhata was a famous Āyurvedic physician from the 6th century C.E. who wrote the Ashtānga Hridayam and the Ashtānga Sangraha. Earlier sages in the oral lineage of Āyurveda were Lord Brahmā, who taught Prajāpati, who passed it to the Ashvin twins. They, in turn, taught Indra, who passed it to Ātreya (6th century B.C.E.), who taught Agnivesa, who in the 5th century B.C.E. wrote the first major Āyurvedic treatise, which is no longer in existence.

Āyurveda incorporates the Shad Darshan, the six systems of Indian philosophy—Sānkhya, Nyāya, Vaisheshika, Mīmāmsa, Yoga, and Vedānta. *Shad* means six. The Sanskrit root of the word *darshan* is *drish*, which means "to see." In this sense darshan is inner vision as well as outer vision. The six systems represent six visions of life. They are ways of orienting with reality.

Table 1: Shad Darshan: The Six Philosophies of Life

Philosophy	Founder
Sānkhya	Kāpila
Nyāya	Gautama
Vaisheshika	Kanāda
Mīmāmsa	Jaimini
Yoga	Patañjali
Vedānta	Bādarāyana

Darshan is translated as direct perception or philosophy, which is love of truth. While darshan is not philosophy, philosophy comes from darshan. Therefore, we translate Shad Darshan as Six Philosophies that Āyurveda accepts for the healing of mankind.

Why do we study the Shad Darshan? Three of these systems—Sānkhya, Nyāya, and Vaisheshika—predominantly deal with the material world. These philosophies try to understand and explain everyday experience on the level of the physical. Knowledge about physical creation was most important to them. Logical reasoning, understanding cause and effect, or experiences one can reduce to cause and effect, are the focus of Nyāya. This system is also concerned with the means of knowing and right knowledge.

Vaisheshika is also focused on the level of the physical world without concern for what created it, where it came from. It is really more a model of physics, of particle interactions, than a philosophy of speculative thought. In contrast, Sānkhya states that we need to consider the origin of the world. Moreover, it is important to see how the theme of microcosm and macrocosm (as above, so below) plays out. In Sānkhya, physiology is expressed as a model of evolving Consciousness. Non-material in nature, Consciousness expresses itself in an evolutionary scheme, as the entire diversity of material creation. These three paradigms—Sānkhya, Vaisheshika, and Nyāya—form a natural grouping for understanding the physical universe.

The other three—Yoga, Mīmāmsa, and Vedānta— observe inner reality as an attempt to understand outer reality. They are concerned more with pure philosophy and are less concerned about understanding the physical interaction of things. Their emphasis is on how we can evolve.

All six systems lead to evolutionary fulfillment and self-realization. What these philosophies are fundamentally trying to do is to alleviate pain and suffering, a common rallying point for all of them. They all want to bring us to a cessation of pain and suffering, which is a way of looking at them in relation to Buddhism. Buddhism and its Four Noble Truths specifically deal with this subject. (see "Buddhism" on page 21) In studying the Shad Darshan, we try to understand "what is" and how to relate to it in order to achieve self-realization.

Sānkhya

The most notable proponent of Sānkhya[2] philosophy was Kāpila, one of the great enlightened rishis (seers). The word Sānkhya comes from *san* and *khya*. San means Truth. Khya means to realize, to know, to understand. Sānkhya is a philosophy to discover and understand the Truth of life. Kāpila discerned 24 principles in the manifestation of the Universe. We will consider each of these principles in detail.

Purusha and Prakruti

The first concept of Sānkhya philosophy that we will consider is *Purusha*. *Pur* means city. *Sheta* means dwelling, living, existing. Purusha is that pure Consciousness that exists, lives, dwells in the city of senses. The body is a city of senses. Many houses gather together to create a city. In the same way we have many senses—auditory, tactile, optic, gustatory, olfactory—with nine gates or openings: seven in the head, and

---

2. The word sānkhya in Sanskrit also means enumeration. In enumeration there are 24 principles of creation. Here we are translating sānkhya as "to know the Truth."

**24 Principles of Creation
According to Sānkhya**

1: Prakruti
2: Mahad (Universal
  Intelligence)
  Buddhi (Individual Intellect)
3: Ahamkāra

***Formed from the Interaction
of Sattva and Rajas***

4: Manas
Sensory Faculties (Jñānendriya):
5: Hearing
6: Touch
7: Vision
8: Taste
9: Smell
Motor Faculties (Karmendriya):
10: Speech
11: Grasping
12: Walking
13: Procreation
14: Elimination

***Formed from the Interaction
of Tamas and Rajas***

Objects of Sensory Perception
  (Tanmātrās):
15: Sound (Shabda)
16: Touch (Sparsha)
17: Form (Rūpa)
18: Taste (Rasa)
19: Odor (Gandha)
Five Elements (Maha Bhūtas):
20: Ether (Ākāsha)
21: Air (Vāyu)
22: Fire (Agni)
23: Water (Āpas)
24: Earth (Pruthivī)

the anus and urethral opening. There are three extra gates in women: the nipples and the vagina. Pure Consciousness dwells within this city of senses. Purusha is the ultimate Truth, the ultimate healing power, the ultimate enlightenment, the transcendental state of being and existence. Purusha is energy and this energy is choiceless, passive awareness. It is formless, colorless, beyond attributes and takes no active part in Creation. Purusha can be called pure Consciousness.

Prakruti is primordial will, primordial matter, creative potential. Prakruti has form, color, and attributes in the field of action. It is Awareness with choice, Divine Will, the One who desires to become many. The universe is the child born out of the womb of Prakruti, the Divine Mother. Prakruti creates all forms in the universe, while Purusha is the witness to this creation. There is no matter without energy but there can be energy without matter. Prakruti cannot exist without Purusha. However, there can be Purusha without Prakruti. Sānkhya says Prakruti is creativity, the feminine energy. Within the womb of Prakruti the whole universe is born. Therefore, Prakruti is the Divine Mother.

The unmanifested state of Purusha and Prakruti is called *Brahman*, the state of pure Awareness, pure Consciousness. Before Prakruti begins to manifest, at the merging point of Purusha and Prakruti, it is *avyakta*, which means unmanifested. Once Prakruti manifests, it is *vyakta*, which means manifestation. The root cause of the entire universe is Prakruti, not Purusha.

In the potential energy of Purusha and the creative will of Prakruti, we find an understanding of the evolution of non-material energy (Purusha/Prakruti, avyakta) into material expression (vyakta). Each progressive step acts as an agent or a cause for the manifestation. The scheme of cause and effect is key to the functioning of creation through the Sānkhya model. This is the journey of Consciousness into matter.

Mahad (Creative Intelligence)

Purusha and Prakruti are together for the purpose of creation. In the presence of Purusha, when Prakruti becomes conscious of Consciousness, Prakruti creates the first expression of creation, which is *Mahad*. Mahad has self-awareness. The meaning of Mahad is supreme intelligence, that which puts everything in its proper place. Even in the single cell there is intelligence and each cell has a unique function. The bone cells choose and utilize calcium, magnesium, zinc, and other minerals. The muscle cells choose protein. There is intelligence and right order in the cells, and that order is cellular intelligence.

The Journey of Consciousness into Matter

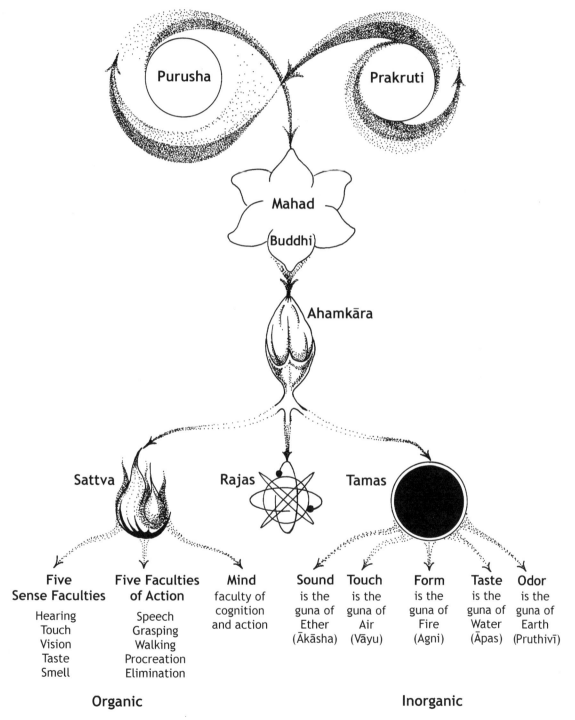

Illustration 1 — The Journey of Consciousness into Matter

That is Mahad. There is communication between cells which is the flow of intelligence called *prāna*, the life force. Mahad is this collective intelligence.

Ahamkāra

Mahad is pure intelligence and from Mahad comes *Ahamkāra*. Ahamkāra means the feeling of "I am," the ego. "I" is the center and where there is a center there is a radius, and where there is a center and a radius there is a circumference. That circumference forms a frontier, the border of consciousness. We all live in the tiny enclosure of consciousness, which is centered upon ahamkāra, the "I former." The question is how a center is formed. When you allow your eyes to focus, in that very looking there is perception. And the moment you identify with an object, there is the birth of "I," the birth of Ahamkāra. In Mahad there is no differentiation. However, Ahamkāra focuses on one thing, making it the center of vision. This center is "I." Ahamkāra is a process of identification based upon previous accumulated experience. But the moment "I" is formed, which is a center created in the consciousness, then that creative intelligence (Mahad) becomes *Buddhi*, which is reasoning capacity, intellect, individual awareness. Mahad is the universal principle. Buddhi is the individual principle.

Sattva, Rajas, Tamas

The pulsation of cosmic prāna causes Consciousness to break up into the three universal qualities (*gunas*) which pervade all Creation—*sattva, rajas, tamas*. Because of the formation of an ego reference point, sattva, rajas and tamas can be perceived as distinct, separate, and defined. Sattva is the pure essence of light, right action, and spiritual purpose. Rajas is the principle of movement, change, excitability. Tamas is inertia, darkness, confusion. These three universal qualities influence both our minds and bodies. On the universal level, sattva is vast, clear space; rajas is atmosphere; and tamas is solid substance. On the individual level, sattva is perception, the knower; rajas is the movement of perception, which becomes the process of attention; and tamas is the precipitation of perception, which is experience, the known. Sattva is the light of Consciousness; it is potential energy. Rajas is kinetic energy. Tamas represents inertia. Without tamas there is no experience. Sattva is the observer. Rajas is observation. Tamas is the object to be observed. Sattva is creative, rajas maintains, tamas is destructive.

Although sattva, rajas and tamas are each present to some degree in every object of creation, some objects arise primarily from sattva and some primarily from tamas. Rajas is the energy which is the momentum of creation. Attention is a combination of sattva and the flow of rajas. Through rajas Consciousness becomes matter.

Sattva is further described by the Sanskrit word *jñānashakti*, which means the energy of cognition, the motive for perception. *Jñana* means perception, knowledge, cognition, intelligence. Rajas is described as *kriyāshakti*, the energy of observation. *Kriya* means action, creativity. Tamas is described as *dravyashakti*, which is material matter, the observed. You wake in the morning because of sattva (jñānashakti). Because of rajas (kriyāshakti) you plan for the entire day. In the evening after a heavy dinner, you feel tamas (dravyashakti), heavy, dull, like going to sleep. Tamas brings sleep, inaction and darkness. The inaction of tamas and the inaction of Purusha are different. The inaction of Purusha is pure Consciousness; the inaction of tamas is unconsciousness, a blind force without awareness, which brings confusion when it causes unconscious action.

Rajas is the active vital force which moves to sattva to create the organic universe, the world of sensory perception. Rajas moves to tamas to create the inorganic universe. Therefore, sattva and tamas are inactive energies that require the active, kinetic force of rajas. As a result of the influence of the three universal qualities, the five *jñānendriya* (sensory pathways), the five *karmendriya* (motor pathways), and the mind are differentiated as part of the organic universe. The five *tanmātrās*, or objects of sensory perception, and the five elements (Ether, Air, Fire, Water, and Earth) are differentiated as part of the inorganic universe. The tanmātrās are the gunas (qualities) of the elements: *shabda* (sound), *sparsha* (touch), *rūpa* (form), *rasa* (taste), and *gandha* (odor or smell).

The five elements are born in the womb of tamas but contain all three gunas. Even the tanmātrās contain all three gunas. Though they are derived from tamas, there are some rajasic and sattvic qualities in the tanmātrās and therefore in the elements. Earth is tamas. Water is tamas and sattva. It seeks its own level, which is tamas, but is transparent, which is sattva. Fire is intense rajas and sattva, Air is rajas but also sattva, while Ether is pure sattva. The elements evolve successively to include their own related tanmātrā and each of the prior tanmātrās. For example, Ether is just shabda tanmātrā, Air is comprised of shabda and sparsha, while Earth is comprised of shabda, sparsha, rūpa, rasa, and gandha. Each element manifests from the addition of its primary tanmātrā to the tanmātrās of the preceding element(s).

We can put our knowledge of the philosophy of Sānkhya into our daily lives and relationships in moment to moment existence. The moment we look at our bodies in the mirror, we start judging. Many of us don't like the face, hair, nose, or color we have. But we are not nose, face, or body; we are the dweller dwelling in this body. We are something higher and nobler. We are Purusha. We are *Shakti*. In this way we can apply the philosophy of Sānkhya in our daily lives for self-healing. We all must heal ourselves.

The same thing applies when your wife is yelling at you or your husband is criticizing and you become upset and angry. You are not anger, you are the watcher of anger. You are not fear, you are the witness of fear. You are not bored or tired, you are the pure observer of the tiredness.

Sānkhya philosophy has changed my life and I'm sure it will also change your life. Self-acceptance and self-love are the first steps to bliss.

Nyāya and Vaisheshika

The philosophies of Nyāya and Vaisheshika are represented by the writings of Gautama and Kanāda, respectively. Nyāya means logic and Vaisheshika means to specify the important aspects of concrete reality. The proponents of Nyāya and Vaisheshika believed in obtaining knowledge through observation and critical logic. They were like modern scientists. They found that certain principles which can be experienced with sensory perception are real—*pratyaksha*, that which can be seen and experienced. *Prahāna* means proof. The proponents of Nyāya and Vaisheshika discovered ways of investigating the truth and they stated that truth could be proven.

Nyāya and Vaisheshika go together. While Vaisheshika speaks about nine causative substances of the universe, called *nava karna dravya*, Nyāya deals with how to think about them—the reasoning. *Nava* means nine, *karna* means causative, *dravya* means substances. These nine causative substances are Ether, Air, Fire, Water, and Earth; the soul, (*ātman*), which is spirit or self; mind, (*manas*); time, (*kāla*); and direction, (*dig*).[3]

Vaisheshika holds to the atomic theory of existence that claims the entire universe is composed of atoms. Vaisheshika believes the union and separation of atoms is guided or directed by the will of the Supreme Being. Ether, Air, Fire, Water, and Earth are eternal atoms. The union of atoms in twos, threes, etc., created universal elements at the time of creation and these atoms will separate at the time of *pralaya*, disintegration or annihilation.

The Four Pramāna–Sources of Valid Knowledge

According to Nyāya, there are three sources of non-valid knowledge: *samshaya* (doubt), *bhrama* (faulty cognition), *tarka* (hypothetical argument), and four sources of valid knowledge:[4]

Pratyaksha (Perception)
Anumāna (Inference)
Upamāna (Comparison)
Shabda (Testimony)

Nyāya states that any reality can be understood by these four methods of understanding, comprehension and perceiving.

Pratyaksha. Nyāya classifies perception as *laukika* (ordinary) and *alaukika* (extraordinary). *Pratyaksha* (perception) is knowledge produced through contact of the senses with objects of the world. This contact must be clear. When in the twilight one perceives a rope as a snake, it is false and invalid perception.

There are five ordinary external perceptions—hearing, touching, seeing, tasting, and smelling. Extraordinary perception is based upon association and intuition and includes perception of the qualities of soul, thought, desire, aversion, pleasure, pain, and cognition.

Āyurveda uses both ordinary and extraordinary perception as diagnostic tools. When a patient has a fever, it is measured with a thermometer. The skin looks red and feels hot. Ordinary pratyaksha is that which can be experienced by direct

---

3. Some scholars describe the elements as composed of atoms, in the sense of irreducible units. In Vaisheshika, the causative substances are atoms and the elements are molecules in the Western sense. Element is the grosser form. Each element is composed of atoms of the same name, but also of the other four atoms, giving rise to molecules. For example, the element Air contains predominately Air and also contains all the other atoms. Fire is composed mainly of Fire and also contains the other atoms. In Sānkhya, the elements are composed of the tanmātrās, which are similar to the causative substances of Vaisheshika, but subtler than atoms. In Sānkhya, Nyāya, and Vaisheshika, the tanmātrās or causative substances are irreducible, but the elements are molecules.
   Note that we use Nyāya as a way of reasoning and understanding experience in what we call the physical universe. The content is Vaisheshika. Therefore, the concept of the elements and atoms belongs under Vaisheshika.
4. The four sources of valid knowledge according to Nyāya are accepted by Āyurveda. However, other philosophies present information that is slightly different.

perception through the senses. Extraordinary perception through association and intuition is developed through persistent yogic and Āyurvedic practice in daily observation.

Anumāna. The second proof is *anumāna*. Anumāna involves inference and cognition based on some previous knowledge or experience. Wherever there is smoke, there will be fire. Ten miles away behind the mountain there is a big cloud of smoke. We have not seen the fire but have previous experience that smoke and fire go together. We have seen people dying. Hence we draw inference that man is mortal. Āyurveda can use inference to see which *dosha* is aggravated. For example, we can say that wherever there is inflammation, there is *pitta*.

Upamāna. The third proof is *upamāna*. Upamāna relies upon comparison. There is a kind of knowledge that comes when one perceives the similarity between the description of an unfamiliar object and something already known. Doctors compare disease processes and pathological conditions as one way of understanding. Āyurveda uses comparison to understand the different diseases in terms of their doshas. For instance, a pitta type cold will show thin, yellow mucus, a sore throat and fever while a *kapha* type cold will present thick, white, copious mucus, chest and bronchial congestion and chills.

Shabda. The fourth pramāna is *shabda*, which means verbal testimony, that which is authentic and truthful. The Bible, the Koran and the Vedas are sacred texts. They are authority, which gives them authenticity and validity. These sacred texts receive the status of authority from people who regard them as authority. These authorities are called *āpta*, those whose thoughts, feelings and speech/actions are consistent. These people have told us that the Vedas are true. X-rays, electrocardiograms and MRIs are also objective observation, shabda. If an ultrasound shows that there are gallstones, we must believe it. The patient is one who knows the truth that he/she has a tummy ache, so we must believe the patient and listen with great respect.

The Elements

We will now consider the five elements or panchamaha bhūtas. The elements as referenced in this section are molecules composed of the atoms or basic substances, which are the first five of the nine causative substances[5] outlined by Vaisheshika.

---

5. The nine dravyas or causative substances are Earth, Water, Fire, Air, Ether, Time, Direction, Soul, and Mind.

Ether. Ether is called *ākāsha* in Sanskrit. It is a mystic word. Ākāsha means all-enclosing, all-pervading, omnipotent, omniscient, omnipresent. All-pervading Ether serves as the common factor or "home" for all objects in the universe.[6] Ether, which is the first expression of Consciousness, is the basic need of the bodily cells. In the development of matter, Ether comes first. Ether is expansive, empty and has no resistance. Ether provides freedom in which to move. Without Ether there is no love or freedom. Āyurveda holds that within Ether there is a pure presence of spiritual energy that manifests as nuclear energy.

> **Attributes of Ether**
> **Gunas** (Qualities): Clear, light, subtle, soft, immeasurable
> **Karmas** (Actions): Vibration, expansion, non-resistance, freedom, love. Descent of intelligence into the heart of the matter.
> **Tanmātrā:** Sound
> **Type of Energy:** Nuclear energy

Air. This same Consciousness, when it moves in a particular direction, becomes Air. Air is called *vāyu*. We translate vāyu as Air but words are not sufficient to convey the deeper meaning. Air is a principle of movement necessary for keeping the body in constant motion and manifests as electrical energy.

> **Attributes of Air**
> **Gunas** (Qualities): Mobile, dry, light, cold, rough, subtle
> **Karmas** (Actions): Movement in a particular direction
> **Tanmātrās:** Sound and touch
> **Type of Energy:** Electrical energy

Prāna is the basic principle of the Air element. It is the flow of Consciousness from one cell to another cell in the form of intelligence. Prāna is the vital life force and is necessary for all subtle and gross movements within the cell, within the system and within the physical body. In other words, sensory stimuli and motor responses are the subtle movements of prāna. Even the movements of the heart, respiration, peristalsis and other involuntary movements are governed by this principle of Air, prāna.

Fire. Where there is movement there is friction and where there is friction there is Fire. So the next manifestation of Awareness is Fire. Fire is called *agni*. All transformative processes are governed by the Fire element. It governs the metabolic processes regulating the transformation of food into energy and is responsible for body temperature and the processes of digestion, absorption and assimilation of food stuffs. Within each of the doors of perception—ears, skin, eyes, tongue, nose—there is a subtle Fire component that is necessary

> **Attributes of Fire**
> **Gunas** (Qualities): Hot, sharp, light, dry, subtle
> **Karmas** (Actions): Brilliance, luminosity, penetration, the radiant flame of intelligence
> **Tanmātrās:** Sound, touch, form
> **Type of Energy:** Radiant energy

---

6. According to Vaisheshika, there are five kinds of atoms: Ether, Air, Fire, Water, and Earth, each having its own qualities. Ākāsha (Ether), the first substance, is the substratum of the quality of sound. There is only one atom of Ether and it is universal. Ākāsha is also translated as space or sound and cannot be perceived directly. It is unlimited, eternal and universal, so it does not have a perceptible dimension. It is formless, so it does not have color. Therefore, Ākāsha cannot be perceived, but it can be inferred as a quality of sound. Ākāsha is not made up of parts and does not depend upon any other substance for existence. It is all-pervading in the sense that it has unlimited dimension and its quality of sound is perceived everywhere.

for sense perception and processing of perception into knowledge.

Fire is carried throughout the body in the blood and plasma as heat. If the blood supply is cut off, that part of the body will be cold. Poor circulation results in cold hands and feet. Fire regulates understanding, comprehension, and selectivity. The Fire element is radiant energy and is present in the body as the flame of attention.

Water. The next element is Water, *āpas*, which is associated with chemical energy. Water is the universal chemical solvent and all biochemical functions are governed by it. Water is necessary in the human body for assimilation and for maintaining electrolyte balance. The plasma in our blood is composed of approximately 90 percent water and this water carries nutrients from one part of the body to the other. Oxygen, food particles and the subtle molecules of minerals are carried from one cell to another cell, from one system to another system, by this continuous river of fluid, the plasma. The body's lymphatic system is also governed by the Water element. Within the medium of Water all the elements maintain their function. This is the Water of Life.

Earth. The solid, dense and hard element is Earth, *pruthivī*, the firm ground for global life. Pruthivī cradles and holds all living creatures of the planet, giving them food and shelter. All solid structures, hard, firm, and compact tissues are derived from the Earth element (e.g., bones, cartilage, nails, hair, teeth, and skin). Earth is associated with mechanical energy.

Attributes of Water
Gunas (Qualities): Cool, liquid, dull, soft, oily, slimy
Karmas (Actions): Downward movement, cleansing, cohesiveness, adhesiveness, percolation
Tanmātrās: Sound, touch, form, taste
Type of Energy: Chemical energy

Attributes of Earth
Gunas (Qualities): heavy, dull, static, dense, hard, gross
Karmas (Actions): Gravitation, downward attraction
Tanmātrās: Sound, touch, form, taste, odor
Type of Energy: Physical, mechanical energy

Table 2: The Elements and Associated Types of Energy

Ākāsha	Ether	nuclear energy
Vāyu	Air	electrical energy
Agni	Fire	radiant energy
Āpas	Water	chemical energy
Pruthivī	Earth	mechanical energy

The five elements normally support life and maintain harmony in the world but, when they are out of balance, they can cause discomfort and threaten life. The predominance of each element changes continuously, modifying temperature, humidity and seasons. People must strive to accommodate these changes in order to survive. Having intelligence, human beings use knowledge of the elements in order to create optimal environmental conditions. For example, they build brick (predominance of Earth element) houses to protect themselves from changes in air, heat, and water.

All the elements are present in each individual but the proportions and combinations vary from person to person. Keeping one's individual qualitative and quantitative balance of these five basic elements is necessary for total health. When your own unique combination of the elements is maintained, your health is good. But when the combination is upset, disease may result. For example, an increased Earth component can result in obesity; increased Water can lead to edema; increased Fire can cause fever, ulcers, and burning sensations such as heartburn, conjunctivitis or burning urination. Subtle changes in the mental faculties may also appear when the equilibrium is upset. For example, an increase of the Air element may cause fear and anxiety; increase of Fire element can lead to anger and hate; increase of Earth may bring depression and dullness. All five elements play an important role in the formation of the structure of the tissues and in maintaining their functions. Relating this to cause and effect—function is the cause, structure is the effect.

The five elements form the basic foundation of Āyurveda out of which come the three doshas—*vāta, pitta, kapha*. Ether and Air together constitute vāta; Fire and Water, pitta; Water and Earth, kapha.

Soul (Ātman)
We have discussed the five elements. Now we will shift our attention to soul, the sixth of the nine causative substances according to Vaisheshika. According to Vaisheshika, soul is eternal; universal; of two kinds, individual and supreme (jivātman and paramātman); inferred; and indivisible. It is a substratum or phenomenon of Consciousness. Consciousness evolves because soul or spirit exists. Individual souls do not perceive other souls but they do infer their existence.

Sānkhya talks about Purusha, which is pure awareness, the highest principle. Modern science takes seriously only what can be seen, measured, or put on the observation table. Ancient Vedic philosophy speaks a great deal about soul as one's true identity and true Self. Self can exist without body, Self can exist without mind. In a deep sleep, one forgets the body and mind but in a dream state, Self still functions through the mind. The Self is still there enjoying the pure presence, the pure existence.

Without that Self, consciousness is not possible. Ātman cannot be seen but it can be experienced. It cannot be measured but one can merge into it. Vaisheshika's definition of ātman is as a material, causative factor of creation.

Mind (Manas)

The seventh causative substance is mind, manas. Mind is universal, atomic or indivisible, and is not directly perceivable. Mind directs experience. It is awareness functioning through the senses. Mind directs awareness to an object or goal and then perceives the outer object.

The content of mind may be either conscious or subconscious. For example, the cellular mind (atomic mind) is subconscious. The subconscious mind working through the autonomic nervous system directs most of our bodily functions. The beating of the heart, the breathing of the lungs, and the movement of liver cells, cells of the intestinal wall, of the ovaries and fallopian tubes, are all under autonomic control, which is the subconscious mind.

Actually, there is no line of demarcation between the conscious and subconscious mind. Mind is one, but it operates on levels that we call conscious and subconscious. For the convenience of understanding we have created this division. Mind is a wonderful vehicle. Meditation is probing into the subconscious. In meditation, thoughts of the past come up, feelings and emotions surface. When we meditate, our cells become aware and conscious of thoughts, of stress being released. We can begin to talk, share, and communicate with each cell.

Time (Kālā)

The next causative substance is time, kālā, which is movement and change. Time is a force that can produce change and we use it as a marker for change. When we measure time, we measure change.

The function of the doshas is also related to the time of day. For example, 5:00 AM or PM is associated with vāta, and 9:00 AM or PM is associated with kapha. The time of the day produces a different style of function. Time is a cause of change, creation, maintenance, and destruction.

The Earth rotates on its axis and also revolves around the sun. When the Earth completes one rotation, it is one day. When the Earth completes one revolution around the sun, it is one year. Chronological time is based upon the movement of the Earth.

Time can be measured in terms of prāna. One prāna is one breath. One breath is one inspiration and one expiration. Fifteen prāna is said to make one minute; 900 prāna, one hour; 21,600 prāna, one day. The faster the rate of respiration, the shorter the span of life. The slower the rate of respiration, the longer the span of life.

There is chronological time and there is psychological time. Thought takes place in psychological time. Since thought builds on memory, and memory is accumulated past experience, time is the movement of the past into the present and the future. Therefore, thought is the linear movement of time, because of the sequential change of events. Psychological time is the movement of thought. If one enters the inner space beyond thought, one goes beyond psychological time.

Direction (Dig)

The last of the nine causative factors is direction, dig. Direction is an important concept in Āyurveda. Up, down, and lateral movements describe *doshic* function and are referred to as *dosha gati*. Internal and external movements also give a sense of direction.

East, west, north, and south, are four directions also used by Āyurveda. East is hot, sharp, bright. It has more solar energy. West is cool and has more feminine, lunar energy. In the northern hemisphere, the more you go to the north, the colder it is. The more you go to the south, the hotter it is. Āyurveda has used direction for healing purposes—for example, selecting the proper directional axis a person should sleep.

Southeast is the direction of Fire, southwest the direction of Earth, northwest the direction of Air and northeast the direction of Water. Ether is the center. This is the natural order of direction and the elements. Therefore, the kitchen should be located in the southeast part of the house in order to take advantage of the Fire element. Earth will bring sound sleep in the southwest portion. Fresh air should enter through the northwest. The Water element is located in the northeast, providing a good space for meditation and an altar. The middle area, Ether, should be left empty.

Arranging a house in this way helps us bring the blessing of all five elements so that we will be blessed by our environment. This Vedic understanding of arrangement is called *vastu shilpa shāstra*.

Directions and the Elements

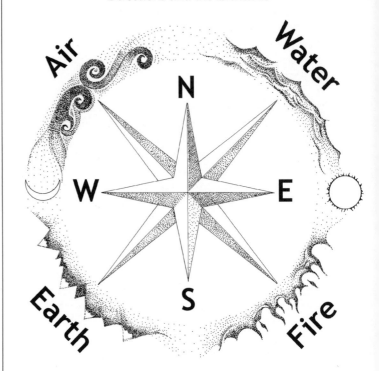

Mīmāmsa

The fourth philosophy is Mīmāmsa, which means to analyze and thoroughly understand the truth. This is a philosophy of attaining freedom through the performance of duty or *dharma* (action in the light of awareness). The proponent of Mīmāmsa was Jaimini, one of the great philosophers. It is a positive way of logic and Mīmāmsa proves that there is a God. Mīmāmsa says that there must be a non-moving mover who moves every object and that non-moving mover is God.

Mīmāmsa emphasizes the teaching of the Vedas from the perspective of rituals. Pūrva Mīmāmsa is based on the initial teachings of the Vedas, while Uttara Mīmāmsa uses the later, higher teachings of Vedānta, which are the Upanishads.

Mīmāmsa believes that the ultimate creator of the universe is God and that God is eternal, timeless, pure existence. It says God is both personal, incarnating in human form to bring peace, love, and order, and impersonal as Brāhma. Mīmāmsa believes in many deities and says that each deity has some significant blessing to offer mankind.

In Mīmāmsa, God as a universal being and as a totality is here in the present. God is reflected in every human being as the sky is reflected in water. In the ocean there is a vast sky. In the river there is a tiny sky. In a small container of water there is a yet smaller reflection. Mīmāmsa says that reflection is incarnation. In some persons the reflection of God is 90 percent. In other persons it may be only 10 percent. Mīmāmsa says that in reality every individual reflects God. Every individual is a complete phenomenon, but the completeness of this individual reflection is difficult to realize. Mīmāmsa says that to understand our individuality, to truly know ourselves, is to know God. Mīmāmsa says there is a lower self, *jīvātman*, and a higher Self, *paramātman*. Through meditation the lower self merges into the higher Self.

The knowledge of Mīmāmsa is vast and cannot be covered in a few brief paragraphs. These teachings include many methods and means of attaining God through rituals, ceremonies, and fasting. Also included are instructions for different ways of *puja* and sacrifice. This philosophy is quite complex. Āyurveda has accepted Mīmāmsa for healing purposes and incorporates rituals such as burning candles, offering flowers, sprinkling holy water, and burning incense, all of which have healing power.

Yoga

The fifth philosophy is Yoga. Yoga means union—the union of the lower self with the higher Self, the union of man with God. It is a practical discipline for knowing the self. Yoga comes from *yuj* that means to unite.

When you control your thought waves, you can go beyond thought. Thought is a barrier, an obstacle, and a block. Yoga is one of the ways to go beyond. Patañjali was the pioneer who organized yogic discipline as a science through his Yoga Sūtras and Āyurveda has accepted this philosophy for healing purposes.

The Yoga system provides a methodology for expanding one's individual consciousness to the universal Consciousness. There are various schools of Yoga—Bhakti Yoga (path of devotion), Jñana Yoga (path of knowledge), Karma Yoga (path of action), etc. Patañjali's Yoga Sūtras gives eight methods to attain enlightenment:

1. Yama (five restraints)
2. Niyama (five observances)
3. Āsana (postures)
4. Prānāyāma (control of the vital force)

5. Pratyāhāra (withdrawal of senses)
6. Dhārana (focusing attention on an object or mantra; one-pointed awareness[7])
7. Dhyāna (meditation; a continuous flow of attention without words or thoughts; moment-to-moment awareness without judgment)
8. Samādhi[8] (balance of body, mind, and consciousness; an expansive state of choiceless, passive awareness; spiritual Bliss)

Patañjali's system has great therapeutic value and discipline. The *yogāsana* is a way of bringing awareness into action in a particular position. Control of the mind is established by quieting and stilling the mind, so that the object of perception becomes the Self. In the broadest sense, Yoga brings attention back to the Self and creates the value of self-referral.

When one sits in the lotus pose, one becomes like a lotus. When in a cobra pose, one becomes like a cobra. When in a tree pose, one becomes like a tree. There is a communion between body, mind and consciousness. Standing on one leg for 10 minutes, 15 minutes, even one hour, will bring *siddhi*, the benefit of that āsana. Every *āsana* has a siddhi, a benefit, which creates biochemical changes in the body. Patañjali made a science of yoga and the ultimate end of yoga is *samādhi*, the merging of the lower self into the higher Self, where body, mind and spirit become one, and that is the state of liberation.

Āyurveda classifies yoga āsanas according to vāta, pitta, and kapha, utilizing yogic science for healing purposes.

Vedānta

The sixth philosophy is Vedānta, which was established by Bādarāyana. *Veda* means knowledge and *anta* means ending, so Vedānta means the ending of knowledge. Knowledge is necessary for learning, inquiring and investigating. But to fully realize life, the merger of the lower self into the higher Self, knowledge becomes a barrier. If one has tremendous knowledge, that knowledge blinds. The person becomes prejudiced and preoccupied with the knowledge. One cannot find God or one's true Self by reading books. We all have to read our own book, which is our daily operating consciousness. We have to read ourselves, our thoughts, emotions, reactions and feelings in every aspect of life and inquire of ourselves what we are.

---

7. This can be likened to the flow of oil on the head in the pañchakarma procedure called *shirodhāra*.
8. "Sama" means balanced, "dhi" means intellect; so samādhi is the state of balanced cognition.

Vedānta is a profound philosophy that Āyurveda has accepted. This philosophy is also referred to as *upanishad*. *Upa* means near, *nishad* means to sit in the vicinity of the enlightened one, the teacher, master, *guru* and listen to him or her without any doubt, delusion or comparison. Vedānta, the entire teaching, is upanishad.

Vedānta uses another word for God called Brāhma, which means the expansion of consciousness. The only thing that exists in Vedānta is Consciousness. There is nothing else. There is a tendency toward dualism in Sānkhya and Vaisheshika. However, in Vedānta there is only one principle, and that is called Consciousness.

Edwin Powell Hubble (1889-1953) was an American astronomer who is considered the founder of extragalactic astronomy and who provided the first evidence of the expansion of the universe. But before Hubble, several thousand years ago, Bādarāyana discovered this same truth and that is why he called the universe *brāhmanda*. Brāhmanda means the golden egg that is expanding. *Anda* means egg, *brah* means expansion—the expanding egg. Bādarāyana also discovered that there is a universal Consciousness in which we all share. We all share in one Consciousness even as we all share the light and that is what Bādarāyana was telling us. Āyurveda has accepted his philosophy for healing purposes.

Buddhism

Later, Āyurveda incorporated the philosophy of Buddhism, founded by Lord Buddha. The essence of Buddha's teachings is condensed within the Four Noble Truths:

1. Suffering exists.
2. There is a cause of suffering.
3. There is cessation of suffering.
4. There is a means to cease suffering.

According to Buddhism there are 12 causes of suffering:

1.	Avidya	Ignorance
2.	Samskāra	Past Impressions
3.	Vignana	Initial Consciousness
4.	Nama Rūpa	Mind/Body
5.	Shadayatana	Six Organs of Cognition
6.	Sparsha	Contact of Senses with Objects
7.	Vedanā	Sensation, Feelings, Pain/Pleasure
8.	Trushna	Thirst to Enjoy
9.	Upadan	Mental Attachment
10.	Bhaka	Becoming
11.	Janma	Birth
12.	Jara Marana	Old Age, Death

And there are eight ways to overcome suffering:

1. Right Perception and Observation
2. Right Thinking
3. Right Speaking
4. Right Conduct
5. Right Living
6. Right Doing
7. Right Mindfulness
8. Right Meditation

Lord Buddha was born on the Indian subcontinent around the 6th or 7th century BCE.[9] He was highly enlightened. He never used the word God. He felt God as a pure Presence, pure Existence. Buddhist philosophy encourages entering into that pure existence by emptying our minds of their contents. Buddha said that in order to hold the contents of our minds and our consciousness, we have had to establish definite borders around them. Containers and contained are the same and we live in the tiny enclosures we call consciousness. Buddha said that if we empty our consciousness of its contents, then we dissolve our borders. At that moment we enter *nirvāna*, which is the state of pure Existence. Buddha called this state nothingness or no-mind state.

We have considered the Shad Darshan, the Six Philosophies, on which Āyurveda is based. We have also discussed Buddhism. The creators of these philosophies were great pioneers and have given us profound insights into the truth of life. Each of these philosophies has contributed to the thought of Āyurveda.

* ❊ Sānkhya gave Āyurveda the theory of evolution and a theory of cause and effect.
* ❊ Nyāya and Vaisheshika gave Āyurveda logical and sequential thinking. The body is a material machine and this machine should be corrected. This approach is reflected in modern physics.
* ❊ Mīmāmsa is about action, the path of life, freedom through performance of duty (dharma). Its teachings include methods and means of attaining God through rituals, ceremonies, and fasting.
* ❊ Vedānta gave profound thinking to Āyurveda about eternal, changeless Brahmā, the ultimate achievement of each human being. To achieve that goal each person needs perfect health.

---

9. There is much scholarly discussion about the exact year of the Buddha's birth. Modern scholars specify dates ranging from 563 to 623 BCE.

* Āyurveda uses Yoga therapeutically and indeed each of these systems has great value.

* And finally, Buddhism. Buddha says everything is going to end. Do not worry about disease, because disease is going to end. Have patience. Buddhist philosophy says there is suffering and a simple way to go beyond suffering is to have patience, to give time for pathogenesis to eradicate itself. That is what Buddhism has given to Āyurveda.

 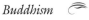

Chapter One

2

Universal Attributes and Doshic Theory

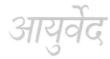

In chapter one we considered the Shad Darshan, the six philosophies, which Āyurveda accepts as a basis for its thought. We also briefly discussed the five elements. In this chapter we will go into greater detail about the elements and come to a better understanding of how these basic principles lie at the heart of Āyurvedic science.

We will first try to understand the inanimate world and will then connect to the animate world through doshic theory. The purpose of this approach is to bridge a model of physics to a model of physiology through gunas (universal attributes) and karmas (actions).

The Five Elements and Their Attributes

The rishis perceived that in the beginning the world existed in an unmanifested state of Consciousness, avyakta—meaning unmanifest. From that state the subtle vibrations of the cosmic, soundless sound Aum manifested. From the subtle vibration of Aum came the Ether or Space element. This ethereal element then began to move and through its subtle movements created the Air element, which is Ether in action. The movement of Air produced friction and through friction heat was generated.

Particles of this heat combined to form intense light and from this light the Fire element emerged. Thus, Ether produced Air and it was Air that further manifested into Fire. The heat of Fire dissolved and liquefied certain ethereal elements, forming Water that then solidified to form the molecules of Earth. In this way, Ether manifested into the four elements of Air, Fire, Water, and Earth.

From Earth, all physical bodies for organic living beings were created, including both the plant and animal kingdoms. Earth was also the origin of all inorganic substances that comprise the mineral kingdom. Thus, out of the womb of the Five Elements all matter was born.

The five basic elements exist in all matter. Water provides the classic example: the solid state of water, ice, is a manifestation of the Earth principle. Latent heat (Fire) in the ice liquefies it, revealing the Water principle. Eventually water turns into steam, expressing the Air principle. The steam disappears into Ether or Space. Thus the five basic elements—Ether, Air, Fire, Water, and Earth—are all present in one substance. All five originated from the energy within Cosmic Consciousness and all five are present in all matter in the universe. Thus, energy and matter are one.

Man is a microcosm of the universe and, therefore, the five basic elements present in all matter also exist within each individual. In the human body, many spaces are aspects of the Ether or Space element. The spaces in the mouth, nose, gastrointestinal tract, respiratory tract, abdomen, thorax, capillaries, and tissues are all examples of Space.

Air is the element of movement. All movements involve Air as an element, because it alone moves everything. Any time there is motion, it means Air is present. The nature of the elements themselves determines the nature of physiology. Within the human body, Air is present in the pulsations of the heart and the expansion and contraction of the lungs. Under a microscope, even a single cell can be seen to move. Response to a stimulus is the movement of afferent and efferent nerve impulses, which are sensory and motor movements respectively. Movements of the nervous system are also governed by the Air principle present in the body.

The third element is Fire. The source of Fire and light in the solar system is the sun. In the human body, the source of Fire is metabolism. Fire works in the digestive system as well as in the gray matter of the brain, where Fire manifests as intelligence. Fire also activates the retina to perceive light.

Therefore, body temperature, digestion, thinking processes, and vision are all functions of bodily Fire. All metabolism and enzyme systems are controlled by this element.

Water, the fourth element, manifests in the body as the secretions of digestive juices, in the mucous membranes and in plasma and cytoplasm. Water is vital for the functioning of all the systems of the body. For example, dehydration resulting from diarrhea and vomiting must be treated immediately to protect the patient's life.

Earth, the fifth element, is also present in the microcosm of the human being. Life is possible on this planet because the Earth holds all living and non-living substances to its solid surface. In the body, all solid structures are derived from Earth.

Table 3: The Senses and the Elements

Jñānendriya (Sensory Faculties)	Sensory Organs	Karmendriya (Faculties of Action)	Motor Organs	Tanmātrās (Objects of the Senses)	Maha Bhūtas (Elements)
Hearing	Ears	Speech	Vocal Cords	Shabda (Sound)	Ether
Tactile perception	Skin	Giving and receiving	Hands	Sparsha (Touch)	Air
Vision	Eyes	Walking	Legs	Rūpa (Form)	Fire
Taste	Tongue	Procreation	Genitals	Rasa (Taste)	Water
Smell	Nose	Excretion	Excretory organs	Gandha (Odor or Smell)	Earth

The Five Elements and Tanmātrās

The five elements manifest in the functioning of the five senses as well as in certain functions of human physiology. Tan means subtle and mātrā means elements. The tanmātrās, the subtle elements, are the objects of the five senses. The five tanmātrās are sound, touch, form, taste, and odor or smell; the five senses are hearing, tactile perception, vision, taste, and smell. The tanmātrās are the ways in which the objective world is sensed. The five elements have functional integrity with the five sensory organs, which allows us to perceive the external environment. Their presence is the reason for the existence of the senses themselves. (see illustration on page 7)

The tanmātrās form the Common Ground for the expression of the objective world and the entire world exists on this Ground. Another meaning of tan is mother, and mātrā also means matter—the mother of matter. The mother of this whole world is the tanmātrās. The tanmātrās are in the womb of the Cosmic Mother, Prakruti. It is this energy that gives rise to the objective five elements. Each element is related primarily to one tanmātrā but can contain a portion of the others as well. Ether comes out of shabda tanmātrā (sound); Air out of shabda and sparsha tanmātrās (sound and touch); Fire out of shabda, sparsha and rūpa tanmātrās (sound, touch and sight); Water out of shabda, sparsha, rūpa and rasa (sound, touch, sight and taste); and Earth out of shabda, sparsha, rūpa, rasa and gandha (sound, touch, form, taste and odor).

These five elements—Ether,[10] Air, Fire, Water, and Earth—are also related to the five organs of action—mouth, hands, feet, genitals and excretory organs—which allow us to respond to the input we receive from the objective world. Ether is the medium through which sound is transmitted and is thus related to the function of hearing. The sensory organ of hearing is the ear. The organ of action associated with the sense of hearing is the mouth and vocal cords, which produce sound.

Air is related to the sense of touch and the sensory organ of touch is the skin. The organ of action related to the sense of touch is the hand. The skin of the hand is especially sensitive and the hand is responsible for the actions of holding, giving, and receiving.

Fire, which manifests as light, heat, and color is related to vision. The sensory organ of vision is the eye. The organ of action related to the sense of vision is the feet. A blind man can walk but his walking has no direction. Eyes give direction to the action of walking.

Water is related to taste. The sensory organ of taste is the tongue. Without water the tongue cannot perceive the different tastes. The related organ of action is the reproductive system. The tongue is closely related in function to the action of the genitals (penis and clitoris). In Āyurveda, the penis and clitoris are considered the lower tongue and the tongue in the mouth is the upper tongue. The person who controls the upper tongue has control over the lower tongue and vice versa.

Earth is related to the sense of smell. The sensory organ of smell is the nose. The organs of action related to the sense of smell are the excretory organs. The nose is related to the anus.

---

10. Ether is the preferred term when referring to the five elements. Space normally refers to physical space.

This relationship is demonstrated by the fact that a person who has constipation or an unclean colon experiences bad breath and a dull sense of smell.

The Basic Attributes of Tridosha—Vāta, Pitta, Kapha

According to Āyurvedic philosophy, the entire cosmos is an interplay of the energies of the five elements—Ether, Air, Fire, Water, Earth. Āyurveda groups the five elements into three basic types of energy or functional principles that are present in everybody and everything. There are no single words in English to describe these principles, so we use the original Sanskrit words vāta, pitta and kapha, called the three doshas or tridosha. Dosha literally means "fault, "impurity," or "mistake." However, that definition is not adequate in this context. Dosha is a specific word used by Charaka, Sushruta, and Vāgbhata. Dosha is organization. As long as the doshas are normal in quality and quantity, they maintain a harmonious psychophysiology. The moment they go out of balance, they corrupt or pollute or vitiate the dhātus (bodily tissues) and then they become dosha (here meaning impurity). Therefore, dosha is that which becomes vitiated and then affects the bodily tissues, leading to disease. But in a healthy way, dosha means three principles that govern psychophysiological response and pathological changes. The doshas—vāta, pitta, and kapha—bind the five elements into living flesh. The concept of support is a natural function of these principles of physiology we call vāta, pitta, kapha. They are the agents of DNA which form the blueprint for the physiology. They are energy complexes; these complexes are known by their attributes, or gunas.

Energy is required to create movement so that fluids and nutrients get to the cells, enabling the body to function. Energy is also necessary to metabolize the nutrients in the cells and is utilized to lubricate and maintain cellular structure. Vāta is the energy of movement, pitta the energy of transformation, digestion or metabolism, and kapha the energy of lubrication and structure.

In Āyurveda, body, mind, and consciousness work together in maintaining balance. They are simply viewed as different facets of one's being. To learn how to balance body, mind, and consciousness requires an understanding of how vāta, pitta and kapha work together. According to Āyurvedic philosophy, the entire cosmos is an interplay of the energies of the five basic elements—Ether, Air, Fire, Water, and Earth. Vāta, pitta and kapha are combinations of the five elements that manifest as patterns in all creation.

Ancient Āyurveda might have classified human beings into five body types based upon the predominant element. But as Ether is essentially inert and Earth is the solid, supporting foundation of creation, these two elements did not lend themselves to a typology as well as did the active, mobile, and changing elements of Air, Fire and Water. Āyurveda incorporates the three active elements as the primary elements in the principle of tridosha.

Every dosha is composed of all five elements. However, two elements are predominant in each.

> Vāta is Air and Ether.
> Pitta is Fire and Water.
> Kapha is Water and Earth.

Vāta, pitta, and kapha are the very foundation of Āyurveda. The concept of the humors or principles—wind, bile, and phlegm—found in the Greek medicine of the past is likely an offspring of Āyurveda.

Vāta. In the body, vāta, principally composed of Ether and Air, is the subtle energy associated with movement. It governs breathing, blinking, muscle and tissue movement, the pulsation of the heart, and all the movements in the cytoplasm and cell membranes. In balance, vāta promotes creativity and flexibility. Out of balance, vāta produces fear, anxiety, and abnormal movements.

Pitta. Principally made up of Fire and Water, pitta expresses itself as the body's metabolic system. It governs digestion, absorption, assimilation, nutrition, metabolism, body temperature—all transformations. In balance, pitta promotes understanding and intelligence. Out of balance, pitta arouses anger, hatred, jealousy, and inflammatory disorders.

Kapha. Kapha is principally a combination of Earth and Water and is the energy that forms the body's structure, and provides the "glue" or cohesion that holds the cells together. Kapha supplies the water for all bodily parts and systems. It lubricates joints, moisturizes the skin and maintains immunity. In balance, kapha is expressed as love, calmness, and forgiveness. Out of balance, it leads to attachment, greed, possessiveness, and congestive disorders.

Attributes (Gunas) and Their Effects on Doshas

Charaka, the great Āyurvedic physician of ancient times, found that all organic and inorganic substances, as well as all thoughts and actions, have definite attributes. These attributes contain potential energy and express the static nature of a substance, while the actions express kinetic energy. Attributes and actions are closely related since the potential energy of the attributes eventually becomes action, or kinetic energy, released when the substance undergoes chemical transformation such as burning or digestion. According to Āyurveda, there are twenty basic attributes.

Charaka categorized these attributes into 10 opposite pairs (e.g., sharp and slow or dull, dry and oily, liquid and dense). These opposite forces function together. Basically, the universe is the manifestation of the two opposites, male and female energy. Actually it is possible to understand the universe in its entirety in terms of the interactions of opposing basic attributes. These pairs of opposites must be understood as having relative relationships—relative to subject, relative to individual and also relative to standard normality. Nothing is absolute.

Table 4: The 20 Attributes and Their Relationship to the Tridosha

Vāta	Pitta	Kapha
Dry	Hot	Heavy
Light	Sharp	Slow / Dull
Cold	Light	Cold
Rough	Liquid	Oily
Subtle	Mobile	Liquid
Mobile	Oily	Slimy / Smooth
Clear		Dense
		Soft
		Static
		Sticky / Cloudy
		Hard
		Gross
Elements of the Tridosha		
Space + Air	Fire + Water	Water + Earth

Vāta, pitta, and kapha each have their own attributes, in fact each of these terms is really only a name for a grouping of attributes. Vāta represents the collection of dry, light, cold, rough, subtle, mobile, and clear qualities. Pitta, similarly, is made up of hot, sharp, light, liquid, mobile and slightly oily qualities. Kapha includes attributes of heavy, slow or dull, cold, oily, liquid, slimy or smooth, dense, soft, static and sticky or cloudy.

In Āyurveda there is a law which states that like increases like. When similar qualities come together, their quantitative expression increases. For example, the summer season has attributes similar to those of pitta—hot, liquid, light, mobile, and penetrating. Therefore, in the summer pitta in the body will be increased. Vāta is light, subtle, dry, mobile, rough, and cold. So, in the fall season, which also exhibits these attributes, vāta will tend to be increased in the human constitution. Kapha is liquid, heavy, cold, sticky and cloudy. In the winter when these characteristics predominate in the external environment, internal kapha tends to be increased.

The concepts governing Āyurvedic pharmacology, therapeutics, and food preparation are based on the 20 attributes. Through an understanding and application of the actions of the attributes, balance of the tridosha can be maintained.

We will now consider each of these attributes and their effects on tridosha. The section called "The Twenty Attributes (Gunas) and Their Effects on the Doshas" on page 283 details these attributes and their actions on the doshas and agni.

Guru (Heavy). The heavy quality increases kapha and decreases vāta and pitta. Guru promotes growth in the body. Meat, cheese, yogurt, and sugar are heavy. Eating heavy foods may cause weight gain. Sleep is also heavy and sleeping for 10 hours leaves a person feeling heavy throughout the day. Eating and not doing much physical activity is heavy. To some extent we need the heavy quality for nourishment, groundedness, centeredness, and stability. However, too much of this quality slows digestion and metabolism, and creates dullness.

Laghu (Light). The light quality increases vāta and pitta and decreases kapha. The opposite of heavy is laghu. This quality makes the body alert and attentive. But too much of this quality creates spaciness, ungroundedness, and instability. It creates insecurity, fear, and anxiety.

Manda (Slow/Dull). The slow quality increases kapha and decreases vāta and pitta. Manda creates sluggishness, slow action, relaxation and dullness, as well as calm, quiet, and silence. Rich and fatty foods induce this quality.

Tīkshna (Sharp). The sharp quality increases vāta and pitta and decreases kapha. The opposite of manda is tīkshna. Sharp qualities are present in cayenne pepper and other spicy foods. Fire is hot and sharp. This quality improves learning, concentration, understanding, appreciation, and comprehension. In excess, it can create ulcers.

Shīta (Cold). The cold quality increases vāta and kapha and decreases pitta. Shīta creates cold, numbness, unconsciousness, contraction, stagnation, fear, and insensitivity in the body. Cold promotes accumulation of mucus, thus raising kapha. The cold quality cools down pitta, slows digestion and reduces immunity. Exposure to cold weather reduces the natural resistance of the throat and may help promote a sore throat, if your internal fire, or agni, is not strong enough to give protection.

Ushna (Hot). The hot quality increases pitta and decreases vāta and kapha. The opposite of cold is ushna. The hot quality stimulates gastric fire, improves circulation, digestion, absorption, and assimilation. It liquefies kapha, as fire melts wax, and calms vāta, because vāta is cold. The hot quality promotes cleansing. If you eat hot curry, your sinuses begin to run, because heat liquefies kapha and removes it from the system. Green chilies and cayenne pepper are hot. Hot causes increase of pitta, and since pitta is hot, it can make a person irritable and angry.

Snigdha (Oily or Unctuous). The oily quality increases pitta and kapha and decreases vāta. Snigdha brings relaxation. It creates smoothness, moisture, lubrication, and vigor. It promotes compassion. Love is oily, liquid, and nourishing because it has the quality of snigdha.

Rūksha (Dry). The dry quality increases vāta and decreases pitta and kapha. The opposite of snigdha is rūksha. It creates dehydration and makes the stool hard and dry, causing constipation. Rūksha stimulates fire, because fire is dry. This quality causes choking, constriction, spasm, and pain. Dry weather causes aggravation of vāta under the skin, causing the skin to become dry, rough and cracked. Fear, nervousness and loneliness are dry. Rūksha creates isolation, separation, and rejection. When a person is lonely, the dry quality is aggravated.

Shlakshna (Slimy/Smooth). The smooth quality increases pitta and kapha and decreases vāta. Cheese and oils increase pitta, avocado and ghee increase kapha. This quality lubricates and makes the body flexible. Shlakshna prevents osteoporosis and arthritic changes.

Khāra (Rough). The rough quality increases vāta and decreases pitta and kapha. The opposite of smooth is khāra. Khāra increases dryness, absorption, and constipation. All raw vegetables are rough and provoke vāta. The rough quality is also present in garbanzo beans, adzuki beans, black beans, and pinto beans. Even after being cooked, they are still rough, astringent, produce gas, and increase vāta.

Sandra (Dense). The dense quality increases kapha and decreases vāta and pitta. Meat and cheese are dense. Sandra increases the compactness of the body and makes a person more grounded. When vāta is provoked, people may crave meat, which brings a feeling of stability. Sandra promotes solidity, density, and strength. The firmness and solidity of healthy muscle tissue is kapha. The dense quality overall is kapha increasing.

Drava (Liquid). The liquid quality increases pitta and kapha and decreases vāta. The opposite of dense is liquid. However, the word liquid doesn't give the total significance. Sandra means dense, highly concentrated, and drava means less concentrated, diluted. For example, water is drava, liquid, diluted. But if you continue adding salt to water, the stage comes when the salt stops dissolving. That salty water is highly concentrated and dense. Kapha has these qualities of dense, liquid and salty. Drava dissolves and liquefies. The liquid quality promotes salivation, compassion, and cohesiveness. Excessive intake of water will cause water retention and increase kapha.

Mrudu (Soft). The soft quality increases pitta and kapha and decreases vāta. Mrudu creates softness, delicacy, relaxation, tenderness, love, and care. It provokes mucus and increases kapha in the system. The soft quality calms vāta, because vāta is rough. Love is soft while anger is hot, sharp and penetrating; fear is dry and rough. Sleeping on a soft water bed increases kapha.

Kathina (Hard). The hard quality increases vāta and decreases pitta. In later stages of disease, it also increases kapha such as when a tumor is formed. The opposite of mrudu is kathina. Kathina increases hardness, strength, rigidity, selfishness, callousness, and insensitivity in the mind. In pneumonia, the lungs become hard. Sleeping on a hard bed increases vāta. Callouses on the hands or feet is kathina.

Sthira (Static). The static quality increases kapha and decreases vāta and pitta. Sthira promotes stability and support. Sitting quietly induces the static quality and brings stability and healing.

Chala (Mobile). The mobile quality increases vāta and pitta and decreases kapha. Chala is the opposite of sthira. Chala promotes motion, shakiness, and restlessness. Our thoughts, feelings and emotions are mobile. Insecurity and shakiness come from mobile quality. The mobile quality increases vāta in the system, while the static quality brings groundedness. Jogging, jumping, and physical activity are examples of chala.

Sūkshma (Subtle). The subtle quality increases vāta and pitta and decreases kapha. Many drugs and herbs are sūkshma, subtle. For example, marijuana increases vāta and pitta and makes a person spacey. Alcohol and aspirin are also subtle and especially increase pitta.

Sthūla (Gross). The gross quality increases kapha and decreases vāta and pitta. Sthūla causes obstruction and obesity. Meat and cheese are gross and increase kapha. The opposite of sūkshma is sthūla.

Vishada (Clear). The clear quality increases vāta and pitta and decreases kapha. Vishada pacifies but creates isolation and diversion. The opposite of āvila is vishada. An excess of clear quality can manifest from too much cleansing, such as excessive enemas or purgatives. Too much cleansing increases vāta and pitta.

Picchila (Sticky). The sticky quality increases kapha and decreases vāta and pitta. Picchila causes cohesiveness in body and mind. In excess, it can cause attachment which is a sign of high kapha. This twentieth guna is sometimes called **āvila (cloudy)**[11]. The cloudy quality increases kapha and decreases vāta and pitta. Āvila causes lack of both clarity and perception. All dairy products are āvila and increase kapha.

Āyurveda uses these 20 qualities as a therapeutic guide, a diagnostic tool, and a clinical barometer in order to pinpoint which quality has provoked vāta, pitta or kapha.

Prakruti: Your Unique Body Type

Each person's combination and proportions of vāta, pitta and kapha are determined by the genetics, diet, lifestyle, and emotions of the parents, among other factors, at the time of conception. The combination of the three doshas, which forms the person's constitution and is set at conception, is called prakruti. Prakruti is simply the unique psychophysical makeup and functional habits of a person.

There are seven possible combinations of vāta, pitta and kapha. For example, a person might be mostly kapha with a secondary characteristic of pitta and a small amount of vāta. In

---

11. The qualities of the twenty gunas are described in more than one way. Picchila is used by some authors and āvila is used by others.

Āyurveda this would be written $V_1 P_2 K_3$. A person might be equally pitta and vāta with a small amount of kapha. This would be written $V_3 P_3 K_1$. The numbers serve to suggest the ranking of each dosha. A few rare individuals are born with a constitution where all three doshas are equal in quality and quantity, $V_3 P_3 K_3$. These people experience good health and excellent digestion. However, the majority of people will have one or two doshas predominant. With proper diet and lifestyle, these people can maintain balance and optimal health. The prakruti, as one's genetic code, does not change during one's lifetime, except in rare cases.

Not every person with the same ratio of doshas in their prakruti is identical. This is because, even though the quantities of the doshas are the same, the qualities express in different ways. For example, a person with V_3 may be more cold while another with the same proportion may be more dry.

Vikruti
There is also a state called *vikruti*, which reveals the present state of the three doshas. If the present state of the doshas is the same as prakruti, that person is balanced and healthy. In a person of excellent health, the proportions of vikruti will be the same as prakruti. But more likely there will be a difference, for vikruti reflects any aspects of diet, lifestyle, emotions, age, environment, etc., that are not in harmony with one's prakruti. An Āyurvedic physician can establish this difference through a variety of procedures that include taking a life history, analyzing the face and tongue, and taking the pulse. It is this difference between prakruti and vikruti that provides the Āyurvedic physician with precise information to formulate a program for restoring health. No matter what the constitution, it is possible to achieve optimal health through proper diet, cooking methods, lifestyle, and an attitude toward life that specifically suits each individual.

There are four general categories which describe prakruti: janma prakruti, deha prakruti, dosha prakruti, and manas prakruti.

Janma Prakruti. Janma prakruti is also called karma prakruti, because it reflects the effects of karmic influences on the constitution. We are bound to birth and death by karmic forces that influence the physical, mental, astral, and causal bodies. The cause of birth is desire. When we take birth (at the moment the soul enters the fetus), the karmic momentum of the individual manifests from the causal to the mental body then to the astral body and finally to the physical body. The resulting individual constitution is janma prakruti. We have chosen our parents through karmic bonds. Moksha (liberation) cannot be attained until all karmic seeds are roasted in the flame of attention, meditation.

Janma prakruti is the genetic prakruti, which is determined at the moment of conception. This genetic prakruti is a combination of the ratios of VPK in the mother and the father at that time. Diet, lifestyle, and mental/emotional factors affecting the parents can influence the qualities of VPK in their sperm and ova.

Deha Prakruti. Deha prakruti is the current bodily prakruti. It includes the fetal prakruti during pregnancy, which is influenced by the mother's diet, lifestyle, environment, and mental/emotional states. Janma (genetic) prakruti can be altered by these maternal influences and long-standing congenital abnormalities may result, which means deha prakruti is different from janma prakruti. For instance, due to aggravation of the doshas in the fetus caused by the mother's diet and lifestyle, the baby could develop cleft palate or spina bifida.

Deha prakruti reflects the dharma associated with a particular birth. Behind every dharma is karma, which is action. Dharma is duty, responsibility. The mother's dharma and actions influence the baby's constitution. The deha prakruti is also a physical expression of the causal, mental, and astral bodies. The physical/psychological makeup reflects the dharma that the individual has taken birth to perform, and the individual will possess abilities that make it possible to fulfill that dharma.

Dosha Prakruti. Dosha prakruti represents the ratio of doshas present at the time of birth, when the baby takes its first breath. The season, time, place, date, and planetary disposition at birth can all affect dosha prakruti. Dosha prakruti is deha prakruti expressed in terms of vāta, pitta, and kapha.

Manas Prakruti. Manas prakruti is a term that defines the mental constitution. Manas prakruti is described in terms of the three gunas—sattva, rajas, tamas. Sattvic qualities of mind are clarity, alertness, attentiveness, love, compassion, and cooperativeness. Rajasic qualities are self-centeredness, selfishness, and restlessness. Rajas is movement; the movement between the observer and the observed, between subject and object. Tamasic qualities express as dullness, gloominess, depression, sadness, and laziness. Tamas is crystallization of experience.

Manas prakruti is also part of your genetic code. Right at the time of fertilization, the sperm and ovum join, carrying vāta, pitta, and kapha from the parents. Similarly, they carry sattva, rajas, and tamas from the cosmic mind. The cosmic mind maintains equilibrium of sattva, rajas, and tamas. Cosmic tamas creates darkness. Cosmic sattva creates the rising of the sun. Cosmic rajas creates the movement of the earth and galaxies. So, in the cosmic mind, sattva, rajas, and tamas are perfectly harmonized, qualitatively and quantitatively. That is why there is order in the cosmos. Nevertheless, at the time of fertilization, an individual soul's past life karma yields the qualities of that karma into an enclosure of jīvātman, a tiny bubble of the ocean of consciousness, which is formed because of a movement of sattva, rajas, and tamas.

Therefore, at fertilization, sattva, rajas, and tamas, in a particular permutation and combination, yield into the consciousness of the fertilized ovum. There is embryonic consciousness and within that consciousness, there are embryonic manas, smruti, buddhi and ahamkāra. In the embryonic smruti, we carry past life memory. In the embryonic buddhi, the embryo has the capacity to discriminate and digest thoughts.

According to Āyurveda, the heart is the seat of the mind. Manas prakruti, the mind, is expressed during the third month of pregnancy when the heart is developing. There is also unmanifest embryonic mind that we may call the subconscious mind. We have a subconscious mind and the cosmos has a subconscious mind. The cosmic subconscious mind is in a pre-Big Bang state. When the Big Bang occurred, the cosmic subconscious became conscious and creation occurred.

In summary, janma prakruti, the genetic code at the time of fertilization, does not change. Deha prakruti can change through the actions of the mother. Similarly, manas prakruti is subject to change. A person who is born with more rajasic quality can see his manas prakruti change to a predominance of sattva through meditation, yoga, contemplation, or the guidance of a spiritual master. The purpose of manas prakruti is to be a springboard, so that you can balance on this springboard and jump into the cosmos. Manas prakruti can be used to make a quantum leap into the cosmic order. It does not matter if you are tamasic. Just say, "Yes, I'm tamasic; that's fine." You can acknowledge this in yourself. Once you know you have tamasic qualities, the tamas begins to change. A mad man does not know that he is mad. The moment he knows he is mad, in that moment his madness goes away. That is the beauty of manas prakruti.

Characteristics of the Vāta Individual

The Sanskrit term vāta is related to the verb *vah*, meaning vehicle, to carry or to move. So vāta is the principle of mobility that regulates all activity in the body, from how many thoughts one might have during a given period to how efficiently food moves through the intestines. The vāta quality is responsible for joy, happiness, creativity, speech, sneezing, and elimination, to name just a few functions. Vāta is in charge of the vital life essence, prāna. Thus when vāta (prāna) leaves the body, life ceases.

Vāta has the qualities or attributes of dry, light, cold, rough, subtle, mobile, and clear, with an astringent taste, and brownish and blackish colors. How these qualities translate into the makeup of the vāta individual is shown in the chart of vāta attributes. Physically, vāta persons have light, flexible bodies and big, protruding teeth. They have small, recessed, dry eyes. With irregular appetite and thirst, they often experience digestive and malabsorption problems. Vāta types tend to be delicate in health, so may have few or no children.

In their behavior, vāta individuals are easily excited. Indeed, they are alert and quick to act without much thinking. They have good imaginations and enjoy daydreaming. Vāta individuals are loving people but may love someone out of fear or loneliness. Fears of darkness, heights and enclosed spaces are not uncommon in vāta individuals. Their faith is flexible and ready to change, but the change does not necessarily last for long. Because of this tendency to change, vāta people may often move furniture or residence to keep from feeling bored. They do not like sitting idle and seek constant action. Due to their active natures, they make good money but spend it on trifles and have difficulty saving. (see "The Attributes of the Vāta Individual" on page 42)

Characteristics of the Pitta Individual

The word pitta is derived from the Sanskrit word *tap*, meaning to heat and to be austere. Pitta represents the Fire principle in the body. Literally everything that enters the body must be digested or "cooked," from the sight of a full moon to a strawberry popped into the mouth. In addition to the gastric fire, pitta also includes the enzymes and amino acids that play a major role in metabolism, and even the neurotransmitters and neuropeptides involved in thinking. Some of pitta's responsibilities are regulating the body heat through chemical transformation of food and giving a person appetite, vitality, learning, and understanding.

Pitta is hot, sharp, light, liquid, spreading, and slightly oily in nature. It is sour, pungent, and bitter to the taste, and has a fleshy smell. It is associated with the colors red and yellow. These qualities are revealed in the body of the pitta person, as shown in the chart of pitta attributes. By virtue of these attributes, pitta people have a sensitive and reactive body with a medium frame and weight. They seldom gain or lose much weight. They may have sharp, yellowish teeth with soft and, at times, bleeding gums. Their eyes are bright but tend to be sensitive to light. Pittas usually have strong appetite and thirst and like cold drinks and sweets.

Pitta types have excellent capability for learning, understanding, and concentrating. They are highly disciplined and excellent leaders. These people are blessed with wisdom, which is sometimes reflected by baldness—so much wisdom indeed that it "burns" off their hair! Pitta individuals never yield an inch from their principles, which sometimes leads them to fanaticism. They may give a wrong answer but with great confidence.

As a matter of fact, they can be judgmental, critical, and perfectionistic, and tend to become angry easily. They love noble professions and often make large amounts of money to spend on luxurious items. They like perfume and jewelry. They may not have a strong sex drive. Overall, the pitta constitution is endowed with moderate strength, much material knowledge, wealth, and a medium span of life. (see "The Attributes of the Pitta Individual" on page 43)

Characteristics of the Kapha Individual
The phrase kapha comes from two Sanskrit roots, *ka* meaning water and *pha* meaning to flourish—that which is flourished by water. Kapha's nature is also Earth, so Earth and Water give kapha its definitive qualities. Kapha comprises all our cells, tissues and organs. Kapha molecules tend to stick together to form dense masses and give the body a chubby shape. Lubrication of joints and organs, strong muscles and bones, cellular secretions, and memory retention are all part of kapha's function.

Water and Earth give kapha the qualities of heavy, slow, cool, oily, liquid, slimy, dense, soft, static, sticky, cloudy, hard, and gross. It has a sweet and salty taste and is white in color. The presentation of these qualities in the kapha constitution is in the table of kapha attributes.

These qualities give a strong and large body frame, large eyes, strong teeth and thick, curly hair to people of kapha constitution. They have thick, smooth, oily and hairy skin. Kapha people have a steady appetite and thirst, but tend to have slow digestion and metabolism. These characteristics often result in weight gain, which kapha people have great difficulty in shedding. At times, cravings for sweet and salt lead to water retention. They love eating, sitting, doing nothing, and sleeping for a long time.

Kapha people are blessed with a deep, stable faith, with love and compassion, and a calm, steady mind. They have good memory, a deep melodious voice, and a monotonous pattern of speech. A kapha person makes and saves money. Extravagances may be spending a little amount on cheese, candy and cakes. An unbalanced kapha suffers from greed, attachment, possessiveness, and laziness. All in all, the healthy kapha individual is endowed with excellent strength, knowledge, peace, love, and longevity, due to a strong constitution. (see "The Attributes of the Kapha Individual" on page 44)

Table 5: The Attributes of the Vāta Individual

Attributes	Manifestations in the Body, Mind & Emotions
Dry	dry skin, hair, lips, tongue; dry colon, tending toward constipation; hoarse voice
Light	light muscles, bones, thin body frame, light, scanty sleep; underweight
Cold	cold hands, cold feet, poor circulation; hates cold and loves hot; stiffness of muscles
Rough	rough, cracked skin, nails, hair, teeth, hands and feet; cracking joints
Subtle	subtle fear, anxiety, insecurity; fine goose-pimples; minute muscle twitching, fine tremors
Mobile	fast walking, talking, doing many things at a time; erratic; restless eyes, eyebrows, hands, feet; unstable joints; many dreams; loves travelling and does not stay at one place; swinging moods, shaky faith, scattered mind
Clear	clairvoyant; understands immediately and forgets immediately; clear, empty mind, experiences void and loneliness
Astringent	dry choking sensation in the throat; gets hiccoughs, burping; loves oily, mushy soups; craving for sweet, sour and salty tastes; tendency toward constipation
Brownish-black	Dark complexion; dark hair and eyes; color of vāta āma, e.g., dark coated tongue

Table 6: The Attributes of the Pitta Individual

Attributes	Manifestations in the Body, Mind & Emotions
Hot	good digestive fire; strong appetite; body temperature tends to be higher than average; hates heat; gray hair with receding hair line or baldness; soft brown hair on the body and face
Sharp	sharp teeth, distinct eyes, pointed nose, tapering chin, heart-shaped face; good absorption and digestion; sharp memory and understanding; intolerance of hard work; irritable; probing mind
Light	light/medium body frame; does not tolerate bright light; fair shiny skin, bright eyes
Liquid	loose liquid stools; soft delicate muscles; excess urine, sweat and thirst
Spreading (mobile)	pitta spreads as rash, acne, or inflammation over the body or affected areas; pitta subjects want to spread their name and fame all over the world
Oily	soft oily skin, hair, feces; may not digest deep-fried food which can cause headache
Sour	sour acid stomach, acidic pH; sensitive teeth; excess salivation
Pungent	heartburn, burning sensations in general; strong feelings of anger and hate
Bitter	bitter taste in the mouth, nausea, vomiting; repulsion toward bitter taste; cynical
Fleshy smell	fetid smell under armpits, mouth, soles of feet; socks smell
Red	red flushed skin, eyes, cheeks and nose; red color aggravates pitta; does not tolerate heat and sunlight; color of pitta without āma
Yellow	yellow eyes, skin, urine and feces; may lead to jaundice, over production of bile; yellow color increases pitta; pale yellow coloring is normal pitta, but dark yellow is color of pitta āma

Table 7: The Attributes of the Kapha Individual

Attributes	Manifestations in the Body, Mind & Emotions
Heavy	heavy bones, muscles, large body frame; tends to be overweight; grounded; deep heavy voice
Slow/Dull	slow walk, talk; slow digestion, metabolism; sluggish gestures
Cool (Cold)	cold clammy skin; steady appetite and thirst with slow metabolism and digestion; repeated cold, congestion and cough
Oily	oily skin, hair and feces; lubricated, unctuous joints and other organs
Liquid	excess salivation; congestion in the chest, sinuses, throat and head
Slimy/Smooth	smooth skin; smoothness of organs; smooth, gentle mind, calm nature
Dense	dense pad of fat; thick skin, hair, nail and feces; plump rounded organs; firmness and solidity of muscles; compact, condensed tissues
Soft	soft pleasing look; love, care, compassion, kindness and forgiveness
Static	loves sitting, sleeping and doing nothing
Sticky	viscous, cohesive quality causes compactness, firmness of joints and organs; loves to hug; is deeply attached in love and relationships
Cloudy	in early morning mind is cloudy and foggy; often desires coffee as a stimulant to start the day
Hard	firm muscles; strength; rigid attitude
Gross	causes obstruction; obesity
Sweet	the anabolic action of sweet taste stimulates sperm formation increasing quantity of semen; abnormal function may cause craving for sweets
Salty	helps digestion and growth, gives energy; maintains osmotic condition; abnormal function may create craving for salt, water retention
White	pale complexion; white mucous; white coating on tongue; color of kapha āma

3

The Doshas
and Their Subtypes

आयुर्वेद

The human body is a biological combination of the five elements—Ether, Air, Fire, Water, and Earth. The combination of Ether and Air form vāta, Fire and Water form pitta, and Water and Earth form kapha. Āyurveda further categorizes each dosha into five subtypes (or *subdoshas*), depending upon their function and location.

Vāta and Its Subtypes

Prāna, the life force in the body, manifests as different vāta systems in the body. Vāta has the attributes of dry, light, cold, rough, subtle, mobile, clear, and astringent taste. Vāta is present throughout the body and is predominant in the head, throat, diaphragm, small intestine, belly button, pelvic girdle, bones, thighs, colon, and heart. It has affinity for and concentrates in these sites. The normal functions of vāta in the body are movement, respiration, and ingestion of food and water. Without ingestion, there is no digestion.

The different functions of vāta relate to their locations within different structures. This process is called Āyurvedic bio-morphology. Vāta is classified as five types: *prāna, udāna, samāna, apāna,* and *vyāna.* According to Āyurvedic anatomy and physiology, the specific sites of these five subtypes of vāta are of great therapeutic value in addressing imbalances of vāta dosha. Prāna is located in the head and the brain; udāna is in the throat and diaphragm; samāna is in the small intestine and belly button; apāna is located in the colon; and vyāna is in the heart.

Table 8: The Subtypes of Vāta

Subtype	Governing Element	Primary Sites	Functions	Direction
Prāna	Ether	Head, Brain	Pūrana: to fill the space	Downward, Inward
Udāna	Air	Diaphragm, Throat	Udvahana: moves upward	Upward
Samāna	Fire	Small Intestine, Navel	Viveka: isolation, separation, splitting	Linear
Apāna	Earth	Colon, Pelvic Cavity	Dhārana: holding	Downward, Outward
Vyāna	Water	Heart, Whole Body	Praspandanam: pulsation, throbbing	Circular, Circulation

All sensations are a creation of prāna and there is no sensation without prāna. When prāna is dropped, sensations are stopped. A touch to the skin is carried to the brain by prāna and then we react to the touch. When prāna reacts in a motor response, it becomes *apāna*. Prāna carries sensory stimuli and apāna carries motor responses. The apāna present in the nervous system is called *sūkshma apāna* or *shakti apāna*.

Movement is circulation—the rhythms of the diaphragm, heart, lungs, and even the gastrointestinal tract. Movements are of two kinds, voluntary and involuntary. Voluntary movements are those under motor control, such as the movements of the biceps, triceps, and other skeletal muscles. Other movements, such as the heartbeat, are involuntary, because they are under the control of the autonomic nervous system. There are certain movements that are both voluntary and involuntary, such as the movement of the diaphragm, but these movements are classified as involuntary. A person can control respiration for a short period but, beyond that, it becomes automatic.

There are five important functions of vāta in the body:

pūrana	to fill the space.
udvahana	to move upward
viveka	isolation, separation, splitting
dhārana	to hold the flow
praspandanam	pulsation, throbbing

Pūrana means to fill the space, as air fills a vacuum. Pūrana is associated with prāna vāyu and fills the spaces of the cells and governs inspiration.

Udvahana is upward movement, which is udāna vāyu.

Viveka means isolation, separation, splitting, as a single cell splits into two cells. Samāna vāyu is associated with viveka. Here viveka means discrimination between essential and non-essential, which is one of the processes of digestion governed by samāna vāyu. Therefore, in the process of digestion samāna splits the foodstuff into essential and non-essential for absorption in the small intestines and at the cellular level.

Dhārana means to hold the flow, as when one inhales and holds the breath, and also means circulation and nutrition. For example, through circulation, vāta carries nutrients to the cells and, by osmosis, the cells are nourished by vāta. That is also dhārana. Dhārana is associated with apāna vāyu, which absorbs minerals and thereby governs the nourishment of the body. If a person has severe diarrhea, the dhārana function is lost. Dhārana is also necessary for the tone of the body.

Spandanam means pulsation and *praspandanam* means continuous pulsation. Praspandanam is movement of the body governed by vyāna vāyu, pulsation. When one feels the throb of the pulse, it is because of vyāna.

The most important site of vāta is pakvāshaya, the colon. From the Āyurvedic point of view, this is a vital site. When vāta is aggravated, the person develops constipation and lower backache. The person also develops pain in the thighs, ringing in the ears, and aches and pains in the bones and joints, as well as tingling and numbness in the skin. Most vāta diseases are treated by injecting oil in the rectum. When the colon is lubricated with oil, vāta calms down.

Vāta is specifically related to *shabdendriya*, the auditory pathways, and *sparshendriya*, the tactile pathways. The ears are constantly open to the air, so one can hear sound through the ears. Similarly, the skin is always exposed to the air and we feel touch through the skin.

Functions of Vāta

All physical movements
Maintenance of life
Communication
Governs the mind, sensory
    perception, and motor functions
    —including speech and muscular
    co-ordination
Movement of thoughts, feelings,
    and nerve impulses
Respiration
Heart function
Circulation
Ingestion
Peristalsis and enzyme secretion
Assimilation and absorption
Elimination of urine, feces, sweat
Menstruation; delivery of baby
Orgasm
Cellular respiration and division
Hearing
Touch
Clarity
Creativity
Joy

Sites of Vāta

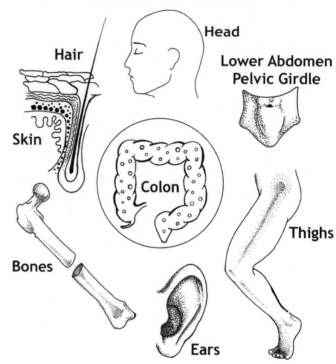

Sites of Vāta:

pakvāshaya	colon
kati	pelvic cavity, waist
sakthi	thighs
mūrdhni	head
asthi	bones
srotra	ears (organs of hearing)
tvak	skin (organ of touch)

The Flow of Prāna

Awareness
(Motionless Prāna)

↓

Perception

↓

Sensations

↓

Feelings

↓

Thoughts

↓

Emotions

We will now go into detail about each of the five subtypes of vāta and examine the function of each one separately.

Prāna Vāyu

Prāna is present in the head and moves downward and inward. It is connected with higher cerebral function. Vāyu[12] and vāta are the same. To say prāna vāyu sounds better than prāna vāta. Prāna vāyu is located in the cranial cavity and it moves in the head. It also moves down to the throat, heart, trachea, lungs, and diaphragm. Because of this movement, prāna is responsible for inhalation. Prāna creates a union of outer cosmic prāna and inner prāna. Prāna is movement of mind, thoughts, feelings, emotions, sensation, and perception. When prāna is motionless, it becomes blissful awareness. So, awareness becomes perception, perception becomes sensation, and sensation becomes feelings. Then thoughts arise and feelings become emotions. This is the natural order.

---

12. Vāyu means air and is used as a synonym for vāta, especially in discussing the subtypes of vāta.

Motionless prāna is Pure Awareness. The moment prāna moves in a particular direction, awareness becomes attention and attention becomes perception. Through perception, prāna creates sensation through which one senses the object of perception. Then sensation becomes feelings and feelings create emotion. Therefore, emotion is the reaction to the flow of prāna and all emotions come from memory.

Indriya means sensation, sense organs, and *chitta* means mind. Feelings, emotions, and awareness are all a part of mind. Prāna moves the mind and prāna becomes mind. If one controls prāna, one can control the mind. Mind is a flow of thought as the river is a flow of water. If thought is clear, the river is clear. If water is dirty, muddy or polluted, the river is polluted. If water is abundant, the river is flooded and swollen. If water is diminished, the river is narrow. As the water, so the river.

Mind is a flow of thoughts. If thought brings fear, the mind becomes fear. If thoughts breed anger, the mind becomes anger. If there is positive thinking, the mind becomes positive. If there is negative thinking, the mind becomes negative. Changing thought is changing the mind. By improving thinking, one will improve the mind and improvement of mind is improvement of man. As the thought, so the mind and as the mind, so the man. Thought is intention. With right thinking, positive thinking, one has right intention, and right intention is right attention. According to modern medicine, thought is a biochemical vehicle but according to Āyurveda, thought is a vibration of prāna. To go beyond thought is the highest *prānāyāma* (breathing pattern).

When prāna is motionless, absolutely still, it is pure, choiceless awareness. Choice is vibration and movement. Therefore, choice becomes desire and desire causes one to choose. By controlling prāna through prānāyāma, one controls the choice and desire and hence the mind. In this way, prāna becomes manas (mind).

Certain signs and symptoms become apparent with an imbalance of prāna vāyu. Palpitation means undue awareness of the heartbeat and is a pranic disorder. Normally, we are not aware of our heartbeat. Palpitation is a physiological and pathological symptom. Imbalance of prāna vāyu can also cause dyspnea, undue awareness of respiration, or breathlessness. Again, breathlessness can be physiological or pathological. Exercise can produce shortness of breath, as can some emotions, such as anger. Pregnancy and obesity can also cause breathlessness. However, dyspnea at rest is a sign of cardiac

Prāna

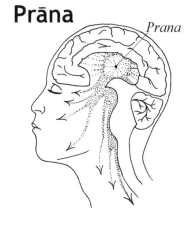

Prana

involvement. If a person has congestive heart failure or right ventricular failure, there is increased cardio-pulmonary action and the person will experience breathlessness at rest.

Other symptoms of prāna vāyu disorders are anxiety, nervousness, fear and anger. Anger is pitta but pitta can disturb prāna vāyu as a psychological manifestation. Inability to focus the mind or concentrate is also a symptom of imbalance of prāna vāyu. Diseases of prāna vāyu imbalance include stroke paralysis, grand mal epilepsy, petit mal epilepsy, sleep apnea, and the tremors of Parkinson's. Respiratory disorders include bronchitis, asthma, and pneumonia, as well as hiccoughs and constant burping.

Udāna Vāyu

The next important vāyu is udāna, which is upward moving energy. Udāna vāyu is located in the diaphragm and moves upward through the lungs, bronchi, trachea, and throat. Udāna also goes up into the brain and stimulates memory. Udāna is the nerve impulse that takes place at the solar plexus and tracheal plexus. It governs the movement of the diaphragm and intercostal muscles, and helps the process of exhalation. Udāna is responsible for speech and expression. A person cannot speak without exhalation.

Prāna vāyu is the energy that brings oxygen into the lungs and udāna vāyu is responsible for exhalation of carbon dioxide. Udāna vāyu helps oxygenation. When oxygenation is good, the person appears fresh and vital. If there is insufficient oxygen, the person suffers from cyanosis and has a purple color. So, udāna vāyu maintains the normal skin color of the complexion because of oxygenation. It is responsible for moving oxygenated blood upward. When a child crawls on the floor and tries to raise its head, that is udāna vāyu. If udāna is weak, the child cannot lift its head or support its neck. Udāna vāyu also helps a person rise from confusion, attachment, and depression. Yogāsanas that stimulate udāna are shoulder stand, cobra pose, and camel pose. These āsanas bring udāna up. If udāna is weak, indulging in actions such as jogging or jumping is like beating a tired horse.

Udāna vāyu disorders create difficulty of speech, such as stuttering or muttering. It creates lack of memory, lack of creativity, and no sense of goal or direction. Suppressed udāna vāyu also creates depression and discoloration of the skin. It can create certain bronchial conditions—hoarseness of voice, asthma, pneumonia and emphysema—as well as blushing and flushing.

Udāna

Udana

Samāna Vāyu

Samāna vāyu is present in the small intestine and navel. It moves the duodenum, jejunum, and ileum. This vāyu provides the stimulus for the secretion of digestive juices. Therefore, samāna vāyu is closely connected with agni (digestive fire). There are agnis in the liver and samāna vāyu provides the energy to secrete the liver enzymes. The bile that is secreted from the liver, along with the liver enzymes, are accumulated in the gallbladder by samāna vāyu. It constricts the gallbladder and pushes the bile from the gallbladder through the bile duct into the duodenum. All of these movements are governed by samāna vāyu.

Samāna

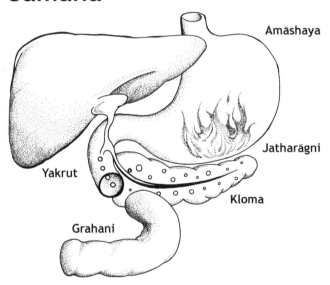

This vāyu plays an important role in creating hunger. When one feels hungry, samāna is awake. Samāna sends a message to prāna asking for food. When one eats, samāna vāyu stimulates the secretion of hydrochloric acid and opens the pyloric valve for movement of foodstuff into the duodenum. Samāna vāyu brings the foodstuff into the cecum, which is called the second stomach. The entire movement around the belly button is samāna vāyu and this movement is linear and outward. Prāna moves downward, udāna moves upward, vyāna moves circular, samāna moves linear, like peristalsis. Hence, samāna vāyu governs digestion, absorption, and assimilation.

The disorders of samāna are loss of appetite, indigestion, increased or decreased peristalsis, bloating, lack of absorption and assimilation, and poor digestion. Therefore, a disorder of samāna vāyu can create malabsorption syndrome.

Apāna Vāyu

The fourth vāyu is apāna. Apāna vāyu is present in the pelvic cavity, in the cecum, ascending colon, transverse colon, descending colon, sigmoid colon, rectum, and urinary tract. Apāna vāyu is also present in the vagina and cervix of a woman and testicles, prostate, and urethra of a man. It moves downward and outward. It regulates the function of the kidneys. The urine is filtered in the kidneys and drop-by-drop is brought down into the bladder. It also stimulates menstruation, defecation, and flatulence. Apāna is motor function working with different segments of the lumbosacral spine. From the lumbosacral spine the message is carried to the bladder to evacuate urine; to the rectum to evacuate feces; to the womb to produce menstruation or delivery of a child. Apāna pushes the child from the womb. If apāna is stuck or weak, labor is delayed.

In addition, apāna vāyu regulates the movement of the sciatic nerve and the lower part of the body. It is also responsible for movement of sperm in the man and the desire to make love. In the woman, apāna stimulates ovulation, regulates menstruation, and during pregnancy apāna nourishes the fetus and moves it during delivery.

During intercourse, apāna of the man and woman merge together and bring the meeting of the sperm and ovum. Apāna is responsible for conception. If apāna is weak, conception is not possible. If apāna vāyu is weak, a woman accumulates fat in the thighs.

Apāna vāyu disorders include constipation or diarrhea; retention of urine or polyuria; no menstruation or profuse menstruation. Pain during menstruation, pain during sex, lower backache, and pain during ovulation are also disorders of this vāyu. Apāna vāyu is responsible for sexual impairment, premature ejaculation or premature orgasm. Strong apāna creates a strong sex drive and weak apāna weakens the sex drive.

Disorders below the belly button are associated with apāna. Disorders at the belly button are samāna. Disorders above the belly button are prāna. Osteoporosis is an apāna vāyu disorder. Apāna vāyu nourishes the bones through the colon mucous membrane and the absorption of minerals.

Apāna

Lumbar Vertebrae
Colon
Sacrum
Bladder
Coccyx
Prostate
Testicle

Vyāna Vāyu

The main function of vyāna vāyu is to maintain cardiac activity, circulation, nutrition and oxygenation of cell tissues and organ systems. Vyāna vāyu is present in the heart and maintains the circulation of arterial blood, venous blood, and lymphatic circulation. Vyāna moves throughout the body. Vyāna is a strong vāyu and all reflex actions, including the corneal reflex, are governed by its energy. It is responsible for the movement of the joints and skeletal muscles through the reflex arc. The reflex arc goes only to the spinal cord and not to the brain, and the spinal cord answers these reflexes.

If vyāna vāyu is affected, the person may have poor circulation and sudden lack of oxygenation, which is called ischemia, lack of oxygen supply to the organs. When coronary arteries are clogged, a person may get ischemic heart disease. If the carotid arteries are clogged, a person may develop ischemic conditions of the brain. When a person suffers a heart attack, blood supply to the heart is blocked and the heart muscle dies, causing the heart to stop beating. In the same way, a heart attack to the brain is called stroke paralysis. Edema, or stagnation of blood in the lower extremities, is another condition caused by poor circulation. All these conditions are vyāna vāyu disorders. When vyāna is affected, prāna is also affected, because these two vāyus have functional integrity.

Pitta and Its Subtypes

In Sanskrit the word pitta comes from *tapa*. Tapa means to heat, to become hot. It also means austerity and concentration. The word pitta means the energy that creates heat in the body. Pitta in the body is a biological combination principally of Fire and Water. The qualities of pitta are hot, sharp, light, liquid, spreading, oily, and sour. Lastly, pitta has a fleshy smell and is pungent and bitter to the taste.

Āmāshaya means stomach. The upper part of the stomach (the lesser curvature) is related to kapha, where more mucus is present. But the lower part of the stomach (the greater curvature) is related to pitta. Pitta is present in the stomach, small intestine, and in the blood, as well as the liver, gallbladder, and spleen[13]. It has affinity for and concentrates in these sites. It is also present in the eyes, sweat, sebaceous secretions, and the gray matter of the brain. Nevertheless, the most important site of pitta for therapeutic purposes is the small intestine.

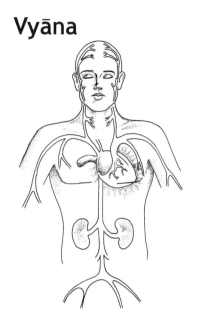

Vyāna

Functions of Pitta
Governs bodily metabolism
Digestion, absorption, assimilation of food
Maintenance of body temperature
Appetite
Thirst
Taste
Color
Luster of eyes, hair, skin, body
Sensitive and reactive body
Intelligence, understanding, comprehension, knowledge
Courage
Ambition
Transformation
Visual perception

---

13. Structurally, the spleen is a large lymphoid tissue, hence it is related to kapha. However, it is also a reservoir of blood and therefore related to pitta functionally and to rakta vaha srotas.

Pitta in the small intestine is present as digestive enzymes; in the stomach as hydrochloric acid, pepsin, and gastric intrinsic factor; in the blood as hemoglobin; in the liver as bile. The spleen is a big reservoir where blood is filtered and pitta is present in the blood. Pitta in the spleen kills bacteria and the parasites of malaria. Color perception by the retina of the eye is governed by pitta. When the body is hot, pitta is released through the sweat as a cooling mechanism. People who do not sweat accumulate fire in the body. At the root of the hair, sebaceous secretions hold the hair tight. If the sebaceous secretions are in excess, the hairs lose their grip and fall out. Pitta people have a problem with hair loss.

Sites of Pitta

nābhi	belly button
grahani	small intestine
āmāshaya	stomach
rakta	blood
yakrut	liver
plīhā	spleen
pittasha	gallbladder
sādhaka	gray matter of the brain
hridayam	heart
tvak	skin
sveda	sweat
lasīkā	sebaceous secretions
vasā	subcutaneous fat
drig	eyes (organs of sight)

Sites of Pitta

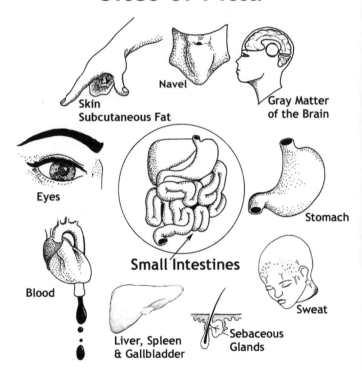

The physiological functions of pitta include digestion of food, maintenance of body temperature, and eyesight. Because eyesight is regulated by pitta, people with pitta prakruti often have poor eyesight. The transparency of the lens and the cornea of the eye are related to pitta, as well as the cone cells of the retina.

Pitta creates flavor in the mouth, taste. Pitta contains agni (digestive fire) and taste is agni. If you have balanced agni, that is, healthy pitta, you have good sense of taste in the mouth. Taste does not lie only in the food, taste lies in your pitta, agni. Agni has fragrance and stimulates the olfactory sense. Appetite is created by pitta but pursuit of appetite is governed by samāna vāyu, which sends a message to prāna that there is too much fire in the stomach. Therefore, appetite is created by pitta, pursued by samāna vāyu, and regulated by prāna vāyu.

The glow of the body, the luster of the eyes, hair, and skin are associated with pitta. Pitta governs intelligence and intellect, and is necessary for understanding and comprehension. Pitta gives knowledge, ambition, and bravery. A pitta body is more sensitive and reactive than a vāta body and the skin is easily sunburned.

Table 9: The Subtypes of Pitta

Subtype	Governing Element	Primary Sites	Functions
Pāchaka	Fire	Small Intestine, Stomach	Digestion, absorption and assimilation of foods
Rañjaka	Water	Liver, Spleen, Intrinsic Factor in Stomach	Produces bile, liver enzymes; gives color to blood
Sādhaka	Ether	Brain (gray matter), Heart	Conscious thinking and emotions; comprehension
Ālochaka	Air	Eyes	Maintains iris color; visual perception
Bhrājaka	Earth	Skin	Maintains skin color, texture and temperature; stereognosis

Pitta is responsible for transformation. There is an apple hanging in the tree. That apple is outside of your body. You pluck the apple and start chewing. The pitta in the stomach digests the apple. The pectin part of the apple is sent to the colon to bind the stool. The sugar part of the apple goes with the blood into the muscles, bones, and even into the reproductive tissue. The transformation of the apple into blood glucose is governed by pitta. When you eat food, that food undergoes the process of digestion, absorption and assimilation, and then the food becomes a part of the cells. The moment water, food, and air molecules enter the cell, they become intelligence. Ultimately, pitta transforms food into pure consciousness.

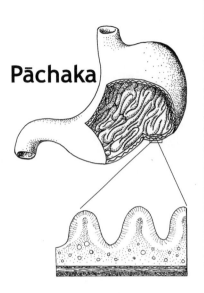

Pāchaka

Pitta is divided into five subtypes—*pāchaka, rañjaka, sādhaka, ālochaka,* and *bhrājaka.* We will now examine more closely the specific functions of each subtype.

Pāchaka Pitta

The pitta present in the stomach and small intestine is called pāchaka pitta. The Sanskrit word pāchaka comes from the root *pach,* which means to digest, absorb, and assimilate. It includes hydrochloric acid, digestive enzymes, and pepsin. The intestinal digestive juice that is secreted from the villi of the small intestine is also pāchaka pitta.

Pāchaka pitta in the stomach digests starch, glucose, and fructose. The initial digestion of protein also begins here through enzymatic actions. Fruits, which are composed of fructose, are easily digested and leave the stomach within one hour. The digestion of starch begins with saliva in the mouth. Some precursors of pāchaka pitta are present in the saliva (salivary amylase or ptylin) and make the saliva acidic.

The pāchaka pitta in the stomach is a part of *jāthara agni.* Jāthara means stomach. This agni is the central fire, gastric fire, and this digestive fire in the stomach is the main agni in the body. When the gastric fire in the stomach is high and there is more secretion of hydrochloric acid and digestive enzymes, the stomach becomes grouchy and creates the sensation of hunger.

Jāthara agni is composed of pāchaka pitta, prāna vāyu, samāna vāyu, and *kledaka kapha,* which we will discuss later. This pitta governs the digestion in the stomach within the first two hours after the ingestion of food. Then the pyloric valve opens and the food passes into the duodenum, the upper part of the small intestine.

The pāchaka pitta in the stomach and the pāchaka pitta in the small intestine work together. The entire small intestine is divided into three parts. The upper part is the duodenum, the middle part is the jejunum, and the lower part is the ileum. The ileum opens into the cecum through the ileocecal valve. The ileum and jejunum are longer than the duodenum. The duodenum is that tiny, strong loop of the small intestine that hugs the head of the pancreas and opens into the stomach through the pyloric wall.

Inside the small intestine there are tiny protuberances called villi and these villi move in waves. Through this movement, the food particles pass through the villi. The moment they contact the villi, samāna vāyu helps to secrete pāchaka pitta, which enters into the particles of food. The hot, sharp, and penetrating qualities of pāchaka pitta break down the food so that the blood vessels of the villi can absorb the nutrients. Essentials from the foodstuff are absorbed and non-essentials for further digestion are sent to the next villi. The villi are constantly working, moving food in one direction.

The end products of digested foodstuff are absorbed through the small capillaries, then enter the blood vessels and are sent to the general circulation. This transformation of foodstuff into the essence of food is called āhāra rasa. Āhāra means food and rasa means juice. Āhāra rasa is chyle, the nutrient precursor or primordial foodstuff.

A disorder of pāchaka pitta may create hyperacidity, hypoglycemia, and craving for sugar. It may also create gastritis, peptic ulcer, indigestion, anorexia, and dyspepsia.

Rañjaka Pitta

Now we will switch our attention to rañjaka pitta, which is mainly present in the liver and spleen. Rañjaka is also present in the stomach as intrinsic factor. The Sanskrit word rañjaka means to give color. Rañjaka pitta in the liver gives color to all tissues. Skin color, hair color and the color of eyes are related to rañjaka pitta. Rañjaka pitta is responsible for erythrogenesis, the creation of red blood cells in the bone marrow, which are mixed with rasa dhātu, the plasma. Thus, rañjaka pitta is responsible for giving color to the blood.

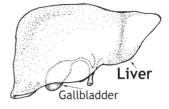

Rañjaka

Liver
Gallbladder

The liver is a complex biochemical lab and a vital organ in the body. A person can live without the spleen, without a kidney or lung, but nobody can live without the liver. The function of rañjaka pitta in the liver is the disintegration of hemoglobin, which produces heme and globin. From heme, bile is produced, and that bile is rañjaka pitta. Its job is to give color to the urine, feces and sweat.

Rañjaka pitta in the stomach is intrinsic factor, which is responsible for the production of blood in the bone marrow. Rañjaka pitta in the spleen kills bacteria and parasites as well as produces some white blood cells (rasa dhātu), so its job is more protective.

There is a functional integrity between the liver, stomach, spleen, and bone marrow. If the function of the liver is affected, the bone marrow will also be affected. If the function of the stomach is affected, it will affect the liver. In a way, the spleen and liver also have functional integrity. The job of the spleen is to filter the blood and to send unwanted, heavy, old red blood cells to the liver; the liver destroys them and separates the hemoglobin from the blood. Then the liver utilizes the hemoglobin that is liberated for the production of bile salts, pigment, and enzymes. Therefore, when the spleen is enlarged the liver may also be enlarged, and vice versa.

The Sanskrit word for liver is *yakrut*. *Ya* means circulation and *krut* means action. The liver has an important function in the digestion of fat and synthesis of proteins through the action of amino acids. It also helps to circulate rañjaka pitta through the hematopoietic system. The rañjaka pitta in the liver and the rañjaka pitta in the stomach (intrinsic factor) enter the circulation and go into the bone marrow. Blood cells are created in the bone marrow but the intrinsic factor—one of the components of the stomach's digestive juice—enables vitamin B_{12} to enter the blood and general circulation, and to go into the bone marrow. There the rañjaka pitta from the stomach (the intrinsic factor and vitamin B_{12}) stimulates erythrogenesis, the creation of red blood cells. The building material of the bone marrow is kapha, but the functional aspect of the production of red blood cells is pitta, governed by *rakta agni* and rañjaka pitta.

When a person undergoes surgery in which part of the stomach is removed, that person often experiences anemia. According to Āyurveda, rañjaka pitta is secreted from the lesser curvature of the stomach. This part of the stomach is the acid bearing area, which secretes hydrochloric acid and intrinsic factor. If the lesser curvature is cut and directly joined to the duodenum, an important portion of the stomach is gone. That person may not secrete sufficient intrinsic factor, which then affects the production of red blood cells, and the result is anemia.

Yakrut is an important seat of fire—the seat of anger, hate, envy, and jealousy. All these emotions need to be processed and metabolized. To metabolize an emotion means to be aware of that emotion. Paying total attention to a feeling or emotion allows the agni of the liver to release it. The anger, fear, or anxiety can then leave with awareness and maturity. Repressed, unmetabolized emotions can create stress in the organs. These emotions want to come out but, if we suppress them, they accumulate in the tissues and lead to disease. Āyurveda does not separate emotions from the organs. We cannot separate body from mind and mind from consciousness.

According to Āyurveda, the agni (fire component) of the liver includes *bhūta agni,* which corresponds on the physical level to the liver enzymes. Bhūta means element or that which manifests as matter. The five basic elements—Ether, Air, Fire, Water, and Earth—are called bhūtas. The flame of jāthara agni goes into the liver and manifests as the agni of these five elements. Whatever food we eat is composed of the five elements. For example, an apple has all five elements, but is composed predominately of Air and Water. Therefore, the apple is crunchy, astringent, and yields gases. The job of bhūta agni is to transform the elements of ingested food into a form the body can use.

There are five bhūta agni: nabhasa agni, the ethereal fire; vāyavya agni, the airy fire; tejo agni, the fiery fire; āpo agni, the watery fire; and pārthiva agni, the earth or mineral fire. These different fire components manifest as specialized enzymes that govern the transformation of unprocessed elements of food into the processed elements of the seven dhātus (tissues).

Five Bhūta Agnis	
Nabhasa Agni	Ether
Vāyavya Agni	Air
Tejo Agni	Fire
Āpo Agni	Water
Pārthiva Agni	Earth

Rañjaka agni is the thermodynamic energy of rañjaka pitta, present in the liver, spleen and stomach. It is the fire component released from the disintegrated red blood cells, and it governs the transformation of rasa into rakta dhātu.

There is a fine line between rañjaka agni, bhūta agni, and rakta agni. Rañjaka agni incorporates bhūta agni. It gives color to rasa dhātu and transforms rasa into immature (asthāyi) rakta dhātu. Bhūta agni is the specialized function of rañjaka agni in the liver that converts food and other substances into their elemental components. Rakta agni does further transformation of asthāyi rakta into mature (sthāyi) rakta dhātu, essential to the maturation of red blood cells. (see "Nutrition and Structure of the Dhātus" on page 104)

Disorders of rañjaka pitta include hepatitis, anemia, chronic fatigue syndrome, and mononucleosis. When kapha disturbs rañjaka pitta, the person may develop gallstones. If kapha is long-standing and lingers in the liver, the person may develop high cholesterol, fatty degeneration of the liver, or steatorrhea (fatty diarrhea).

There is a relationship between rañjaka pitta and ālochaka pitta, the pitta associated with the eyes. If the sclera is yellow, it is due to a disorder of rañjaka pitta and ālochaka pitta. The eyes and liver are connected, and toxicity in the liver may create visual disturbance. Photophobia is sensitivity to light due to toxicity in the liver. The same thing happens if a person drinks too much alcohol. When the liver metabolizes alcohol, excess pitta is produced. Visual perception on a subtle level is also affected, because a rañjaka pitta disorder may even affect the sādhaka pitta of the brain.

Sādhaka

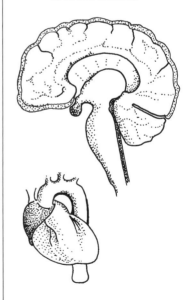

Sādhaka Pitta
Sādhaka pitta is present in the gray matter of the brain as certain neurotransmitters, and in the heart as part of the cardiac plexus or the heart chakra. It is responsible for knowledge,

understanding, comprehension, and appreciation. It transforms sensations into feelings and emotions. It also creates the feeling of "I am" that is ego. In Vedic philosophy the ego is not a bad thing. A person must have self-confidence, self-esteem, and that self-esteem is called ego, ahamkāra. Self-esteem is essential for survival and growth.

Prāna vāyu, sādhaka pitta, and tarpaka kapha are important in brain function. We have not yet studied kapha. There is a sensitive film of white matter over the brain that is called *tarpaka kapha*. Within that sensitive film of white matter, every visual, olfactory, and tactile experience is recorded and this recording is done by prāna. Nevertheless, the ink that is used to record the experience is sādhaka pitta.

Sādhaka pitta also transforms physical sound into nerve impulse, which is carried to the center of hearing where every sound, as a nerve impulse, is transformed, cooked, digested, and translated into meaning. Meaning is feeling. The word "love" creates certain feelings in one's heart. Love cannot be described but pure essence of love can be felt. If you say that anything that cannot be described does not exist, that means you have lost feeling. Feeling is called ESP—extrasensory perception. Sādhaka pitta, which is present in the brain cells as a specialized neuro-chemical substance, creates ESP, the important sixth sense.

We have studied that prāna is a flow of awareness and this flow of intelligence is neuro-electricity that is moving through the nerves and delivering a message. Though messenger molecules are RNA molecules, prāna brings the message from DNA to RNA. So there is a functional relationship between DNA molecules, which create new cells, and RNA molecules, which are the messengers. Prāna brings the message.

Past memory and experience is stored in the RNA/DNA molecules. In the process of recognition, sādhaka pitta penetrates the memory and chooses a particular file from the vast hologram of RNA/DNA molecules. This is a function of buddhi, the intellect. The memory, smruti, provides past information. The mind is called manas and its function is to process both external and internal sensory experiences. The "I" memory is ahamkāra, "I am." The intellect, memory, mind, and prāna work together in the presence of this "I am."

Ego is necessary. The "I am" is the center within our consciousness. When we realize that we exist, it is because of the intervention of memory, thought, and feelings. When everything is flowing, we still exist but we are not aware that we exist—for example, in deep sleep. So, sādhaka pitta creates the feeling that "I exist." We exist in time as a function. Looking is a function, as is listening and breathing. Therefore, function is a moment of time. When one function is looking at another function, then we are aware that we exist. Sādhaka pitta creates that bridge of one function recognizing another function. Because of that recognition, we feel that "I exist."

Truth is eternal, changeless existence. Truth is universal, absolute, vast and immeasurable. Truth is in every individual. There is truth in perception, sensation, memory, feeling, and emotion, and there is truth in ahamkāra. However, absolute, unconditional Truth is within you as soul, spirit.

There is a vast difference between reality and Truth. Reality is a product of mind. Reality in this room is different to reality in another room, because reality is a product of time and space. In other words, Truth that is confined by time and space becomes reality. The moment a person has contact with the Truth, which is sensory contact, it becomes reality. Personal truth becomes reality. Truth is abstract; reality is personal. The universal reality is Truth. The individual truth is reality. Truth is absolutely beautiful but reality is sometimes bitter. Once you swallow the sweet truth, you should also be able to swallow the bitter reality.

When that reality acts, it becomes actuality. The word "actual" comes from the root "act." Actuality means that which is acting now. Anything that touches the senses becomes actual. Therefore, actuality is a product of the senses. The pencil in someone's hand is actual to that person at that time. Therefore, it is also reality to them. When you look at them holding the pencil, it is your reality, but only when you touch it does it become actual to you. The moment Truth becomes perceivable, it becomes actual. When one is walking and suddenly Truth comes, it comes through the window and everyone is aware of it. It is palpable, actual.

So what is the relationship between Truth, reality, and actuality? Reality has to pass through actuality, or actuality must come in close contact with reality, in order to realize Truth. So Truth is unconditional, universal absolute. The moment a person experiences that, it becomes personal reality. As long as a person is in the dream, dream is reality. When he comes out of the dream, reality changes, because reality is bound by time and space. Truth is not.

In that sense, awareness is Truth, consciousness is reality, and perception is actuality. So perception has to pass through consciousness in order to reach awareness, which means actuality has to go through reality in order to reach the Truth.

This transformation is governed by sādhaka pitta. It is sādhaka pitta that bridges this function of looking and listening with total existence. Then existence becomes actual. When we internalize actuality, or reality, it becomes Truth. Truth has a relationship with reality and actuality, but actuality and reality may not have a relationship to the Truth, because the bridge between actuality and reality of Truth is sādhaka pitta. Therefore, we can only have a clear relationship with Truth if sādhaka pitta is healthy. Sādhaka pitta is necessary for the transformation of an object into pure experience. When experience is recorded in the brain cells, it becomes memory and memory is knowledge. This knowledge is a material process.

There are two kinds of knowledge: knowledge from memory and knowledge from direct perception. The knowledge from direct perception is the blissful awakening of pure intelligence, and knowledge from memory is only information. Insight comes from direct perception without interference of information. This is also an important function of sādhaka pitta.

The pitta present in the nervous system that is responsible for all neuro-chemical changes is sādhaka pitta. The gray matter of the brain regulates the temperature of neurons and that is also sādhaka pitta. It is sādhaka pitta that helps to transform molecules of food, water, and air into a biological cellular component called cytoplasm. The content of cytoplasm is further transformed into awareness by subtle cellular metabolic activity because of sādhaka pitta. All biochemical neurotransmitters, which are necessary to maintain higher cerebral activity, fall under sādhaka pitta. The unprocessed cytoplasmic content becomes emotion. Every thought, feeling, and emotion should be processed into intelligence. That which is not processed is crystallized and stored in the connective tissue.

Sādhaka pitta is present in the heart. Here the word heart means the heart chakra, the cardiac plexus. Sādhaka pitta in the heart metabolizes and processes feelings and emotions. Therefore, the heart is the seat of love and compassion. In principle, love is God. In practice, love is feeling and emotion. In actuality, love is compassion, understanding, sharing, and caring. All these manifestations of love are due to sādhaka pitta present in the heart. Every thought and feeling is a biochemical reaction. To make complex neuro-chemistry a simple phenomenon is to understand the function of sādhaka pitta in the heart.

Ālochaka Pitta

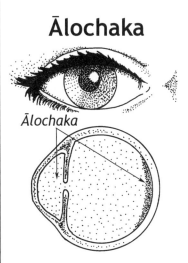

The next important pitta is ālochaka pitta. Ālochaka pitta is present in the eye and governs the luster, color, and translucence of the eye. It is present in the cornea to maintain transference and translucence. It is present in the iris to maintain color and in the lens to maintain transference. It is also present in the vitreous humor and in the cone and rod cells.

Ālochaka pitta is necessary for optical perception. It maintains the temperature of the eyeball, the color of the iris, color vision, and vision of light. When you look at an object, that image is formed on the retina and absorbed by the sharp quality of ālochaka pitta into the optic nerve. Then prāna vāyu carries that image to the mind for interpretation. Ālochaka pitta maintains visual perception and three-dimensional vision. If you have only one eye, what you see is a flat picture. Binocular vision, with two eyes, is three-dimensional. One of the important functions of ālochaka pitta, along with prāna, is accommodation (ability to focus), which means the constriction or dilation of the pupil, so that appropriate light is allowed to enter and fall on the retina for clear perception of an object.

There are certain enzymes present in the retina that are necessary for photosynthesis. These enzymes and neuropeptides transform the optical image into the optical sensation. One of these is rhodopsin, the physical expression of ālochaka pitta in the eye. Ālochaka pitta is responsible for generating the visual impulse, which prāna then carries to the mind, to buddhi, where interpretation of the impulse is accomplished by sādhaka pitta. So, ālochaka pitta meets sādhaka pitta in buddhi, where interpretation of visual perception takes place. This meeting point is in the occipital cortex, the posterior (back) portion of the head. If there is trauma at this meeting point, a person may become blind.

The anterior (front) chamber of the eye is located between the iris and the cornea and is filled with aqueous humor, a pitta liquid. The posterior chamber of the eye is located between the lens and retina and is filled with vitreous humor, a kapha liquid. If there are crystals suspended within the vitreous humor, one sees floaters. The fluid of the anterior chamber goes into the posterior chamber, and this circulation is governed by blood vessels and lymphatics. If something is clogging that flow, the circulation stops and the person accumulates water in the anterior chamber as well as the posterior chamber. That increase in ocular pressure is called glaucoma, a kapha disorder,

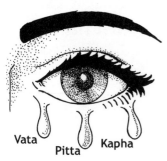

Vata
Pitta Kapha

Cold	Hot	Sweet
Astringent	Sour	Cool
Bitter	Salty	Love
Grief	Pungent	Compassion
Sadness	Anger	Scanty
Loneliness	Hate	
Fear	Frustration	
Supressed	Abundant	

Bhrājaka

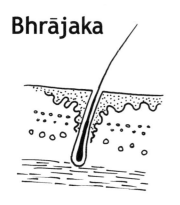

discussed later. The eyes are predominantly made up of pitta but can be adversely affected by kapha.

Ālochaka pitta is also associated with emotions. Different emotions bring a different chemistry to the tears. Tears of joy and love are sweet, scanty, and cool, and come from the lateral (outer) side of the eye. Tears of anger come from the center of the eye and are sour to the taste, and hot. Tears of frustration, grief, sadness, and fear come from the medial (inner) side and are bitter and astringent to the taste.

Disorders of ālochaka pitta can create changes in the eyes, leading to shortsightedness or farsightedness. If ālochaka pitta is increased, it may create conjunctivitis, styes, iritis, burning sensation in the eye, and photophobia (light sensitivity). The root cause of an ālochaka pitta disorder is suppressed tears and avoidance of seeing reality.

Your eyes have the capacity to see the truth. When you look without judgment, without interference of thought and mind, the eyes become the windows of God and you can perceive the Truth. If your thought and mind interfere, then you perceive reality, because reality is a product of your mind. We need sensitive ālochaka pitta that can perceive the truth of reality, the truth of actuality. When you perceive the Truth, there is love, clarity, compassion, and pure awareness.

Bhrājaka Pitta

The skin is the main site of bhrājaka pitta. This pitta keeps the skin warm and is responsible for normal complexion and luster. It also helps in the processing of oils, pastes, and medications applied externally to the skin. When we apply, for instance, sandalwood or ginger paste, the agni principle of bhrājaka absorbs and assimilates the substance. The skin is a gate or door that is kept functional by bhrājaka pitta.

The fire component of bhrājaka pitta is called bhrājaka agni, which maintains the tactile sense of touch, pain, temperature, and stereognosis. Gnosis means knowledge. Diagnosis means after knowledge. After observing, you come to a conclusion, a diagnosis. Prognosis means before knowledge, whether the patient will be cured or not. Stereognosis is three-dimensional, tactile perception. A blind man can recognize a coin or a key by touch, because the skin has the capacity to feel the size, shape, and surface of an object. This knowledge is called stereognosis, touch with comprehension of qualities.

Bhrājaka pitta works in connection with rañjaka pitta and pāchaka pitta. Skin care is important in Āyurveda. Oil is absorbed through the skin and the quality of the oil penetrates deeply into the connective tissue all the way to the bone. The medium that carries and absorbs that oil is bhrājaka pitta.

Abnormal bhrājaka pitta may result in skin conditions such as eczema, dermatitis, acne, and anesthesia—loss of sense of touch, tingling, and numbness. The skin is connected to the liver and to all the internal organs. Underneath the skin, there is connective tissue and within that connective tissue, we accumulate unresolved anger, fear, and stress. When we experience anger, the skin becomes hot and flushed.

The connection between this outer manifestation of the skin and the emotions is established through prāna. The skin is breathing prāna. If a person becomes angry and the skin becomes flushed, subcutaneous breathing is stopped. When a person experiences stress or anxiety, breathing is constricted and shallow, and the skin becomes pale.

Kapha and Its Subtypes

Ka means water and *pha* means flourishing. That which is flourished by water is kapha, the water component. Another name for kapha is *shleshma*. The root of shleshma is *shlish*, which means "to hug." Kapha molecules hug together and create a compact mass.

The molecules of kapha are basically derived from Water and Earth. The qualities of kapha are heavy, slow/dull, cold, oily, liquid, slimy/smooth, dense, soft, static, sticky, cloudy, hard, and gross. Predominantly, they have a sweet and salty taste, so these tastes increase kapha. Vāta molecules, being catabolic (degenerative) and centrifugal, tend to disperse or scatter. Kapha molecules are anabolic (growth promoting) and centripetal, so they tend to coagulate or fall together to the center. Kapha molecules adhere together and create bigger and bigger molecules. Vāta is invisible because it is subtle and minute. Kapha is gross, the opposite of subtle, and can therefore be easily seen. All cells, tissues, and organs are composed of kapha, so kapha is represented by substantial structures in the body.

Kapha is predominantly present in the lymph and in the blood as plasma. Plasma contains more than 90 percent water. A primary site of kapha is the lungs and respiratory tract. It is also present in semen, muscles, fat, connective tissue, and the brain. Kapha is white in color and lymph, semen, plasma, certain muscles, and even the myelin sheath are white, as well as the white matter of the brain. Anything white is kapha, including white blood cells.

Sites of Kapha

Sites of Kapha	
phuphusa	lungs
āmāshaya	stomach
kloma	pancreas
shira	white matter of brain
shushumna jala	cerebrospinal fluid
rasa	plasma
sandhi	joints
gandha	sinuses
nasā	nose (organ of smell)
jihva	tongue (organ of taste)

Kapha molecules make up the main body mass and give shape and form to the body's cells, tissues, organs, and systems. If kapha is depleted by pitta or vāta, then kapha undergoes emaciation due to the hypermetabolic effects of excess pitta or the catabolic action of excess vāta. If kapha accumulates to create a compact mass, it may create a tumor such as lymphoma, myoma, osteoma, or fibrocystic changes in the breasts. Things stick together and accumulate because of kapha.

One example of kapha is the myelin sheath around the axons of certain nerves. When pitta burns the kapha molecules of the sheath, it creates optic neuritis or auditory neuritis, or it results in demyelinating disorders such as multiple sclerosis (MS). MS occurs when pitta burns the myelin sheath, which is kapha, creating space for vāta to enter the lesion. Therefore, an MS patient has vāta symptoms, such as weakness, fatigue, exhaustion, and tremors, and does not tolerate heat, because of high pitta. So MS is a demyelination disorder caused by pitta, exacerbated by vāta and affecting kapha.

Dense, hard kapha molecules create compact bones and the heavy and stable qualities of kapha are responsible for strength, stability, and firmness of the bones and muscles. The white of the eye, called the sclera, is kapha. The kapha present in the white of the eye and vitreous humor (the fluid behind the lens of the eye), the spinal meninges, and cerebrospinal fluid are all kapha. As mentioned earlier, the aqueous humor (the fluid in front of the lens of the eye) in the anterior (front) chamber of the eye is ālochaka pitta. This fluid is transparent, shiny, and bright. The vitreous humor in the posterior (back) chamber is kapha. If the aqueous humor becomes clouded by kapha, the person develops cataracts. Salivation is also kapha, as are gastric mucous secretions and the fluid in the pleural space and around the heart. Kapha is responsible for maintaining all bodily fluids, including intracellular fluid (within the cells) and the extracellular fluid between cells.

The gray matter of the brain is about 80 to 85 percent water and that water component is kapha. However, the functions of the gray matter that maintain the temperature of the neuron, the comprehension and understanding of sensory perception, and the motor responses are governed by sādhaka pitta. Understanding of optical perception takes place in the cerebral cortex. There is a motor and sensory area within the gray matter that governs the understanding of the tactile sensations of touch, pain, temperature, stereognosis, and motor responses. These are governed by sādhaka pitta via prāna vāyu, but the structure of the gray matter and the structure and functions of the white matter are tarpaka kapha.

Through its oily and slimy qualities, kapha lubricates the space between the cells and organs to relieve friction. Its oily and liquid qualities lubricate the joints and muscle tendons. Kapha molecules in the body are heavy and oily, and produce muscles that are strong and powerful. Skinny muscles are a sign of a vāta imbalance.

Anabolic changes are governed by kapha. Metabolic changes are pitta. Catabolic changes are vāta. In catabolism, vāta molecules, due to their dry, light, and rough qualities, break down the kapha molecules and create degenerative changes. The result is destruction, degenerative arthritis, and faster aging. Therefore, vāta people look older. Pitta people look mature. Kapha people look young. Even at the age of 50, a kapha person appears to be 30. At the age of 50, a vāta individual looks 60. Even at the age of 25, a pitta individual can look mature, because of a receding hairline and gray hair. Kapha's anabolic changes are responsible for growth, the

Functions of Kapha
Lubrication
Nourishment
Support and stability
Groundedness
Growth
Gaseous exchange in lungs
Gastric secretions (liquid medium)
Water electrolyte balance
Fat regulation
Strength and stamina
Energy
Sleep
Repair and Regeneration
Memory retention
Contentment
Forgiveness
Compassion
Taste perception
Olfactory perception (smell)

development of the body, healing wounds, the creation of new cells, and repair of ulcers. If kapha in the stomach is lacking and there is high pitta, an ulcer may result. The oily, unctuous molecules of kapha can heal the ulcer.

Table 10: The Subtypes of Kapha

Subtype	Governing Element	Primary Sites	Functions
Kledaka	Fire	Stomach; Gastrointestinal Tract	Gastric secretion; digestion and absorption; nourishes rasa
Avalambaka	Air	Lungs; Pleural Cavity; Heart; Respiratory Tract; Spine	Support; holds emotions; supports all kapha systems
Bodhaka	Water	Oral cavity	Salivary secretions; taste; swallowing; speech
Tarpaka	Ether	Brain (white matter); Myelin Sheath; Cerebrospinal Fluid	Subconscious thinking and emotions; memory
Shleshaka	Earth	Joints	Lubricates joints (synovial fluid); nourishes bones

Kapha molecules in the semen create abundant sperm and fertility, while excess pitta molecules in the semen create medium to scanty sperm. Too many vāta molecules in the semen create oligospermia, a deficient amount of spermatozoa in the seminal fluid, or azoospermia, absence of spermatozoa. One of the causes of infertility is excess vāta or pitta molecules in the semen. However, if a person has abundant kapha molecules in the semen, one drop is sufficient to conceive.

In the human body, there are five types of kapha—*kledaka, avalambaka, bodhaka, tarpaka,* and *shleshaka.* We will now switch our attention to the first of these five types, kledaka kapha.

Kledaka Kapha

Kledaka kapha is present in the gastrointestinal tract. It is liquid, soft, slightly oily, and slimy. This kapha creates a protective lining as the gastric mucous membrane. This membrane can be destroyed when food is consumed. Cayenne pepper, curry pepper, and alcohol dissolve the mucous membrane. Within 72 hours, kledaka kapha provides a fresh, new mucosal lining to protect the wall of the stomach.

The moment food enters the stomach, it is broken down into smaller and smaller pieces so that kapha molecules mix with each molecule of food. Then hydrochloric acid, digestive enzymes, pepsin, etc., go into the molecules of food via the molecules of kledaka kapha. Kledaka kapha, which is liquid, creates a medium for cooking in the stomach. In cooking rice or grain, we add water and water distributes the heat around the molecules of food. In the same way, kledaka kapha, by its liquid quality, helps the digestive enzymes to move equally around a molecule of food, so that molecular digestion is possible.

The pyloric valve also has a mucous lining, created by the heavy quality of kapha, which helps the pyloric valve to stay tightly shut. Kapha is stable, so the stable quality helps the pyloric valve to close tightly and remain stable. After digestion in the stomach, the hot quality of pitta and the mobile quality of prāna and samāna vāta help to open the pyloric valve. From there, the foodstuff flows into the duodenum. Vāta is the impulse of the autonomic system; vāta opens the pyloric valve and starts the flow into the duodenum. Then bile, which is rañjaka pitta from the liver, also comes into the duodenum.

Kledaka kapha is absorbed from the stomach wall into the blood vessels. At this point, kledaka kapha enters plasma and nourishes the kapha of the entire body. In that way, kledaka kapha is the mother of all kapha systems in the body. The word *kleda* means liquefication, hydration. Kledaka kapha maintains hydration of the cells and tissues. This kapha provides energy to a person after consuming food, because its sweet taste causes the blood sugar to rise.

Lack of kledaka kapha and *excess* of pāchaka pitta in the stomach create gastric irritation leading to gastritis (inflammation of the stomach lining). If a person drinks hard liquor, kledaka kapha is burned and the next day the person may have alcoholic gastritis. Kledaka kapha is depleted and pāchaka pitta is provoked. Gastritis can create nausea, vomiting, and stomach ache, which is a sign that kledaka kapha is lacking. Drinking milk and eating a bland diet can restore kledaka kapha. The sweet and slimy qualities of kledaka kapha create a thin film on the wall of the stomach, protecting it from the hydrochloric acid.

Hydrochloric acid and digestive enzymes digest protein, but it is easy for them to also digest the wall of the stomach, because the stomach wall is a form of protein. When the fire (of hydrochloric acid and digestive enzymes) starts digesting the stomach, a gastric ulcer is formed. Sometimes the sharp quality of fire is so high that it penetrates the gastric mucous membrane

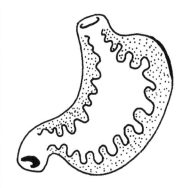

Kledaka

and the musculature of the stomach, creating a hole or perforation.

The stomach is divided into the greater curvature and the lesser curvature. The lesser curvature is the acid bearing area that secretes more hydrochloric acid and other digestive juices, which are pāchaka pitta. The greater curvature, or fundus, produces more kledaka kapha. The lesser curvature of the stomach is near the liver, a pitta organ. The greater curvature is near the spleen, whose function is to filter blood.

How a person sleeps is important. Sleeping on the left side suppresses kapha and builds pitta. The greater curvature of the stomach goes down and the lesser curvature is pressed toward the liver, creating more acid secretion. People who sleep on the left side can increase digestive fire but may have hyperacidity. People who sleep on the right side can calm pitta but might induce kapha aggravation, leading to sinus congestion. Sleeping on the right side brings more spleen energy, while sleeping on the left side suppresses spleen energy and builds more liver energy. When you sleep on the right side, the stomach empties earlier, because the pyloric valve is on the right. However, the food leaving the stomach may not be fully digested. Optimally, one should wait three or more hours after a meal before going to sleep so the stomach has emptied completely.

When the quality of kledaka kapha is balanced, it brings contentment, satisfaction, and a need for smaller amounts of food. When the quality of kledaka kapha is vitiated, a person must eat large quantities of food to build satisfaction. By eating too much, the stomach is expanded and an expanded stomach demands more food to reach its optimal satisfaction. When a person has nervousness, anxiety, insecurity, loneliness, grief, or sadness, kledaka kapha reacts to these emotions by becoming sticky, thick, and demanding more food.

The stomach is like a balloon. With large quantities of food, it will expand. If less is consumed, the stomach wall will shrink. Satisfaction comes by stretching the muscle wall, and kledaka kapha brings that contentment. By eating too much, the stomach is expanded and more food is required to bring that satisfaction. Therefore, kledaka kapha disorders include obesity, obsessive eating habits, hyperglycemia, diabetes, and high cholesterol, which are excess kledaka, as well as hypoglycemia and peptic ulcer, both due to insufficient kledaka kapha.

Avalambaka Kapha
Avalambaka kapha is an important kapha that supports all kapha systems in the body, functionally as well as

Avalambaka

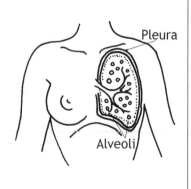

Pleura

Alveoli

structurally. It includes the spine as well as the lungs and heart. It carries pranic energy from the lungs to every cell, tissue, and organ. Kledaka kapha and avalambaka kapha have functional integrity. Without kledaka kapha, avalambaka kapha cannot do anything. Avalambaka kapha is present in the respiratory and cardiovascular systems, in the trachea, bronchi, and bronchioles. It is in the pleural space as pleural fluid, in the pericardial space as pericardial fluid, and in the bronchi and bronchioles as bronchial secretions. Because of its liquid quality, avalambaka kapha helps with gaseous exchange by removing unwanted carbon dioxide from the alveoli so that oxygen can enter. In addition, avalambaka kapha provides the liquid quality within the pulmonary trunk so that oxygenated blood can be carried to the heart. Avalambaka kapha protects the lungs and alveoli, and maintains the tone of the muscular layer of the bronchi. In addition, as pericardial fluid it protects the heart muscle. Avalambaka kapha from the lungs goes into the alveoli and from the alveoli goes into the blood and so enters the heart. It is supportive to both the respiratory and cardiovascular systems.

Another job of avalambaka kapha is to maintain the permeability of the alveoli. The alveoli are delicate and their tone must be maintained. The unctuous quality of avalambaka kapha keeps the alveoli moist. Liquid and sticky qualities of this kapha maintain the lumen of the bronchi.

Avalambaka kapha also supports the intracostal muscles and ribs. In emphysema, the ribs remain expanded, the intracostal space is widened and the chest looks like a barrel due to the drying up of avalambaka kapha. Avalambaka creates confidence, courage, and ability to face problems so that the chest is expanded. When the chest is contracted, the person is not able to cope with challenges.

Psychologically, avalambaka kapha is associated with support, love, and compassion. When there is excessive grief and sadness, avalambaka kapha becomes sticky, and lung function is affected. The lungs are the seat of grief and sadness. The inferior quality of avalambaka kapha may create pulmonary changes and collapse of the bronchial lumen. Bronchitis, asthma, bronchiectasis, pneumonia, and emphysema are all due to dysfunction of avalambaka kapha.

Bodhaka Kapha

The next important subtype of kapha is bodhaka kapha. The Sanskrit word bodhaka comes from *bodhana*, which means to make known. It is located in the mouth and is represented by saliva, which is liquid, sticky, sweet, and slightly unctuous. The

Bodhaka

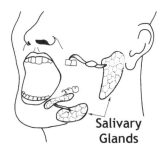

Salivary Glands

liquid quality of bodhaka kapha keeps the mouth wet and soft. Saliva in the mouth prevents friction between the soft tissues of the tongue and palate. We have two types of palate, the hard palate and the soft palate. The hard palate is a bony dome and the soft palate is a soft mobile structure. The tongue moves freely in the oral cavity without sticking to the palate, because of the liquid and unctuous qualities of bodhaka kapha.

There are six salivary glands with ducts that open in the sides of the cheeks. At the base of the tongue, there are two salivary glands, called the sublingual salivary glands. There are also two submandibular salivary glands, and two parotid salivary glands situated below and in front of each ear. We swallow saliva and keep the esophagus lubricated. There is a constant need for saliva to keep the oral cavity moist and lubricated, as well. If the tongue becomes dry, we cannot talk. The thick and unctuous qualities moisten the vocal cords so that the sound coming through the vocal cords is effortless. Saliva is related to bodhaka kapha. One of the functions of bodhaka kapha is to help speech. Bodhaka kapha also helps to nourish rasa dhātu.

The agni of bodhaka kapha, called bodhaka agni, is responsible for maintaining the oral temperature. Any substance that goes into the mouth causes secretion of bodhaka kapha. Bodhaka kapha also lubricates the tonsils, pharynx, and vocal cords. The epiglottis is well lubricated by bodhaka kapha so that foodstuffs can slide over the epiglottis directly into the esophagus without entering the trachea. The pharynx leads to the esophagus and the larynx leads to the lungs. This space within the throat is moistened, and the posterior wall of the pharynx is also well lubricated, by bodhaka kapha.

This kapha is called bodhaka because it helps to receive the knowledge of the taste of food. Each taste bud on the tongue is made of many cells and each cell is covered with bodhaka kapha. These taste buds send the message about taste to the brain. The tongue has many grooves formed by the taste buds.

The tip of the tongue contains taste buds that perceive the sweet taste. On either side, the taste buds perceive more sour taste. The central part perceives the bitter taste. In front of bitter in the central part is pungent. On either side in the central area is the salty taste. The last portion in the back of the tongue is where the astringent taste is perceived.

A moderate amount of sweet taste stimulates the thyroid as well as the pancreas, but an excess sweet foods can weaken

Areas of Six Tastes on the Tongue

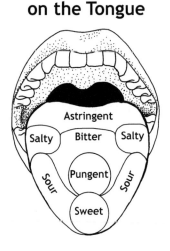

these organs. A patient with bronchitis or pneumonia should not eat sour food, because it may increase pulmonary congestion. Pungent taste stimulates the stomach and small intestines, while salty taste affects the kidneys. An excessive amount of salt is not good for someone with high blood pressure, because it can create edema and kidney stress. Bitter taste affects the liver, spleen, and pancreas, and astringent is related to the colon.

The tongue is made up of muscle tissue and blood tissue, and is directly connected to the plasma. In a state of dehydration, the tongue becomes dry. Many disorders can be diagnosed just by looking at the tongue, because the tongue is a mirror of all the organs of the body.

The papillae on the back of the tongue are special buds that secrete a special quality of bodhaka kapha to maintain the flora of the pharynx. The tonsils also secrete a specialized bodhaka kapha. The tonsil is a protective gland. When the tonsil becomes septic it means bodhaka kapha is deranged, and septic tonsillitis may create myocarditis (inflammation of the heart muscle) or arthritis. A disorder of bodhaka kapha can affect the entire kapha system—kledaka kapha in the stomach, avalambaka kapha in the lungs and heart, tarpaka kapha in the brain, and shleshaka kapha in the joints.

Bodhaka kapha is sweet and bacteria can easily grow in the mouth if there is an excess of sweet taste. If the teeth are not brushed at night, the next morning the oral cavity will be a kingdom of bacteria. Receding gums can become a problem due to infection deep in the pockets of the gums. Take care of your bodhaka kapha before you go to bed by carefully cleaning your mouth.

Triphala tea maintains the normal attributes of bodhaka kapha. It can help viscous, thick bodhaka kapha become thin and liquid. Take half a teaspoon of triphala and place it in a glass of hot water for one minute. Let it cool and strain it. Then swish it in your mouth. Healthy saliva is thin and unhealthy saliva is thick. Thick saliva indicates dental calculi, diabetes, worms, or Parkinson's disease. If a child drools on a pillow while sleeping, it is a sign that the child may have worms, because the presence of worms in the colon stimulates bodhaka kapha secretion. Excess saliva or a sticky mouth may also indicate dehydration or pre-diabetes, because stickiness of the mouth is due to sweet saliva. In a 24-hour period, we swallow about one pint of saliva and in this way bodhaka kapha nourishes kledaka kapha. In addition, through saliva bodhaka kapha helps to maintain water electrolyte balance.

Saliva has healing properties. Cats and dogs heal their wounds by licking the wound. The saliva helps to create granulation tissue, which is necessary for healing an ulcer. Healthy saliva kills bacteria and speeds healing, because of its antiseptic properties.

The digestion of starch begins in the mouth. When food is chewed, the food mixes with the enzymes present in the saliva and bodhaka kapha helps to move the food down into the stomach to mix it with kledaka kapha. Kledaka kapha works in conjunction with bodhaka kapha in the digestion of protein, starch, and carbohydrates.

Tarpaka Kapha

The Sanskrit word *tarpana* means to nourish, to retain, to record. It also means contentment. Tarpaka kapha is predominantly present in the white matter of the brain. It is thick, sticky, slimy, and soft. Tarpaka nourishes the brain cells.

Tarpaka

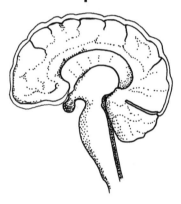

The liquid qualities of tarpaka kapha are present in the meninges and cerebrospinal fluid, which surround the soft brain tissue and the spinal cord. Tarpaka kapha, as cerebrospinal fluid, is slightly sweet because of glucose and slightly salty because of minerals. Because of the sweet and salty tastes, it helps to nourish the nerve cells. Tarpaka kapha brings energy to rasa dhātu (plasma) by way of the sweet and salty tastes, creating a feeling of happiness. If a crying child is given sugar, he becomes happy and stops crying.

Another important site of tarpaka kapha is the myelin sheath, a protective sheath surrounding most nerve cells. One of the functions of tarpaka kapha as the myelin sheath is to protect the impulse that goes from one neuron to another neuron, which is governed by prāna vāyu. But the entire nerve tissue, which is made up of protein substance, is tarpaka kapha. Tarpaka kapha provides a sensitive film to the neuron where every experience is recorded. That is the meaning of tarpana: to retain or record.

Tarpaka kapha lubricates the sinuses and nasal cavities and is present in the spinal cord, where it governs the reflex arc. The tarpaka kapha in the spinal cord acts as a medium for the completion of the circuit for the reflex arc. If batteries are dry, nothing happens. So tarpaka kapha in the spinal cord acts like a battery solution.

Perception is the movement of awareness, but that movement of awareness to the outer object is carried by prāna. When awareness moves, it becomes attention. Sādhaka pitta gives the fire of understanding, absorption, comprehension, recognition, identification, and evaluation. Prāna carries sensory perception and motor movement. In this case, prāna is also the writer that records every good, bad, or ugly experience on the film of tarpaka kapha and tarpaka kapha is a big recording file. Tarpaka kapha is associated with the astral body and within the matrix of the astral body past life experiences are stored.

We carry the memory of our parents' illnesses within the DNA molecules, which is tarpaka kapha. If a person's grandfather had diabetes, tarpaka kapha carries that memory of diabetes in the person's cells. We seek security by retaining memories and tarpaka kapha performs this task. When a child burns his hand in a fire, that memory is recorded. Now when he sees fire, he knows not to play with the flame. There is safety and security in biological memory, which is absolutely necessary for safety. If I touch fire, it will burn me. If I put my finger into the electric socket, it will give me a shock. If I rub a knife over my skin, it will cut my skin. These biological memories are necessary as a protective mechanism.

We also have psychological memories of childhood suffering. Father, mother, brother, or sister may have been abusive and we carry that psychological memory as a non-healing ulcer. Whatever treatment received from parents or teachers during the first seven years of life, stays with us through life and shapes our personality. This treatment may create psychological problems in teenage or adult years. There is nothing wrong with biological memory of disease or injury but psychological memory of abuse can be damaging.

Psychological memory of hurt or insult changes one's personality. Psychological memory comes from desire for protection but it affects the psyche and mind. If a father has abused his daughter, the daughter has that deep-seated psychological memory and may not feel comfortable with a man. She may feel more comfortable with a woman. The same is true with a boy. If his mother abuses a boy, he has memory of the psychological trauma not only toward his mother but also toward any woman. Psychological memories are associated with sexual energy, male and female, to sex organs, relationships, and emotions. Biological memories are associated with organs and tissues.

We need both factual and biological memory. However, is it necessary to record insult or hurt? In a way, our hurt is our choice, and we create our own hurt. We can change today just by bringing more awareness to our action and thinking. Thought is a discharge of tarpaka kapha, so thought is a biochemical and neuro-electrical vehicle that is passing through the matrix of tarpaka kapha. If we are aware of that vehicle, it will send the proper message to our cells.

Tarpaka kapha may work at both the conscious and subconscious levels. There is no clear line of demarcation between conscious and subconscious. The subconscious can become conscious and the conscious can be dumped into the subconscious. When a child is abused and cannot remember the abuse, it is in the deep matrix of tarpaka kapha. Meditation and counseling dig into tarpaka kapha, and then prāna brings all the good, bad, and ugly memories to the surface.

Clarity of sensory perception and spirituality go together. When tarpaka kapha is of inferior quality, it reduces sensitivity. An inferior quality of tarpaka kapha brings an image that interferes with clarity of observation. Looking at an object through a past memory clouds the eye because we are screening it through a past image.

Tarpaka kapha helps to create neurological time, which is stimulus and response. Psychological time is thought. There is no space without time. Time is space and space is distance. There is a distance between you and me and this distance creates separation. You become observer and I become observed. There is always physical distance between the object and the observer but I am talking about psychological distance. So time and space are one. Where there is time, there is division. To look at an object without time means to look at an object without distance. To look at an object without distance means to look without separation, to discover that the observer is the observed. If a person can do this, transformation is possible. Transformation is mutation and mutation is purification of tarpaka kapha. However, our tarpaka kapha is gooey and not ready to change. Our thoughts are crystallized, and grief and sadness are stuck in the deep matrix of tarpaka kapha, where we carry those wounds in the subconscious mind. If tarpaka kapha becomes thick and firm, there is crystallization, rigidity, and callousness, which create confusion. Confusion is conclusion and this conclusion is judgment that is stored in tarpaka kapha. The quality of tarpaka kapha can be changed today simply by observing without distance. To observe without distance means to observe the essence, and that essence is the pure space of existence.

Within tarpaka kapha there is a space beyond time and aging, which can be reached through sensitive awareness. Within that space, a person will no longer live in the past. To live in the present means to live in a timeless space. To live now means to live in eternity. To live in your relationships with these qualities of tarpaka kapha is to live with God.

Heaven is not a geographical place. It is a quality of consciousness. We can make our life heaven. The superior quality of tarpaka kapha makes relationships new. To nourish the rejuvenation of relationship means to rejuvenate the tarpaka kapha of the brain cells. Every moment is a moment of God, a moment of bliss, beauty, and love. When we live with now, in that very moment tarpaka kapha changes and the transformation of tarpaka kapha is the transformation of the person.

Do not live in the past. Change cannot happen in the past and we cannot change the past. The past is dead and gone. The root cause of lack of communication is interference from the past in the present. Relationship is a mirror and in that mirror of relationship, we learn about our hidden subconscious motives. Relationships are not for judgment or criticism but for self-learning, self-inquiry, and self-investigation. The real school is relationship and in the mirror of relationship, tarpaka kapha undergoes change.

A tarpaka kapha disorder can create various physical disorders such as stroke paralysis, Parkinson's disease, or brain tumors. Concussion, compression, or contusion may affect tarpaka kapha and change the entire personality. A blow on the head may traumatize tarpaka kapha, causing the person to lose memory.

Shleshaka Kapha

The last kapha is shleshaka. Shleshaka kapha is thick, sticky, liquid, oily and slimy. It is present all over the body, and especially in the joint spaces, where two bones come together. It lubricates the joints and nourishes the articular (joint) surfaces and cartilages to promote easy movement.

One of the important functions of shleshaka kapha is to support the skeletal system and to strengthen the ligaments. If shleshaka kapha loses its unctuous and liquid qualities, it ceases to nourish the joint. When the joint cracks and pops, it indicates a lack of shleshaka kapha. When the kapha molecules are dried up, vāta enters the joint. Vāta is rough, so the bone surface of the joint becomes dry and rough. Sometimes crystals of calcium begin accumulating in the joint space, creating pain and stiffness.

Disorders of shleshaka kapha include degenerative arthritis and rheumatoid arthritis. Excessive jogging can be

Shleshaka

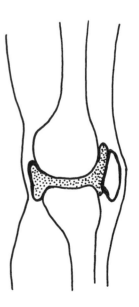

stressful to the joint. Vigorous exercise can change the quality of shleshaka kapha and hurt the joint. As a person ages, he or she may develop arthritis. The best forms of exercise are yoga, aerobic water exercises, Tai Chi, brisk walking, and swimming. Exercise is for circulation and is important each day. Sweating exercise detoxifies the system. A person should exercise to half his capacity, just until sweat comes to the forehead, under the armpits and along the vertebral column. The length of time will vary according to the individual and will increase as strength is built. This type of exercise using only half energy is necessary for the maintenance of physiological functions of vital organs, such as the heart, liver, kidneys, and lungs. Vigorous exercise beyond this capacity may lead to dehydration and can cause constipation. It may also affect the joints, leading to sciatica or arthritis.

When you exercise, watch for profuse sweating, breathing difficulty, a need to breathe through the mouth and tightness in chest area. When any of these three symptoms appear, it is a indication to slow down or stop.

Summary

So the five elements are the building blocks for all matter, and the doshas organize the elements for their functions in the human body. We can think of the doshas as organizational principles that govern the elements in their physiological functions. Each dosha has two predominant elements according to the nature of that dosha's functions. For example, pitta organizes fire and water for the functions of metabolism and digestion in the body. The fire element integrates with the water element in the body and becomes a biochemical fire. It takes the form of chemicals like hydrochloric acid and digestive enzymes, using the water element as a medium to come into contact with the food particles in the process of digestion.

Digestion is the main function of pitta. Everywhere that there is pitta, digestion is taking place, whether in the stomach, intestines, liver, brain, heart, eyes, or skin. The subdoshas describe the different locations and specializations of each dosha's primary functions. Although each dosha is comprised of two main elements, its specialized functions in specific locations may require that the dosha make use of the other elements as well. Hence some subdoshas are governed by an element other than the two primary elements associated with the parent dosha.

Subdosha theory helps us understand the more specific functional relationships between the doshas and the elements.

By understanding this we can see a more complete picture of how the doshas clothe themselves in the five elements to perform their functions in the human body.

Chapter Three

4

Agni
The Digestive Fire

आयुर्वेद

Agni, the Digestive Fire

Agni is the Fire element, which governs all transformation. The primary function of agni is the digestion, absorption, assimilation, and transformation of food and sensations into energy. If you worship agni, you will be blessed with perfect health. Agni is the main source of life. Without agni, life is not possible. In Āyurveda, we say a man is as old as his agni. If agni is in optimal condition, a person's immune system is healthy. When the metabolic fire is robust, a person can live a long, healthy life. When agni becomes slow, the person's health deteriorates. When this vital fire is extinguished, death soon follows. Have you ever touched a dead body? Dead bodies are cold because there is no agni. A living body is warm. A yogi in samādhi and a dead person look alike. In both, the heart and the breath stop. In samādhi, a person looks unconscious and the pupils are dilated. But there is one difference: even in deep samādhi, the body is warm due to agni, whereas a dead body is dead cold.

Agni also relates to maturation. An unbaked clay pot does not last long, but if you bake the pot, it becomes solid and can last a long time. The function of agni is not only digestion, but also to bring maturation to the tissues. The tone of each tissue (dhātu) is maintained by its agni. The word tonic comes from tone, and most tonics kindle agni. The concept of tonics is very old in Āyurveda, and tonification of the tissues is maintained by agni. If we maintain balanced agni, we can live a long and healthy life. Āyurveda is the science of the longevity and one of its important therapies is *rasāyana chikitsā* (rejuvenation therapy). Rasāyana literally means to enter into the rasa dhātu[14] (plasma) and thereby to kindle agni.

The concept of agni is very old, dating back to the Vedic deities. The main three deities in recent times are Brahmā the creator, Vishnu the sustainer, and Shiva the destroyer. If you study the ancient Vedic literature, there are other deities, including *Indra*, who is cosmic prāna, and a deity of fire called *Agnideva*. Agni, the transformative energy, is the mouth of the gods, the mouth of consciousness, the sacrificial fire. If we say that God is pure awareness, then agni is the mouth of pure awareness. Even awareness is nourished by agni, which is a bridge between lower consciousness and higher consciousness. Agni is a bridge between the human lower self and the divine self, *Para Brahman*. Agni is the expression of Purusha as concentrated, condensed awareness, which becomes the flame of light, the flame of attention.

There is agni when we burn a candle or a ghee lamp. Agni is physical fire, but the energy of the physical fire is Agnideva. There is a beautiful picture of Agnideva in Vedic mythology. He has two faces; one is creation, the other is destruction. The creation of new cells is governed by agni and destruction of old cells is also governed by agni. Agnideva has three tongues, and symbolically these are the three gunas: sattva, rajas, and tamas. They also represent the three doshas: vāta, pitta, and kapha. So agni is a dynamic, radiant energy and the force behind the functional integrity of these three gunas and three doshas. The god, Agnideva, is also shown as having seven *shākhā* (extremities), which are the seven dhātus. Each dhātu has its own agni component. Agnideva has three legs: one leg is the physical body, the second is the mental body, the mind, and the third is consciousness. Thus, agni represents the unified functioning of these various energies and structures.

In Āyurvedic philosophy, the creation of universal life is governed by *soma, sūrya,* and *anila.* Soma means the moon,

---

14. See "Dhātus" on page 103 for a full explanation of the bodily tissues (dhātus).

sūrya means the sun, and anila is cosmic prāna, the atmosphere. An individual life is governed by their three representatives. Soma in the cosmos is the moon, but in the microcosm—the body—its representative is kapha dosha. Sūrya in our solar system is the sun, but the source of light and heat in the body is pitta dosha. Lastly anila, the atmosphere, the cosmic prāna, is represented in the body by vāta dosha. So kapha, pitta, and vāta govern individual microcosmic life while soma, sūrya, and anila govern universal or global life. Agni is the biological fire that is the bridge between individual life and cosmic life; a bridge between body, mind, and consciousness. That which enters into the body, the heart, and cellular consciousness is called agni. Vedic philosophy calls this "*agni nārāyana.*" "*Nara*" means human being; "*ayan*" means to enter into (the body and consciousness).

Āyurvedic medicine focuses on the quality and status of agni. Āyurvedic internal medicine is called *kāya chikitsā*, or treatment of diseases affecting the body, mind, and consciousness. Kāya means body and chikitsā means therapy. Kāya comes from *kā*, which means earth, and *ya* meaning circulation; so kāya is that in which nutrients circulate. Agni performs the role of maintaining that circulation in conjunction with the three doshas. If our agni is robust and healthy it brings fragrance to life. When agni is imbalanced, the opposite occurs. When a person has a foul smell or bad breath, that indicates impaired agni. Such a person may use perfume, but there is a perfume in your body, a fragrance of the body, which is agni.

Agni and the Five Elements
All organic and inorganic substances are derived from the five basic elements. Ether is space, nuclear energy, the first expression of consciousness. Air, electrical energy, is the principle of movement, and governs all sensory and motor movements. Water is a universal chemical solvent and in the human body it is present in plasma, cytoplasm, cerebrospinal fluid, vitreous humor, glandular secretions, saliva, pleural secretions, gastric mucosal secretions, and in sweat and urine. Earth is represented by the minerals and hard structures in the body.

Agni is the Fire element, which is radiant energy, and it manifests as body temperature, digestive enzymes, amino acids, and all metabolic activities. Agni in this solar system has its root in the luminous, radiant heat coming from the sun, but there is also dormant, latent heat in the planet. This fire in the earth is called *vaishvānala*. There is also fire in water called *vadavanala*. (*Anala*, used here as a suffix, means agni). The fire in the womb of the earth comes up during volcanic eruptions. There is potential fire in wood, in the ocean, and in the atmosphere. There is also fire in the human body. This fire is centered in the stomach and is called *jāthara agni* (gastric fire).

The Latin word "ignis," from which the English word "ignite" is derived, has a common root with the Sanskrit word "agni." Agni means that which ignites, which is fire.

A **wareness:** each cell is a center of awareness. That awareness is governed by agni.

G **overnor:** of digestion, assimilation, and transformation of matter into energy. Agni also governs the structural and functional activities of all cells and tissues.

N **utrition:** of all bodily tissues; also neutralization of toxins (āma) in the tissues.

I **ntelligence:** cellular intelligence and cellular selectivity and choice.

The Role of Agni in Digestion

The concept of digestion in Āyurvedic medicine is comprehensive. Digestion can be compared to the external preparation and cooking of food. The basic requirements for this are a fireplace or stove, a pot, fuel, air, fire, water, food (the raw material), and an organizer. The same things are needed for internal cooking or digestion. The fireplace represents the *grahani* (small intestine), and the fire is jāthara agni. The cooking pot is the stomach. The fuel is yesterday's digested food, which gives its energy to the wall of the intestines to discharge digestive enzymes. These enzymes are the fuel that kindles agni. The ventilating air is the electrical energy required to conduct the heat, which is samāna vāyu, while the water is the gastric mucosal secretions in the stomach, kledaka kapha. The person or organizer is prāna, which governs all these processes. Without the organizer (prāna), nothing can happen.

The molecules of fire enter the pot and kindle the fire latent within the water, and then the fire within the food. Dormant solar energy in food becomes activated by external agni. The water in the pot (kapha) helps the uniform distribution of fire to each grain. The hotter molecules are light and rise up, while the cold molecules are heavy and go down. Circulation and churning happens in the stomach. Every molecule of agni that enters into the water comes in contact with the molecules of

Digestion
as preparing and cooking food

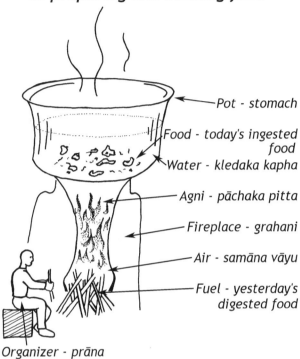

Pot - stomach

Food - today's ingested food

Water - kledaka kapha

Agni - pāchaka pitta

Fireplace - grahani

Air - samāna vāyu

Fuel - yesterday's digested food

Organizer - prāna

food and thus molecular digestion takes place and cooks the food. This process makes prāna available for release.

Our food contains life energy that can only be utilized by the body through digestion. Food has to be transformed into absorbable substances that can nourish the tissues. This can occur partly by external cooking, but whether it is cooked or raw food, we still have to digest it inside the body. If you eat uncooked rice, the prāna is dormant and our system cannot digest it. A cow can digest raw rice because it has very strong, robust agni. But our agni is not like that of a cow. Certain foods, such as lettuce, parsley, and sprouts, have their prāna readily available for the body to digest, so we can eat them raw. However grains, unsprouted legumes, and many vegetables need cooking to make the prāna, which is latent in the food, available to the human body. Many different enzymes are responsible for this transformation and Āyurveda uses the term agni to describe these enzymes and metabolic processes. Without agni, it would be impossible to digest any food or sensory experience.

Normal Functions of Agni

Pakti - digestion, absorption, and assimilation of food and sensory experience; yields nutrition, knowledge, and understanding.

Darshana - responsible for visual perception.

Mātroshna - mātrā means measure; ushna means temperature. Agni maintains normal temperature.

Prakruti varna - maintains constitution and color complexion.

Shauryam - gives confidence, courage, and fearlessness.

Harsha - creates joy, cheerfulness, laughter, and contentment.

Prasāda - provides mental clarity; brings wholeness.

Rāga - creates affection, interest, enthusiasm, colorful quality.

Dhātu poshanam - tissue nutrition.

Ojah kāra - production of ojas; necessary for immunity.

Tejah kāra - production of tejas; necessary for maintenance of semi-permeability of membranes and cellular metabolic activity.

Prānakāra - production and utilization of prāna (vital life force) in respiration and cellular breathing.

Buddhi - provides reasoning capacity of the mind; logical thinking; discrimination.

Medhākāra - maintains intelligence and the flow of cellular communication.

Dhairyam - gives patience, stability, and confidence.

Dīrgham - maintains the span of life

Prabhā - creates healthy glow and luster

Bala - provides strength and vitality.

Agni does *pakti*, which means digestion. This includes digestion of food (carbohydrates, proteins, fat, etc.) plus digestion of sensory perception. Sound, touch, sight, taste, and smell all undergo the process of digestion. By digesting sensory perception, agni gives us knowledge and understanding. The opposite of pakti is *apakti*, which means abnormal digestive function. (The Sanskrit prefix "a" denotes "opposite.") Apakti means indigestion, which can cause bloating, constipation, and diarrhea, as well as confusion and repression of emotions.

Darshanam means visual perception. Ālochaka agni, present in the retina, the cornea, and the lens, is responsible for visual perception. Abnormal function is *adarshanam*, which means impaired visual perception. It may be corneal opacity, cataract, glaucoma, or iritis.

Next is *mātroshna*. Mātrā means dose or measure, ushna is temperature. So mātroshna is measured, normal body temperature. Its abnormal function is *amātroshna*, abnormal heat. This may be hypothermia (decreased body temperature) or it may be pyrexia (increased body temperature).

The next function is *prakruti varna*. Prakruti means normal constitution; varna means color complexion. To maintain normal color complexion is the function of agni. A vāta person tends to have brown color; a pitta person can have red color complexion; and a kapha person tends to be pale white in color. When agni is imbalanced, the person will have *vikruti varna*, which is abnormal color. If there is vāta imbalance there may be blackish discoloration, increased pitta can lead to yellow discoloration, and kapha abnormality can create extreme paleness.

Shauryam means bravery, courage, or fearlessness, all of which come from normal agni. If agni is abnormal there is *ashauryam*, creating fear and anxiety. To face a problem in a relationship, we need healthy agni. Healthy agni gives the courage, confidence, and fearlessness needed to face problems. If agni is impaired, the person has no courage and will run away from the situation.

Healthy agni creates *harsha*, which is joy, happiness, contentment, cheerfulness. When a person laughs his agni is healthy. When agni is abnormal there may be *aharsha*. Aharsha means unhappiness, grief, sadness, and depression. There is no depression without suppressed agni. If your agni is healthy, not only in the stomach but in the liver, kidney, brain, and the entire body, there is no reason to have depression. Agni governs secretion of neurotransmitters and neuro-chemical synthesis of sensation and perception, which becomes understanding. This understanding is higher cerebral activity and comes from healthy sādhaka pitta. If sādhaka agni is low, the result can be chemical depression.

The next function of sama (balanced) agni is *prasāda*. Prasāda means clarity and purity, and it yields comprehension, mental lucidity, consistency, and holiness. The person becomes whole, content. Prasāda also means holy food. When we offer prasāda to Lord Ganesha or Krishna or Shiva, we take some for ourself as a holy, wholesome food from God. The opposite of prasāda is *vishāda*, which is confusion and inconsistency. A person who is whole will behave with the same quality of clarity, compassion, and love whether at work or at home. When agni is abnormal a person will be one thing at work and totally different at home. This creates confusion, which is vishāda.

Rāga means affection, interest, and enthusiasm. Agni gives a person a balanced attraction to life, to relationships, and to food. Your life becomes charming and colorful; there is a great interest to live. When agni is imbalanced, it creates *virāga*. Virāga means repulsion, a flat effect. Some people are so poor, they live on the footpath or under a bridge. They have no social security, no insurance, nothing but sky above and earth below, yet they have such a great enthusiasm to live. That is a sign of robust agni. On the other hand, people may have everything: a house, a car, even a swimming pool. Yet when their agni is imbalanced, they may have virāga, which is repulsion and depression, creating withdrawal from life.

The next important function of agni is *dhātu poshanam*, which is tissue nutrition. All seven dhātus are nourished by dhātu agni. If dhātu agni is high, it causes *dhātu kārshyana*, which means tissue emaciation, and if it is too low, it causes excessive amounts of the unprocessed *dhātu*.

Another function of agni is *ojah kāra*. *Kāra* is creation or production, so it means production of ojas. The end product of digestion at a cellular or tissue level is ojas. Ojas is a biological substance, necessary for maintaining immunity. Abnormal function is *ojohāra*, depletion of ojas, which is diminished immunity. The person becomes sick and susceptible to infections. Agni is responsible for maintaining immunity and those people who have AIDS or other autoimmune disorders have impaired agni.

The next function of agni is *tejah kāra*, which means production of tejas. Tejas is necessary for maintaining semi-permeability of capillaries and cell membranes, so that molecules can enter the cell. The energy that maintains cellular metabolic activity is tejas. *Tejohāra* is depletion of tejas, which can affect cell permeability, resulting in loss of sodium, potassium, glucose and so forth. It is due to impaired agni.

Prāna is responsible for cellular respiration, which is also governed by agni in the cell membrane. At this subtle level, ojas, tejas and prāna work together to govern gaseous exchange, metabolic activity, and immunity. *Prānakāra* means agni creates optimal prāna, which is vital life energy. Its abnormal function is *prānahāra*. In this case, prāna is depleted and the person may go into shock.

The next important function of agni is *buddhikāra*, which is reasoning capacity. It is created by healthy sādhaka agni. When agni is impaired, causing *buddhihāra*, a person has a lack of discriminative power and indecisiveness. Decision-making capacity and decisiveness are functions of agni.

Medhākāra is next. *Medhā* means intelligence. (Don't confuse medhā with meda dhātu, fat tissue.) Cellular intelligence is necessary for communication between two cells. When cells communicate, they maintain their health. If communication is blocked, a cell becomes isolated. An isolated cell is a lonely cell, and such a confused cell can undergo malignant changes, which can lead to cancer. The abnormal function of agni can cause *medhāhāra*, lack of intelligence. In patients of cancer, their cellular agni is drastically affected and cellular intelligence is clogged.

Next is *dhairyam*. *Dhru* means to hold, and *dhairyam* means patience. Patience is very important. Patience means to live now, whereas impatience means to live in the future. One of the abnormal functions of agni is *adhīrata*, impatience. Some people live in the future and want to complete their work as quickly as possible. On a subtle level this is from impaired function of agni. Healthy agni gives one plenty of time, but pitta people whose agni is intensified have very little patience. Impatience makes a person aggressive, competitive, and violent. Interestingly, the opposite of impatience is sloppiness. When agni is low, a person does not care about time; if there is a deadline, he will always be late. That is also imbalanced agni. So laziness and impatience are both abnormal functions of agni, and patience is a normal, balanced function of agni.

Dīrgham is the appropriate span of life. Balanced agni maintains a long span of life. Diminished agni can ultimately create untimely death; the person loses the capacity to digest the experiences of life.

Next is *prabhā*. Agni gives a person a healthy glow and luster. The opposite of this is *chāyā*, which is shadow. Diminished agni gives a person a shadowy appearance, which can show up in the skin tone.

The final function of agni is *bala,* strength. Poor agni creates the opposite of bala, which is *kshaya*, decay or decrease.

The Doshas and Agni

Agni is hot, sharp, dry, light, mobile, and subtle. Vāta gives dry, light, mobile, and subtle qualities to agni, and pitta gives hot and sharp gunas. However, the qualities of kapha are totally opposite to those of agni. Kapha is heavy, dull/slow, cold, oily, slimy, gross, cloudy, and static, all of which slow the action of agni.

In the body, there is no agni without pitta and there is no pitta without agni. Pitta is a container and agni is the content. Relatively speaking, pitta is matter and agni is the energy. At a more subtle level, agni is matter and tejas is the pure essence of agni. So one could say that pitta is the gross matter, agni is the energy or subtle matter, and within agni is the subtler energy of tejas.

All three doshas can affect agni when they are aggravated. Vāta, by its cold quality, can decrease agni, but can also kindle agni by the dry, light, mobile, and subtle qualities. Agni affected by vāta is called *vishama agni*, irregular agni. Vāta can quickly slow agni but can also quickly kindle it. Agni affected by kapha is called *manda agni*, slow or dull agni. It will often produce long-standing effects and can be slow to return to balance. Pitta can both increase or decrease agni. Agni affected by an increase of the hot and sharp qualities of pitta is called *tīkshna agni*, sharp agni. However, if pitta is increased by liquid or oily qualities, it can lead to manda agni. Pitta, when increased by the liquid quality, becomes like hot water. Pouring hot water on a fire slows the fire and can even snuff it out, so pitta can also slow agni.

So vāta aggravation creates vishama agni, increased pitta can create tīkshna agni, and aggravated kapha causes manda agni. However it also works the other way around. Vishama agni leads to vāta disorders, tīkshna agni to pitta disorders, and manda agni to kapha problems. Cause becomes effect and effect becomes cause.

Many factors, such as detrimental lifestyle, diet, bad food combining and repressed emotions, can cause the bodily doshas to become aggravated. This soon disturbs agni, with the result that food cannot be properly digested. The undigested food turns into a morbid, toxic sticky substance, called *āma*. Āma is the root cause of many diseases. The presence of āma in the system leads to fatigue, and a feeling of heaviness. It may induce constipation, indigestion, gases, diarrhea, bad breath, perverted taste, and mental confusion. The tongue gets a thick coating and there may be generalized body ache and stiffness. Because of the critical importance of agni in maintaining health, it is important to have balanced agni, called *sama agni*.

The Four Varieties of Agni

Sama Agni (balanced metabolism). When all the doshas are in balance according to the constitution, then agni maintains its state of equilibrium and provides a balanced metabolism. A person having balanced agni can eat almost any type of food in any season without any adverse signs and symptoms. Digestion, absorption and elimination are all normal. This is the state of perfect health. Neither food nor environment upsets those people with the gift of sama agni. They have a calm, quiet, loving mind, and great clarity of awareness and bliss. Good health, longevity, surplus of ojas, tejas and prāna, and good immunity are all virtues of balanced agni.

Vishama Agni (irregular metabolism). As a result of aggravated vāta, agni can undergo drastic changes. It becomes erratic and produces irregular appetite, variable digestion, abdominal distention, indigestion, gases, constipation, and colicky pain. Even a small quantity of food turns into gas. At times, it may lead to diarrhea, a feeling of heaviness after eating, and gurgling of the intestines. The individual may get dry skin, cracking joints, sciatica, low backache, or insomnia. Emotionally this can result in anxiety, insecurity, fear, and other neurological or mental problems. The person can get cravings for fried and hot, spicy food. The cold quality of vāta slows down agni, and the mobile quality makes it fluctuate, resulting in irregular metabolism. Eventually āma is produced and can be seen on the tongue as a brownish-black coating. Dry mouth, receding gums, muscle spasm, and most other vāta disorders take place because there is vishama agni.

Tīkshna Agni (sharp; hypermetabolism). Due to the hot, sharp, and penetrating attributes of pitta, agni can become intense when pitta dosha is increased. This causes hyper-metabolism. In this condition, the person has the desire to frequently eat large quantities of food. After digestion, one gets dry throat, lips, and palate, as well as heartburn, hot flashes, and acid indigestion. The liquid, sour and hot qualities of pitta may produce hyperacidity, gastritis, hypoglycemia, colitis, diarrhea, and dysentery. Pain in the liver, nausea, vomiting and various inflammatory conditions may occur. Tīkshna agni in some may lead to anger, hate and envy. The person becomes judgmental or critical toward everyone and everything. The subject can have intense cravings for sweets. According to Āyurveda, most pitta disorders have their origin in tīkshna agni.

Manda Agni (dull; hypometabolism). The water and earth molecules of kapha dosha are heavy, slow and cool, which inhibit the light, sharp, and hot qualities of agni. As a result, excess kapha can cause agni to become dull, leading to slow metabolism. A person with manda agni can fast on only water for a few days and still put on five pounds in weight. The individual with this type of agni cannot digest even a normal diet properly. Even without eating, there is heaviness in the stomach, cold, congestion and cough. Over-salivation, loss of appetite, allergies, nausea, and mucoid vomiting can result. Some people may show edema, obesity, hypertension, and diabetes. There will be lethargy, excessive sleep, cold clammy skin, and generalized weakness of the body. Mentally there can be attachment, greed, and possessiveness. The subject may have a strong craving for hot, sharp, dry and spicy food. Almost all kapha ailments are rooted in manda agni.

Table 11: The Four Varieties of Agni

Sama agni	Balanced; tridoshic
Vishama agni	Irregular, usually associated with vāta
Tīkshna agni	Sharp; usually associated with pitta
Manda agni	Dull/slow; usually associated with kapha

The 40 Main Types of Agni

Digestion, assimilation and absorption occur throughout the body, from the immediate absorption that happens in the mouth when chewing to the subtle digestion that feeds each cell of the body. For this reason, Āyurveda has defined more than 40 kinds of agni related to these processes. This section will explain the 40 primary types of agni found in the body.

The Subtypes of Agni

There is one vāta in the body, but for convenience of understanding we categorize it into five subtypes, because of differences in function and structure. In the same way, as a whole, *deha* (bodily) *agni* is the one agni present everywhere, but for better understanding we classify it into subtypes. There are thirteen main agnis, and the most important is jāthara agni, the central fire in the digestive system. Included in this thirteen are five elemental agnis in the liver, called bhūta agni, and seven dhātu agnis, one for each tissue. There are an additional 27 agnis that we will outline in this chapter. (see "The 40 Main Types of Agni" on page 285) Ultimately all types of agni lead to *Brahman agni* or *dhyāna agni*, which is the fire of attention. Keeping in mind the many other kinds of agni, we will begin by looking at jāthara agni.

Jāthara agni is also called *koshta agni, kāya agni,* or *maha agni,* as well as *antara* (internal) *agni*. These are all synonyms. Let us stick to one name, jāthara agni. It is the central fire and it includes agni in the *āmāshaya* (stomach) and grahani (small intestine). Jāthara agni is the functional integrity between the agni components of kledaka kapha, pāchaka pitta, rañjaka pitta, prāna vāyu, and samāna vāyu. It includes gastric mucus secretions (kledaka), the stimuli from the hunger center in the brain (prāna vāyu), peristalsis and opening of the pyloric valve (prāna and samāna vāyu), and the various gastric and intestinal enzymes (pāchaka pitta).

Jāthara agni governs initial digestion. Once we chew and swallow food, it comes into the stomach and kledaka kapha liquefies the food. This stimulates the secretion of hydrochloric acid (HCl) and digestive enzymes, and rennin for coagulation of milk, along with other enzymes. The digestion of carbohydrates, proteins, and fats starts in the stomach and the stomach absorbs water, glucose, alcohol and saline through the stomach wall. The stomach also excretes toxins and stimulates the gastro-colic and gastro-salivary reflexes with the help of prāna vāyu, samāna vāyu, and udāna vāyu.

From a medical standpoint, jāthara agni is very important because it is the gate or doorway of the digestive system. Any physical substance that passes through this gate or that is absorbed through the skin on its way into the body has a much better chance of being digested than something absorbed through other means. Intravenous or intramuscular injections of medicines are not digested by agni. Āyurveda says that any medicine given orally, sublingually, or externally on the skin is

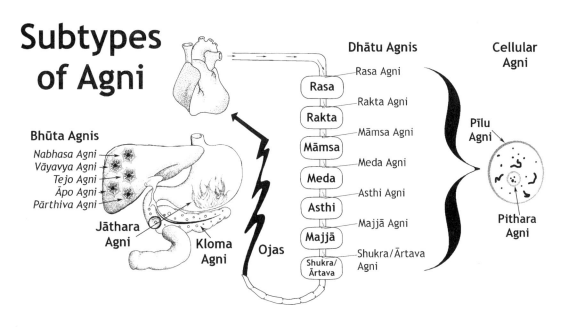

Subtypes of Agni

Bhūta Agnis

Nabhasa Agni
Vāyavya Agni
Tejo Agni
Āpo Agni
Pārthiva Agni

Jāthara Agni

Kloma Agni

Ojos

Dhātu Agnis

Rasa — Rasa Agni
Rakta — Rakta Agni
Māmsa — Māmsa Agni
Meda — Meda Agni
Asthi — Asthi Agni
Majjā — Majjā Agni
Shukra/Ārtava — Shukra/Ārtava Agni

Cellular Agni

Pīlu Agni

Pithara Agni

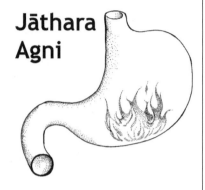

Jāthara Agni

digested by agni, which means the medicine is processed and it can work at the cellular level. Even when a medicine penetrates the skin or fascia, digestion happens through bhrājaka agni, and then through bhūta agni.

When you directly inject medicines such as penicillin or tetracycline intramuscularly or intravenously, there is a risk of severe reactions. Why do people get reactions? Because undigested food or medicine is perceived by the immune system as a foreign body. Agni does not want to accept any foreign body, so it becomes irritable and this irritation of the agni manifests as anaphylactic shock or vasovagal shock. If agni is seriously disturbed, a person's life is in danger. Why are people allergic to certain drugs? Because the drugs are not predigested by one's own agni. The best route of administration is oral because then bodhaka agni and jāthara agni act on the medicine instead of the medicine going directly to the dhātu agni and cellular agni. There are certain highly powerful drugs that cause reactions even when taken orally. Any reaction to a drug is due to the severe reaction of agni and of pitta. Agni will be disturbed first and this will create high pitta, which is shown in the body as diarrhea, rashes, acne, and other pitta disorders.

Kloma agni. *Kloma* means the pancreas. Kloma also refers to the choroid plexuses in the brain, which secrete cerebrospinal fluid. *Kloma agni* governs digestion of sweet taste via the pancreas and water regulation in the body, through the choroid plexuses. Even water has to be digested. Undigested water damages the kidneys and can accumulate under the skin as edema. Sweet taste has Earth and Water components, and the Water in the sweet taste is regulated by kloma agni. Kloma agni operates during the salty phase of digestion. Salty taste has a buffering action and is very important in digestion of carbohydrates and fats.

Bhūta agni is the agni (fire component) of the liver, which manifests as the liver enzymes. Bhūta means element or "that which manifests as matter." The five basic elements—Ether, Air, Fire, Water, and Earth—are present in our food as well as in all other substances. According to Āyurveda, the flame of jāthara agni goes into the liver and manifests as the agni relating to these five elements. There are five bhūta agnis: *Nabhasa agni,* the fire component of Ether; *Vāyavya agni,* the fire component of Air; *Tejo agni,* the fire component of Fire; *Āpo agni,* the fire component of Water; and *Pārthiva agni,* the fire component of Earth.

The liver is both an excretory and secretory organ. It secretes bile and excretes unwanted toxic materials, including heavy metals and bacteria. Bile is rañjaka pitta. It is yellowish-green in color, liquid, oily, bitter and pungent, and is alkaline. It contains inorganic salts and pigmentation. Bile helps excretion by stimulating peristaltic movement, and the pigments give color to the stools. Bile salts reduce surface tension and act as a buffer, thereby emulsifying (breaking down) fat and controlling cholesterol levels. The liver also maintains the acid-alkali balance in the body. Bhūta agni is involved in the elemental metabolism of all substances. However, there are two other types of agni also present in the liver, rañjaka agni and rakta agni, and there is a fine line between the functions of these agnis and those of bhūta agni. Rañjaka agni is the fire component of rañjaka pitta, released from disintegrated red blood cells. It governs the transformation of rasa dhātu into asthāyi (immature) rakta dhātu and contains bhūta agni. Rakta agni transforms asthāyi rakta into sthāyi (mature) rakta dhātu. (see "Rakta Dhātu: the Blood Tissue" on page 113)

Initial digestion begins in the mouth and proceeds in the stomach, where jāthara agni continues to break down the food. It progresses to the duodenum (with kloma agni), into the jejunum, the ileum, and on into the colon, with *pākvāshaya* (colon) *agni*. Throughout this process of digestion, nutrients are absorbed through the villi of the small intestine and, along with glucose and alcohol absorbed directly from the stomach, enter the venous hepatic portal system. This hepatic circulatory system carries the molecules to the liver for further processing by bhūta agni. The bhūta agnis transform the five elements of food into the five biologically available elements of the body that are circulated to the bodily tissues. This process can be studied at the cellular level. Nabhasa agni maintains the shape of cells, vāyavya agni regulates cellular respiration, and tejo agni maintains cellular metabolic activity. Āpo agni maintains the cytoplasm, and pārthiva agni governs mineral regulation. The bhūta agnis yield the twenty gunas (qualities) from the foods and thoughts we consume and these in turn nourish the body and mind. Nabhasa agni yields clear, light, subtle, and soft qualities; vāyavya agni yields mobile, dry, light, cold, rough, and subtle qualities; tejo agni yields hot, sharp, light, dry, and subtle qualities; āpo agni yields liquid, cold, oily, dull, soft, and smooth qualities; and pārthiva agni yields heavy, dull, static, hard, gross, and dense qualities.

Any food we eat is composed of all five elements. For example, an apple has all five elements, but is predominately Air and Water. The apple is crunchy, astringent, and yields gases, due to the Air element, and is juicy due to the Water

> **Functions of Bhūta Agni**
>
> To convert the five elements from food and water into biologically available forms of these elements.
> To nourish cellular consciousness through these five elements.
> To nourish immunity through ojas, tejas, and prāna.
> To stimulate the dhātu agnis and nourish the seven dhātus.
> To manifest the liver enzymes.

element. However it also has a particular form due to the Ether element. It ripens due to the Fire element, and it has minerals, which are Earth element. The job of bhūta agni is to transform these elements of ingested food into a form the body can use, so they can become the biological elements of the seven dhātus. For instance, pārthiva agni transforms the *prithivī* (Earth) element of a food, which is heavy, dull, static, hard, gross, and dense, into biological Earth element, with the help of the dhātu agni at the tissue level and pīlu agni at the cell membranes.

All seven dhātus are nourished through the bhūta agnis. The Water and Earth agnis yield the qualities of Water and Earth into rasa dhātu, the blood plasma. The liver is a large reservoir of blood and plays an important role in regulating blood volume through erythrogenesis (generation of red blood cells). The Fire, Water, and Earth agnis play an important role in the production of rakta dhātu, the red blood cells. Another interesting function of the liver is to nourish māmsa dhātu through conversion of glucose into glycogen, which is stored in the muscles, and through protein metabolism. Māmsa is nourished by Earth, Water, and Fire agnis in the liver. Therefore muscle strength, power, and nourishment are governed by bhūta agni with the help of māmsa agni.

Alcohol and fats are metabolized in the liver. Often people do not eat food excessively high in fat or cholesterol, yet their cholesterol is high because of impaired bhūta agni. One function of the liver is to process and store fat (meda dhātu) and it is bhūta agni that stimulates meda agni to nourish meda dhātu. An imbalance in this process will sometimes show up in the body as high cholesterol. The bhūta agnis nourish asthi dhātu by mineral metabolism and, with vitamin B12 and gastric intrinsic factor, they help the production of red blood cells in the bone marrow, which is majjā dhātu. Finally, through hormone metabolism, the bhūta agnis nourish majjā and shukra/ārtava dhātus. If you look at all these functions of the liver, based upon modern medicine, and the Āyurvedic concept of bhūta agni working in conjunction with the dhātu agnis, you will see the connections. A patient with liver disease can have any of these functions affected. The person can be anemic and become jaundiced, resulting in muscle wasting and emaciation. The bones can become porous and there is often sexual debility.

Jatru agni. There are two schools of thought about *jatru agni*. One says this refers to *ūrdhva* (upper) *jatru granthi* (the thyroid gland), which maintains metabolism. Another says it is *adha* (lower) *jatru granthi* (the thymus gland), which maintains immunity. I like to make it simple and say jatru agni refers to both. These glands of the endocrine system are part of majjā dhātu, so they are related to the chakra system. Jatru agni in the thymus gland maintains immunity by producing ojas. Jatru agni in the thyroid is important for regulating cellular metabolic activity. The thyroid is a bridge between bhūta agni and the seven tissues, maintaining the functional integrity of the bhūta agni and dhātu agni. The agni present within the thyroid relates to T3 and T4 (thyroxin) hormones and it kindles agni at the cellular level. Cellular metabolic activities are governed by jatru agni and, if jatru agni in the thyroid is sluggish, a person's metabolism becomes slow and they easily put on weight. If jatru agni is hyperactive, a person loses weight in the beginning, but the increased appetite can make the person eat a lot and their weight can vary. If there are certain repressed emotions, such as grief, or sadness, these can also impair the function of the thyroid gland.

Dhātu agni. Every dhātu has its agni component. The metabolic fire of rasa dhātu is rasa agni, and that of rakta is rakta agni. Similarly, there are māmsa agni, meda agni, asthi agni, majjā agni and shukra/ārtava agni. *Dhātu agni* can correspond to amino acids and special enzymes necessary for nutrition of the respective tissues. All metabolic transformations of the tissues are governed by the seven dhātu agnis. The food for each dhātu agni is the unprocessed dhātu component called asthāyi dhātu. Asthāyi means immature or unprocessed. The unprocessed tissues are food for the processed tissues and each dhātu agni transforms unprocessed, immature tissue into processed, mature tissue called sthāyi dhātu. This concept of dhātu nutrition is discussed in detail in Chapters 5 and 9.

Between two dhātus there is a membranous structure called *dhātu dhara kalā,* which separates one dhātu from another. A *srotas* is a channel and it is made up of its own related dhātu (tissue). Within this specialized *kalā*, the dhātu agni, ojas, tejas, and prāna govern the functions of that particular dhātu. *Sroto agni* is the name given to the agni of a particular srotas and it maintains the functional activity of the channel. Sroto agni is part and parcel of the dhātu agni present in the root of each of the seven srotāmsi related to the seven dhātus, and in the case of the three channels to eliminate wastes from the body, it is the same as the mala agnis (see below). So at the root of rasa vaha srotas, in the rasa dhara kalā, is rasa dhātu agni; at the root of rakta vaha srotas is rakta dhātu agni; and so forth. Similarly, at the root of *purisha vaha srotas*, in the purisha dhara kalā, is *purisha agni*, and likewise for the other malas.

Pīlu agni. The digestive fire in a cell membrane is called *pīlu agni*. Pīlu means atom, so this is micro-digestion. Pīlu agni maintains the semi-permeability of the cell membrane. Outside the cell are molecules of food, water, and air that have been broken down into their elemental components by bhūta agni. They then pass through pīlu agni in the cell membrane, into the cell and become a part of the living cell. This transformation of extra-cellular nutrients into intra-cellular content is the function of pīlu agni. In conjunction with bhūta agni, it transforms the extra-cellular nutrients into the twenty gunas (qualities), which are related to the main amino acids. Pīlu agni is the same as dhātu agni, but viewed from the cellular level. Another way of saying this is that dhātu agni is the sum of all the pīlu agnis in all cells that comprise a particular type of tissue. For instance, rasa agni is comprised of the total pīlu agni in all plasma cells in the body.

The Amino Acids and 20 Gunas

Manifestation of the 20 gunas in the cell where food nourishes consciousness.

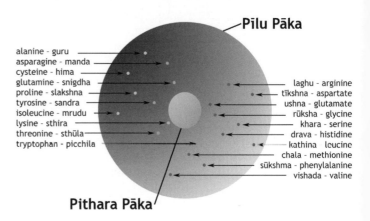

Pīlu Pāka

alanine - guru
asparagine - manda
cysteine - hima
glutamine - snigdha
proline - slakshna
tyrosine - sandra
isoleucine - mrudu
lysine - sthira
threonine - sthūla
tryptophan - picchila

laghu - arginine
tīkshna - aspartate
ushna - glutamate
rūksha - glycine
khara - serine
drava - histidine
kathina - leucine
chala - methionine
sūkshma - phenylalanine
vishada - valine

Pithara Pāka

Every cell is a center of consciousness through which there is a flow of intelligence for communication. These qualities direct the flow, structure and nature of cellular activity, which is anu srotas.

The Ether, Air, Fire, Water, and Earth components of bhūta agni are based in the liver, but they operate throughout the body at the cellular level. Each element nourishes its respective tanmātrā through its gunas (qualities), due to the actions of bhūta agni and pīlu and pithara agni. For instance, Ether element nourishes shabda (sound) through its light, clear, and subtle qualities. These gunas are represented by amino acids at the physical level. Amino acids are the building blocks of protein and the end product of protein digestion. Peptides are organic compounds containing two or more amino acids and production of peptides relates to the sensory pathways. These peptides are chained together by the tanmātrās. Pārthiva (Earth) agni nourishes smell by producing various peptides that relate to the olfactory sense. Āpo (Water) agni nourishes taste; tejo (Fire) agni nourishes vision; vāyavya (Air) agni nourishes touch; and nabhasa (Ether) agni nourishes sound. So at the level of cellular digestion, the bhūta agnis and pīlu agni nourish the senses. From jāthara agni to bhūta agni to dhātu, pīlu, and pithara agnis, food becomes gunas (qualities), food nourishes the mind and senses, and food becomes consciousness.

Pithara agni. Inside a cell, in the nuclear membrane, there is *pithara agni*. Pithara agni further processes the contents within the cytoplasm, nourishing genes and even the RNA and DNA. The qualities induced into a cell, either externally from food or internally from one's consciousness, relate to the amino acids that comprise the proteins formed by the genetic material (DNA and RNA). Pithara means parents. In other words, our genes are carriers of heredity from our parents found within the cell nuclei. Pithara agni is the genetic agni that transforms the cytoplasmic content of food into consciousness. Pīlu agni nourishes the cells and pithara agni nourishes the mind and consciousness at a cellular level and maintains the genetic code, which is prakruti.

Even consciousness needs to be nourished. At the cellular level, food becomes consciousness. Consciousness is the substratum of the mind, the senses, and their objects (sound, touch, form, taste, and smell). The mind is the senses and is nourished by pīlu agni and pithara agni, with the help of bhūta agni, at a very subtle cellular level. Āyurveda classifies food as sattvic, rajasic and tamasic according to the affects they produce on the mind. Tamasic foods include meat, eggs, mushrooms, garlic, and stale foods. They make the mind dull and heavy. Rajasic foods include hot, spicy, and fermented food, including pickles and chutneys, as well as most grains and legumes. They make the senses agitated and the mind hyperactive. Sattvic foods include many fresh vegetables and fruits, certain grains, and some other easily digestible foods. They induce clarity, compassion, and love and thus balance the mind. Sattvic, rajasic, and tamasic qualities are yielded into consciousness by pithara agni.

Indriya agni. These specialized agnis are related to the five senses. Indriya means the doors of perception, which are the five sensory pathways. These are the auditory sense (sound), the tactile sense (touch), the visual sense (vision), the gustatory sense (taste), and olfactory sense (smell). In each of these sensory pathways, there is *indriya agni,* which relates to enzymes and neurotransmitters. The indriya agnis digest, absorb, assimilate, and transform sensory perception into knowledge. Therefore, *you recognize the sight of a tree and the sound of a bird.*

The agni component of sādhaka pitta is sādhaka agni and the indriya (sensory) agnis are a specialized component of sādhaka agni. The bhūta agnis break down the elemental components of food, then the indriya agnis further transform the five elements into their tanmātrā (sensory object) components to nourish sādhaka pitta and the five tanmātrās in the mind. The digestion of sensory perception by the related indriya agni occurs in the brain and sādhaka pitta is nourished by the knowledge it yields. For example if we smell something, gandha agni digests the odor, which is gandha tanmātrā in the object, and brings the knowledge of that smell to sādhaka pitta. However if indriya agni is impaired, there is impairment of sensory perception. For instance, if shabda agni becomes low, as it often does in old age, the person cannot hear very well.

Dosha agni. The agni concept is so well-defined that even the subtypes of the doshas have their own agni components. Vāta has prāna agni, vyāna agni, udāna agni, samāna agni and apāna agni. The same thing is true for pitta. There is pāchaka agni, rañjaka agni, sādhaka agni, ālochaka agni, and bhrājaka agni. Kapha has kledaka agni, avalambaka agni, bodhaka agni, tarpaka agni, and shleshaka agni. The bhūta agnis from the liver maintain the functional aspects of each dosha, through the agni components of the subdoshas. For example, nabhasa agni nourishes prāna vāyu, because prāna is Etheric. Vāyavya agni stimulates udāna, which is related to the Air element. Tejo agni controls samāna, which is related to the Fire element. Āpo agni governs vyāna, which is Water, and pārthiva agni governs apāna vāyu, related to Earth. Along the same lines, nabhasa agni also governs sādhaka pitta and tarpaka kapha. Vāyavya agni nourishes ālochaka pitta and avalambaka kapha, while tejo agni regulates pāchaka pitta and kledaka kapha. Āpo agni governs rañjaka pitta and bodhaka kapha, and pārthiva agni nourishes bhrājaka pitta and shleshaka kapha.

We need to keep all types of agni in balance, so that we remain healthy and happy. Kāya chikitsā, or internal medicine, is basically the treatment of agni because agni is fundamental to health. Whether you are using herbs, doing pañchakarma, or fasting, you are treating agni through the subtypes of the doshas.

Mala agni. There are also three *mala agnis*, for the three excreta. The first is *mūtra agni*, governing excretion of urine. The second is purisha agni, governing excretion of feces. The third is *sveda agni*, governing sweat. Each mala agni is located in the kalā (membranous structure) that surrounds the channels of elimination. Mūtra agni is found in the bladder and urinary system. Excess liquid is carried to the kidneys, where it is filtered through the glomeruli and eliminated via the bladder. Mūtra agni operates in all these sites and maintains the glomeruli threshold, acid-alkali balance of urine, and specific gravity of urine. The function of purisha agni is to absorb liquids and minerals, make the stools well formed, and maintain the temperature of the feces. It gives color to the stools—yellow if pitta, dark for vāta, and pale in the case of kapha. Sveda agni regulates body temperature, maintains the moisture, softness, oiliness, and acid-alkali balance of the skin, and helps to govern the water-electrolyte balance in the body.

Summary
Agni works at many levels. Agni as a whole is regulated by jāthara agni. At a systemic level, agni works in the GI tract as digestive enzymes, hydrochloric acid, pepsin, rennin, gastric intrinsic factor, and so on. Jāthara agni does grosser digestion and creates three mala—urine, feces and sweat—which each have their own agni to carry out their excretory functions. Kloma agni in the pancreas works in conjunction with bhūta agni from the liver and further governs the digestion of proteins, carbohydrates, and fats. The elements of the food—Ether, Air, Fire, Water, and Earth—are transformed into the biological elements by the five bhūta agnis, and the nutrition of the tissues and cells is governed by dhātu agni. On a tissue level, bhūta agnis nourish dhātu agni. On a cellular level, bhūta agni nourishes pīlu agni. Jatru agni is a bridge between bhūta agni and the various dhātu and pīlu agnis. Sensory perception is governed by indriya agnis, and the functions of vāta, pitta, and kapha are governed by their respective dosha agnis. Lastly, cellular metabolic activities are governed by pīlu agni and pithara agni. Agni is the governing principle that operates throughout the digestive process and transforms food and sensations into consciousness.

5

Dhātus
The Seven Bodily Tissues

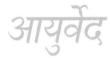

Introduction

The Sanskrit word *dhā* means holding, placing, containing, causing. Dhātu means tissue, that which holds the organ together, the constructing, cementing material of the body. The body is made up of atoms. Many atoms gather together to create molecules, and many molecules come together to create tissues of blood, muscle, bone, etc.

In this chapter we will be discussing these tissues in terms of structure and function, with particular attention to their precursor states, their mature states and volume, their superior states, their inferior and superior by-products, and the agni involved in these transformative processes. There will also be a discussion about disorders of the dhātu at the end of each section.

There are seven *dhātus* (bodily tissues): *rasa, rakta, māmsa, meda, asthi, majjā,* and *shukra/ārtava*. Rasa means the juice of life, which is exemplified by plasma or serum. Rakta is the color red and is also red blood cells, the liquid tissue, or blood. The Western concept of blood includes plasma, but in Āyurveda blood means the red blood cells (RBC). Māmsa is muscle tissue. Meda is adipose tissue, fat or lipid. Asthi is bones and cartilage. Majjā includes bone marrow, nerve tissue, and connective tissue. Shukra is the male reproductive tissue and ārtava is the female reproductive tissue.

Table 12: The Seven Dhātus

Dhātus	Bodily Tissue(s)
Rasa	plasma (serum, white blood cells, lymphatic system)
Rakta	red blood cells
Māmsa	muscle
Meda	adipose tissue / fat
Asthi	bones and cartilage
Majjā	marrow, nerve tissue, connective tissue
Shukra	male reproductive tissue
Ārtava	female reproductive tissue

Nutrition and Structure of the Dhātus

When we consume food, it undergoes the process of digestion in the stomach, small intestine and colon. This process is governed by jāthara agni, the central digestive fire, and bhūta agni, the digestive principle present in the liver. From the introduction of food into the body and its first stages of digestion within the bloodstream all the way through the final stage of tissue formation of the reproductive tissue, the quality of the body's tissues is governed by the factors mentioned above: the digestive capacity, quantity, quality, structure and function of each dhātu.

The nourishment of the tissues of the body actually occurs in stages through each of the dhātus successively. The nutrition of each dhātu is governed by agni or digestive fire; and every dhātu has its own *dhātu agni*. This fire principle of every dhātu must be strong in order to maintain the physiological functions of that dhātu. If one dhātu agni is adversely affected, it will gradually affect the others; however, not necessarily in sequence.

As each dhātu receives the nutrients, it processes and digests these nutrients and produces two results. One result is the mature, fully formed tissue and the other is a precursor or immature, raw form of nutrition for the next level of tissue formation. There are two types or stages of dhātu—*asthāyi* and *sthāyi*. Asthāyi means unstable, immature or unprocessed; sthāyi means stable, mature or processed. Asthāyi, as the unprocessed form of dhātu, circulates throughout the body, while sthāyi is firmly placed in substance and form. Asthāyi can also be called *poshaka*, which means nourisher because it nourishes the mature tissue. Sthāyi is known as *poshya*, meaning that which is nourished.

Dhātu dhara kalā is the membranous structure that holds a dhātu. *Dhara* means holding, *kalā* means membranous structure. One function of kalā is to separate two tissues from one another to give them form and make them distinct. Kalā is the mother of the dhātu because it holds and nourishes the dhātu. The dhātu agnis are present within the kalā and transform raw, unprocessed dhātu into processed, formed dhātu. Therefore *rasa dhātu* has *rasa dhara kalā* and *rasa dhātu agni*, *rakta dhātu* has *rakta dhara kalā* and *rakta dhātu agni*, and so on. Within the kalā of each dhātu there is also *dhātu ojas*, *dhātu tejas*, and *dhātu prāna*. They maintain the function of kalā. On one side of the kalā there is asthāyi dhātu (unprocessed dhātu). Kalā helps to transform this asthāyi dhātu into sthāyi dhātu (processed dhātu), with its dhātu agni, ojas, tejas, and prāna.

The capillaries collect the end product of digested food, *āhāra rasa*, from the gastrointestinal tract and move it into general circulation. *Āhāra* means food and *rasa* means juice or essence. The end product of digested food is āhāra rasa, the "essence of food" or nutrient precursor. Āhāra rasa is the post-digestive dhātu precursor, which we can call chyle. Chyle is the milk-like, alkaline product of digestion that is carried from the intestines by the lymphatic system into the bloodstream. It is produced by jāthara agni and bhūta agni and is the precursor for the nourishment of all the dhātus.

Within five days, this nutrient precursor (āhāra rasa) becomes mature rasa dhātu and *asthāyi rakta*, the second dhātu. Then rasa is transformed into *sthāyi rakta* from *asthāyi rakta dhātu*. It is rasa that nourishes rakta and all successive dhātus. From the initial formation of āhāra rasa, it takes 10 days to create mature *rakta dhātu*. There are seven dhātus and each stage of dhātu nutrition takes an additional five days. Seven multiplied by five is 35 days, so rasa dhātu becomes mature shukra or ārtava dhātu (reproductive tissue and the seventh dhātu) in 35 days.

Dhātu By-products

In this transformation of immature dhātu (asthāyi dhātu) into mature dhātu (sthāyi dhātu), three types of products are created for each dhātu. The first is *sāra*, which means pure essence. This is the pure, stabilized, mature tissue (sthāyi dhātu) itself. The other two are by-products. The superior by-product is called *upadhātu*, and the inferior by-product is called *mala*. Mala is also known as *kitta*, which means inferior.

In the West we have translated *mala* as waste product. We do not have an understanding for the value of it. Mala is a process that we often try to reduce to one word. However, it is a series of events that enable nutrition as well as the elimination of waste. Mala is more than an impurity and each mala has a nutritive function.

As an example of the by-products of a dhātu, the sāra of rasa dhātu is the pure sthāyi rasa; the superior by-products of rasa are the top layer of the skin, lactation, and menstruation; and the inferior by-product of rasa is *poshaka kapha* (*kleda* or mucus). Poshaka means nourishing, so poshaka kapha nourishes all kapha systems. Every dhātu has each of these three types of products.

When a person has a particular dhātu that is fully mature and of superior quality is it called *dhātu sāra*. The concept of sāra indicates the superior and obvious expression of that tissue's presence. In other words, the superior qualities associated with a particular dhātu will clearly express themselves. Because form follows function, this physical manifestation of the tissue indicates that the function is quite strong in that area.

Disorders of the Dhātus

Disorders of a dhātu are caused by the entry of a dosha into the dhātu. This can cause quantitative or qualitative changes in the dhātu. Qualitative change is called *dhātu dushti*. Either asthāyi (immature) or sthāyi (mature) dhātu (tissue) can be affected. *Asthāyi dhātu dushti* manifests as an acute condition. *Sthāyi dhātu dushti* is usually longer lasting. Increased quantity of a dhātu is called *dhātu vruddhi*. Decreased quantity is *dhātu kshaya*.

Dhātu dushti can be defined as the qualitative changes that take place within the dhātu due to the aggravated qualities of a dosha. Present in both the dosha and the dhātu, the attributes or gunas (see chapter 2) are the factors that change. When the aggravated dosha enters the dhātu, the qualities it carries affect the qualities of the dhātu. For instance, if vāta enters rasa dhātu; it carries the qualities of dry, light, and rough. The inherent attributes of rasa dhātu include oily, heavy, and smooth. Ideally, your diet and lifestyle would support the attributes of rasa dhātu. The effect of vāta entering rasa dhātu could include dry, rough skin, emaciation, and dizziness.

Quantitative changes refer to an increase or decrease in the dhātu. When any dosha—vāta, pitta, or kapha—goes into a dhātu, it affects the nutrition of the dhātu as well as the dhātu agni. When it causes slow agni, there is undue production of that dhātu. Therefore, the dhātu is increased in quantity, called dhātu vruddhi. Alternatively, if there is high agni, there is decreased production of the dhātu, called dhātu kshaya.

In both these conditions there can also be qualitative changes in the dhātu, called dhātu dushti. But dhātu dushti can occur without quantitative changes being present, due to variable agni. When these changes affect the asthāyi (immature) dhātu, they tend to be acute disorders. However, when any dosha goes into a sthāyi (mature) dhātu, it usually creates a chronic condition. Qualitative changes in the sthāyi dhātu caused by the entry of the dosha creates sthāyi dhātu dushti.

Asthāyi conditions can be treated simply as a vāta, pitta, or kapha imbalance, but when sthāyi dhātu is affected, a chronic condition may persist for years because the mature, fully formed dhātu (tissue) is affected. Both the excess dosha and affected dhātu need to be treated. Pañchakarma is important in treating a chronic condition, as it eliminates excess doshas, helps to kindle dhātu agni, and improves the quality of both sthāyi dhātu and asthāyi dhātu. See "The Seven Bodily Tissues (Sapta Dhātu)" on page 284 for more information on the dhātus.

Rasa Dhātu: the Plasma Tissue

Rasa dhātu is the first and foremost juice of all life—from the amoeba to the human being—and is associated with plasma. Āhāra rasa is the asthāyi form of rasa dhātu, forms within 12 hours of the intake of food, and is the source of nutrition for every cell and bodily tissue. Rasa agni, the fire principle of rasa, transforms āhāra rasa into sthāyi rasa (mature rasa) and asthāyi rakta (immature rakta). This transformation, from food to plasma, takes five days.

Within rasa dhātu are the five elements—Ether, Air, Fire, Water, and Earth—and six tastes—sweet, sour, salty, bitter, pungent, and astringent. Rasa has mainly sweet and salty tastes, but the other four tastes are minutely and subtly present. Within rasa there are also the three gunas—sattva, rajas, tamas. All these elements, tastes and gunas are nourished by rasa agni.

Rasa dhātu contains both hot and cold molecules. The hot molecules are red blood cells and the cold molecules are white blood cells. Rasa—which includes white blood cells—and rakta (red blood cells) function together. White blood cells and red blood cells bathe and breathe in plasma, which is rasa dhātu. Plasma also includes blood serum and lymph, the circulating fluid of the lymphatic system. In fact, the entire lymphatic system is part of rasa dhātu.

Eight important qualities are also present in rasa dhātu. The qualities look like kapha—liquid, oily, slimy, cool, heavy, soft, slow, and sticky. Rasa dhātu is mixed with kledaka kapha from the stomach. Kledaka kapha, vyāna vāyu, and a small amount of pāchaka pitta are present in rasa dhātu. Because of the presence of vyāna vāyu, rasa dhātu is mobile, active, and keeps flowing. Pāchaka pitta gives rasa a yellowish color. Without pāchaka pitta, which contains agni, the transformation of asthāyi into sthāyi rasa is impossible.

The superior quality of rasa dhātu—rasa sāra—is responsible for clear perception, clarity, faith, love, and trust. When the quality of rasa dhātu is superfine, it brings music and perfume to life. Another meaning of rasa is musical melody. When music is playing, you automatically begin moving your body, because rasa dhātu is dancing with the music.

Rasa also means mercury. Superfine mercury is considered the semen of Shiva. Mercury is the heaviest metal and it gives longevity. There is much confusion about mercury in the Western world. Modern technology says mercury is a poison. It is toxic to the body and can kill a person. Mercury poisoning creates blackening of the teeth, profuse bleeding, and depression of bone marrow production. But if it is "purified," the poison can become *amrita*, nectar. Indian alchemy uses mercury for enlightenment, realization, and longevity. Purified mercury must be humanized, made ready for human consumption, through a long procedure.

The function of rasa dhātu is *prīnana*, which means nutrition. The ancient rishis declared the amount of rasa in the body to be nine *añjali*, which is approximately seven quarts. This amount may vary from person to person, depending on diet, water intake, and body weight and size. If the amount is increased or decreased, it can create problems or disease.

By-products of Rasa Dhātu

The superior by-products of rasa are the top layer of the skin, lactation and menstruation. After a woman delivers a child, it takes three to four days for her to develop milk, because rasa dhātu takes that amount of time to create lactation. The inferior by-product, or mala, is poshaka kapha.

When rasa dhātu is fully mature and has superior quality, it is called rasa sāra. A person with rasa sāra has beautiful, soft, smooth skin. The hair is soft and wavy. The skin has good complexion, uniform color, with no moles or pimples. Such skin is absolutely healthy. A rasa sāra person has strength and stamina, great love, compassion, and profound faith. The concept of sāra indicates the superior and obvious expression of that tissue's presence.

Negative emotions such as anxiety, fear, nervousness, and insecurity flow within rasa dhātu. These emotions create biochemical changes that circulate in the body and are stressors related to the aging process. The resulting molecules move around in rasa dhātu and seek weak spots in which they stagnate.

The qualities of these negative emotions can alter the qualities of the doshas, resulting in doshic imbalance and leading to biochemical changes. For example, fear can make vāta more cold and dry, anxiety can make it more mobile, while loneliness may be responsible for excess clear, spacey quality. Similarly, anger can increase the hot and sharp qualities of pitta; hate can increase the bitter quality, and jealousy the sara (creeping) quality. For kapha, attachment enhances sticky and oily qualities; greed can increase sweet and salty tastes, and possessiveness the heavy guna, which can lead to depression.

Faith improves the quality of rasa dhātu and the moment rasa dhātu is adversely affected, your faith is also affected. You begin doubting and become skeptical. There is a difference between faith and belief. Belief is personal. What you believe binds you and blinds you. Belief creates groupism and leads to division. The disease process begins in the mind, in your belief system. However, faith is universal, because God is universal and truth is universal. Faith is love and trust, and it can move mountains. The moment you lose your faith, you will change the quality of your rasa dhātu. Many people in the modern world are losing faith. For example, people believe in their nationality, and nationalism is a belief system that is the root cause of division between one person and another. The global rasa dhātu, the cosmic prāna, is deranged.

Disorders of Rasa Dhātu

Lack of taste or a perverted taste in the mouth is a disorder of rasa dhātu, because taste is a function of rasa dhātu. If a person has a salty or sweet taste in the mouth, that taste comes from rasa dhātu and indicates that rasa dhātu is affected.

Lack of faith, lack of clarity, and nausea are also common symptoms of imbalanced rasa. Excess salivation, heaviness, stupor, generalized body ache, water retention, and swelling are all kapha symptoms associated with rasa. One may think that anemia is connected to rakta dhātu. However, before rakta dhātu is affected, a person often looks pale because of increased rasa dhātu. The body retains water, and rings and clothes become tight. If a woman in her premenstrual period develops symptoms of water retention, tender, swollen breasts, and a feeling of heaviness, her rasa dhātu is adversely affected.

Sexual debility is another disorder of rasa. Rasa dhātu nourishes shukra (male reproductive tissue), so a man with imbalanced rasa may have improper erection or premature ejaculation, as well as low libido. Inferior rasa dhātu can create wrinkling of the skin, emaciation and weight loss, causing a person to appear older. Low rasa agni leads to cold hands and feet. All of these conditions are rasa dushti, as if the person has lost the vigor, vitality, and ability to do anything. Rasa dushti may also create severe dehydration, leading to dry tongue, lips and skin, as well as dizziness. If a person is irritated by loud noise, his rasa dhātu is affected.

Causes of Rasa Disorders
Heavy food
Cold food and drinks
Overeating
Oily or fried food
Leftover food
Excess sugar, salt, or pickles
Hydrophilous substances, such as yogurt, cheese, cucumber, watermelon, and sea salt
Incompatible food combining
Too much thinking
Worries, anxiety, and lack of faith
Bacteria (*krumi*)
Excess bodily *āma*

Table 13: Signs and Symptoms of Rasa Disorders

Rasa Vruddhi (*Increased Rasa Dhātu*)	Rasa Kshaya (*Decreased Rasa Dhātu*)	Rasa Dushti (*Disturbed Rasa Dhātu*)
Lymphatic and venous congestion	Anemia	Lack of taste/ perverted taste
Repeated colds, bronchial & sinus congestion	Dehydration	Lack of faith
Water retention (edema), swelling	Dizziness	Lack of clarity & perception
Excess salivation	Dry skin	Fatigue
Feeling of heaviness in the heart	Emaciation	Nausea
Pallor	Excess thirst	Stupor
	Fatigue	Generalized pain and body-ache
	Hypersensitivity to sound	Fever
	Palpitations	
	Shock	

Fever

Fever is caused by the entry of vāta, pitta, or kapha together with āma (toxins) into rasa dhātu. According to Āyurveda, there are many different kinds of fever. Fever is classified as mono, dual, or triple doshic. Triple doshic fever can be compared with septicemia (pathogenic bacteria in the blood) in modern medicine. During fever there is low appetite, because agni from the gastrointestinal tract is pushed into rasa dhātu, depleting the fire in the stomach. However there is too much fire in rasa dhātu, resulting in an internal feeling of heat, and that fire also goes into the mental faculties, creating anger.

Fever of kapha type begins with low agni and toxins moving from the stomach to rasa dhātu. Kapha fever has runny nose, cold, congestion, and cough. Fever may be vāta type, beginning in the colon with constipation, leading to shivering, body ache, insomnia, and anxiety. Pitta fever starts in the small intestine and causes high temperature, temporal headache, nausea and irritability. There is photophobia (sensitivity to light) and sometimes diarrhea or dysentery (inflammation of colon mucous membrane). However, rasa dhātu has kapha characteristics and any fever that goes into rasa creates some kapha symptoms. Hence kapha-type colds and fever are most common but with vāta provocation there will be less congestion, with pitta aggravation more inflammation, and with increased kapha, more congestion.

Decreased and Increased Rasa Dhātu

When rasa dhātu is depleted, it is called rasa kshaya. One of the causes of chronic fatigue syndrome is depleted rasa. Decreased rasa dhātu creates vāta symptoms, including dehydration. Imbalanced rasa is associated with deep-seated grief and sadness, which are primarily vāta emotions. If there is long-standing, lingering vāta dosha in rasa dhātu, then rasa may be so depleted that a woman will have breasts that are undeveloped and small, due to the chronic effect of vāta dosha. Shatāvarī ghee applied to the breasts and taken internally may improve the size of the breasts within six months to one year. On the other hand, if there is long-standing kapha dosha in rasa dhātu, the breasts will be unduly enlarged and pendular. The size and shape of the breasts depend upon the quality of rasa dhātu. If there is excess vāta in rasa, a woman's menstruation will also be affected, even leading to cessation of menses.

The quality and attributes of rasa dhātu are responsible for the growth of breast tissue and for maintaining ovulation and menstruation. In one case I saw, a 30-year-old woman had no menstruation for 12 years. Her breasts were totally absent and she had hairs around the nipple. This is a sign of endometriosis, of vāta going into the rasa dhātu and pushing kapha into the womb, creating fibrous tissues. If there is excess vāta in rasa dhātu and a woman has pain during ovulation, one tablespoon of aloe vera gel with a pinch of black pepper will kindle rasa agni and help to normalize ovulation.

Premenstrual syndrome or premenopausal syndrome is also associated with rasa dhātu. For this, give 500 mg shatāvarī with guduchi. These herbs aid the transformation of unprocessed rasa dhātu into processed rasa. If rasa agni is low, there is undue production of rasa dhātu. If rasa agni is high, rasa dhātu becomes dry. So increased agni decreases the sthāyi rasa dhātu, its by-products—lactation, menstruation and poshaka kapha—and asthāyi rakta dhātu. Decreased agni increases the sthāyi rasa dhātu, its by-products and asthāyi rakta dhātu. There is no problem in the dhātu unless there is a problem with agni. Herbs that kindle rasa agni include shatāvarī, ginger, holy basil, and lemongrass.

To treat rasa dhātu depletion, soak five fresh dates in warm water overnight. The next day, remove the seeds, put the dates in a blender with one-half cup warm milk and blend. Drink this date shake in the early morning and take no other food for two hours. Dates are nourishing and strengthening for rasa dhātu. If there is an allergy to milk, use rice milk, almond milk, or plain water. For another nourishing drink, take one cup of grape juice and add a pinch each of cardamom, ginger, and saffron.

If rasa is increased, perhaps to 11 añjali, it is called rasa vruddhi. Increased rasa creates lymphatic congestion, edema, swelling, excess salivation, heaviness, and stupor, all of which are kapha symptoms. Rasa is easily affected by kapha, because the by-product of rasa is kapha. Lymphatic stagnation, lymphatic congestion, edema, and breast congestion are all kapha disorders. If pitta goes into rasa dhātu, the person can develop acne, hives, rashes, urticaria, and fever. When vāta enters rasa dhātu, there is dryness, fatigue, and emaciation.

To keep rasa healthy, drink at least five to seven cups of water each day, apart from other fluids. The exact amount varies according to constitution, diet, lifestyle, physical activity, job, weather, and season. Kapha should drink approximately four to five cups daily, pitta five to seven, and vāta six to eight. A pitta person may require more, especially in summer, because there is so much heat in the body. A skinny vāta person may take less, but must be careful not to dehydrate. Insufficient water will deplete rasa dhātu. Use plain water, warm or room temperature, not iced. Ice water is one of the causes of rasa dushti. Ice slows the movement of the srotas (pathway), slows agni and produces āma (toxins). Anything below body temperature is a shock to the system, and ice water is a shock to the stomach and digestive fire.

Every thought and emotion causes biochemical changes in the blood and plasma, and rasa dhātu reflects this. A person can slow the aging process by improving the quality of rasa dhātu. Human beings are as old as their rasa. Āyurveda in a true sense is the science of longevity, and a long, healthy life is possible by changing attitude, thinking, and by bringing a new quality into rasa dhātu. Even at the age of 90 a person's lips and cheeks can be juicy and full of vitality, and can have a youthful and beautiful appearance.

Rakta Dhātu: the Blood Tissue

Although rasa and rakta dhātus are integrated and function together, they are considered separate systems in Āyurvedic theory. From āhāra rasa (the nutrient precursor), it takes five days for sthāyi rasa dhātu to be formed. Sthāyi (mature) rasa and asthāyi (raw) rakta are formed at the same time. After 10 days, sthāyi rakta is formed.

Rakta dhātu is the red blood cells in the heart and blood vessels, and it provides a bridge between the body's internal and external environments by carrying nutrients to the tissues. It transports nutrients from the gastrointestinal tract, prāna from the lungs, and vyāna from the heart to the cells of the body. The waste products from the cells in the form of carbon dioxide are carried to the lungs. Other waste products are carried by the blood to other excretory organs and are related to apāna vāyu.

Āyurvedic and Western concepts of blood are different. In the West, blood includes both red blood cells and plasma. Āyurveda divides the two into rasa (plasma) and rakta (red blood cells). Rasa and rakta dhātus transport specific hormones (agni) from endocrine glands to the target tissues. The endocrine system is associated with majjā dhātu, the nerve tissue, which we will discuss later. All cells are bathed in rasa/rakta dhātu to provide a stable liquid composition, according to the individual prakruti. Rasa and rakta dhātus regulate temperature by distributing heat from the skeletal muscles and active organs to all body parts. This distribution of heat is an important function of rasa and rakta dhātus together.

In addition, while rasa dhātu provides nutrition (prīnana), rakta dhātu provides life function (*jīvana*) and gives oxygen to every cell, a function of prāna. Thus, rakta dhātu provides vital life support for cellular activities. Rañjaka pitta is present in rakta dhātu, as is prāna vāyu and vyāna vāyu, and together they are responsible for circulation.

Red Blood Cells

When the red blood cell is young and fresh, it is flexible. It passes through small capillaries and carries oxygen and prāna from the lungs to the peripheral and deep connective tissues, where the life of every cell is maintained. Every cell breathes via red blood cells, the hemoglobin. When hemoglobin combines with oxygen, it forms oxyhemoglobin. Prāna, the life energy, flows through the red blood cells. Red blood cells are biconcave, shaped like a ring but thin at the center and thick at the periphery. They are elastic and flexible, so they can easily pass through the capillaries and make contact with every cell. Because of their thin center, they yield oxygen easily, which is the jīvana (life-giving) function of rakta dhātu.

In the human body, every cell is a center of awareness, and that awareness is maintained by red blood cells. The flow of awareness is called prāna, intelligence. According to Āyurveda, oxygen is the food of prāna, but oxygen is not prāna. You can pour oxygen into a dead body but it will not bring back life. Prāna uses oxygen, but oxygen is not prāna. Please bear in mind that every cell has electromagnetic energy, and this electromagnetic energy maintains the permeability of the cell membrane. Through those tiny holes of the cell membrane, the lifeless (without consciousness) molecules of food, water and air are transformed into the living cell. This transformation is accomplished by prāna with the help of tejas.

Rakta dhātu is formed in the yolk sac of the liver and spleen of an embryo. For that reason, five thousand years ago Āyurvedic yogis said that the root of rakta dhātu is the liver and spleen. After the infant is born and the lungs begin breathing, the liver and spleen stop producing red blood cells and that function is transmitted to the cells of the bone marrow, which has functions of both rakta and majjā dhātus.

Blood vessels are created by amino acids and enzymes, known as rakta agni, that are already present in the blood. If a blood vessel is cut, new branches will form via a process called anastomosis.

The individual quantity of blood varies according to body height and weight, prakruti (constitution), lifestyle and whether a person is vegetarian or non-vegetarian. But the total amount of rakta dhātu in the healthy human being is eight añjali, which is approximately 5.2 quarts (5 liters). Rakta dhātu (the red blood cells) is flowing along with the nine añjali of rasa dhātu (plasma).

If blood is placed in a test tube, molecules of rakta dhātu will settle at the bottom. The upper part is rasa dhātu (plasma or serum). Water is liquid, and rasa dhātu is mainly comprised of water. Its contents include proteins (kapha molecules), amino acids (pitta molecules), agni, vitamins, nutrients, hormones, electrolytes—such as sodium and potassium, which are electrically charged atoms, and cellular waste (āma). All these are present in the serum.

The red blood cell contains rañjaka pitta. It contains iron, called *lohita*, and has a red color because of iron oxide. The red blood cell, combined with oxygen to create oxyhemoglobin, carries vital life support to other cells and yields prāna to every cell in the body.

The life of a red blood cell is about 120 days. As the cell grows old, it becomes fragile, because the agni of rakta dhātu begins disintegrating the old cell. Stress and other use factors cause them to break apart. That destruction takes place in the liver. From the iron content of the disintegrated red blood cells, a modified rañjaka pitta is prepared. One of the components is biliverdin, which is formed from the oxidation of bilirubin by rañjaka agni and rakta agni in the liver, then excreted into the bile. The kapha part, the globin, of the disintegrated hemoglobin, nourishes the liver and maintains immunity. If a person has insufficient globin in the liver, he is more likely to develop hepatitis. All this is governed by rakta agni.

Asthāyi rakta dhātu is carried to the bone marrow by vyāna vāyu and the liver recycles iron from disintegrated red blood cells back to the bone marrow to produce new red blood cells. So rakta agni and bhūta agni combine with majjā dhātu agni to create new red blood cells.

If a pitta woman carries a pitta fetus, there may be too much rañjaka agni in the liver of the infant. Some of these infants are born with premature hepatic cells, because of the pitta prakruti in the mother and a pitta provoking diet during pregnancy. These premature hepatic cells cannot process bilirubin into bile. So the bilirubin, instead of going into the bile, goes into the blood. Within the first seven days the baby may develop a physiological jaundice, called icterus neonaturum, which means jaundice in the newly born child. Putting the baby under a blue light will help the immature hepatic cells to mature, and these mature hepatic cells can then begin the proper processing of bilirubin back into the bile, which frees the baby from the jaundice. This process takes a week to several weeks. Blue light heals the liver and calms bhūta agni and rañjaka pitta, which is in excess in this condition.

Rañjaka pitta is represented by bile, which includes bile pigments from the heme component of disintegrated hemoglobin. Rañjaka agni is the fire component released from the disintegrated red blood cells, and it is the main source of bhūta agni. Bhūta agnis are the specialized liver enzymes that govern the transformation of unprocessed elements of food into processed elements of the tissues. Rañjaka agni gives color to rasa dhātu and transforms rasa into asthāyi rakta dhātu. However, it is rakta agni that does further transformation of asthāyi rakta into sthāyi rakta dhātu.

Rakta agni is present in the red bone marrow, as well as the liver and spleen, which are the root of rakta vaha srotas, the channel relating to red blood cells. In the embryo, rakta agni produces new red blood cells in the liver and spleen. Once the baby is born, rakta agni is predominantly present in the red bone marrow, which takes over the job of erythrogenesis, the production of new red blood cells. The function of rakta agni in the liver is then to work in conjunction with rañjaka agni to destroy old red blood cells; in the spleen, it is to filter the bacteria and parasites. The role of rakta agni in the bone marrow is to produce the new red blood cells. There are certain enzymes within rakta dhātu that create new capillaries, a process called anastomosis, and these enzymes are components of rakta agni.

By-products of Rakta Dhātu
The superior by-products of rakta dhātu are sirā (blood vessels) and *kandara* (small tendons and sinews, such as the hamstring muscles). The inferior by-product of rakta is bile, *poshaka pitta*, and that pitta nourishes all pitta systems in the body.

The concept of waste in Āyurveda is different from western ideas. Bile has a vital role in the body. Even the presence of feces has a function and supports the colon. Too much cleansing with colonics will cause the colon to lose its tone. Sweat is also a waste product, but sweat gives softness and oiliness to the skin by retaining sebaceous secretions.

Rakta dhātu is hot, sour, and slightly pungent to the taste. Rasa dhātu has all six tastes—sweet, sour, salty, pungent, bitter, and astringent—but rakta dhātu is predominantly sour and has a metallic taste because of hemoglobin.

Rakta dhātu gives energy, life, warmth, and color to the complexion. Healthy blood gives longevity. Rakta has a typical fleshy smell and is associated with *spanda dhamanī* (pulsating arteries), due to the presence of prāna, the vital life force. It is one of the life giving and life taking tissues. If an artery is cut, the person will bleed to death. Blood is life and life is blood. In a way, consciousness is flowing through the blood and every red blood cell is a vibrant, conscious molecule. For that reason, there is spirit in the blood.

The superfine molecules of rakta nourish the brain to yield comprehension, understanding, and biological strength to the body. These superfine molecules (via their oxygen carrying capacity) fight against infection as an oxidative burst from the immune system and create immunity through ojas.

When rakta dhātu is optimal, it is called *rakta sāra*. A person with rakta sāra has a healthy complexion and warm, delicate skin, with rosy cheeks, red lips, and lustrous eyes. He has pink nails, a pink glans penis, and pink hands and feet. A rakta sāra person is sensitive and reactive and doesn't tolerate the hot sun. This type of person is happy and bright, but may be judgmental, critical, and a perfectionist. In a way, this person has a highly developed pitta personality, with happiness, joy, wisdom, intelligence, and brilliance. In addition, rakta sāra promotes longevity. These are the superfine qualities of rakta dhātu.

Disorders of Rakta Dhātu

Rakta dhātu is affected by hot, spicy food, alcohol and tobacco, excess sour, salty and oily foods, and by too much sun and heat. Anger, hate, and envy are hot and sharp emotions. Hence, they affect pitta in rakta dhātu, which is rañjaka pitta.

When rakta is increased, called *rakta vruddhi*, a person develops pitta symptoms, such as bleeding from any of the natural openings. High altitude and dry weather can crack the nasal and mucous membranes. That is vāta. But without high altitude or dry weather, bleeding is caused by pitta. All inflammatory conditions—repeated infections, conjunctivitis, bleeding piles, hemorrhoids, and canker sores on the mouth or tongue—are due to increased pitta and this generally affects rakta.

Erysipelas is an acute inflammatory condition that shifts from one place to another place on the body. At one moment a person will have a rash and itching on the neck, and within a short time the entire hand will be swollen. Splenomegaly (enlarged spleen), hepatomegaly (enlarged liver), hypertension

---

Causes of Rakta Disorders

Hot, spicy food
Excess sugar and salt
Sour foods, such as yogurt, cheese, pickles or fermented foods
Oily or fried food
Incompatible food combining
Tobacco, alcohol, marijuana, and other drugs
Loss of blood
Deficiency of iron or vitamin B12
Excessive exposure to the sun
Working near a fire or in hot conditions
Exposure to radiation
Emotional factors, such as repressed anger, hate, envy, and aggressiveness
Bacteria (krumi)
Liver and Spleen diseases

(high blood pressure), and a sudden aversion to meat are other symptoms connected with an acute condition. A person may decide to be a vegetarian, but when a meat eater suddenly develops nausea toward meat, rakta is increased and the liver is affected. Consuming meat three times a day will make rakta hot and heavy. Increased rakta dhātu may also create undue anger and hate.

Polycythemia is a classic picture of increased rakta dhātu. The hands and cheeks are flushed. Increased tejas can burn the immunity and the person may develop an autoimmune disease called lupus. In lupus the cheeks become red and a person's ojas is depleted. Because of increased rakta dhātu, there is high pitta, leading to high tejas that burns ojas.

Table 14: Signs and Symptoms of Rakta Disorders

Rakta Vruddhi (*Increased Rakta Dhātu*)	Rakta Kshaya (*Decreased Rakta Dhātu*)
Polycythemia	Anemia
Fullness of blood vessels	Emptiness of blood vessels
Bleeding tendencies	Pale skin, conjunctiva, lips,
Skin conditions such as: rash,	tongue, and nails
urticaria, acne, dermatitis,	Dry, rough, cracked skin
eczema, erysipelas	Breathlessness on exertion
Hypertension	Craving for iron
Red, warm hands and feet	Craving for hot spicy foods, sour,
Red eyes	citrus fruit, or meat
Enlarged liver or spleen	Cold hands and feet
	Loss of luster
	Lack of enthusiasm

When rakta dhātu is decreased, called *rakta kshaya*, the person appears pale and has symptoms of pallor, palpitation, and breathlessness. In addition, a person loses interest and enthusiasm for life. Decreased rakta creates cold hands and feet, while increased rakta creates hot hands and feet. In decreased rakta, there will be either increased vāta or increased kapha symptoms. In decreased rakta, the person may develop edema or swelling because of kapha. The skin becomes dry, rough, cracked, pale, and cold, and the person has a craving for sour things. Children eat clay when they are lacking in iron, because of decreased rakta dhātu. These important symptoms indicate decreased rakta.

Rakta dushti manifests as eczema, psoriasis, or chronic dermatitis, as well as bleeding from the skin and gums.

Repeated boils, acne, hives, rashes, urticaria, and profuse menstrual flow are also indications. The person easily bruises and the skin has a bluish color.

Herpes comes under rakta dushti and pitta type of chronic fatigue syndrome is due to rakta dushti in the liver. Hepatic dysfunction (liver dysfunction), mononucleosis, hepatitis, splenitis, and appendicitis, as well as discoloration of the skin, are rakta dushti. Some people have visible blood vessels on the nose because of chronic alcoholism. Because of chronic vāta dushti in the blood, the skin develops age spots and freckles. Blood clots are a dushti of rakta, as well as varicose (enlarged) veins and thrombophlebitis (inflammation of a vein with a blood clot). AIDS is also classified as rakta dushti.

One of the most important treatments in Āyurveda is *rakta moksha*, bloodletting, an ancient treatment for the purification of blood. That's why Lord Dhanvantari has a leech in his hand.[15] Leeches are being used in the West therapeutically in over 2000 cases annually, especially for reattaching digits. Bloodletting is good for increased rakta and also for many rakta dushti conditions.

What is the difference between rakta dushti and increased rakta? When a dosha goes into asthāyi rakta dhātu and slows down dhātu agni, it affects the nutrition of rakta and creates increased raw rakta dhātu. This is an acute disorder. If any dosha goes into sthāyi rakta, then it creates a chronic condition, such as psoriasis or sickle cell anemia. Rakta dushti refers to qualitative disturbance, resulting from the effects of a dosha in rakta dhātu. When sthāyi dhātu is affected, it causes a chronic dushti condition. Pañchakarma is important in treating a chronic condition. It helps to kindle dhātu agni and improves the quality of both sthāyi dhātu and asthāyi dhātu. Rakta moksha is the specific form of pañchakarma that targets rakta dhātu.

Every second, millions of red blood cells are born and every second a similar number of cells are dying. A cell born at this moment will continue to live and circulate in your body for 110 to 120 days. After that time, the cell goes into the liver to die. But we never cry for the dead cell. Right from the mother's womb, we carry billions and billions of red blood cells. Out of those billions, in every moment, one third of those cells die, one third are born again and one third continue in their tasks.

---

15. Lord Dhanvantari is a mythological figure thought to have given Āyurveda to Sushruta. He is a key figure for Āyurvedic knowledge. In his four hands, Lord Dhanvantari carries the tools of healing in Āyurvedic medicine: a leech, a vessel of *amrit*, a conch shell, and a spear of light.

High blood sugar, high triglycerides, and high cholesterol in the blood can create a heart attack, high blood pressure, or stroke paralysis. Triglycerides are a sugar component. When liver enzymes do not process glucose into glycogen, that unprocessed glucose develops in the blood as triglycerides and may make the blood thick and viscous. Thickened blood moves with resistance and may create a blood clot. It deposits kapha molecules, fat molecules, on the walls of the blood vessels, causing the narrowing and clogging of the artery. Diabetes is increased sugar in the blood, which involves rakta dushti.

Table 15: Blood Types Correlated to the Doshas

Blood Type	Dosha	Holds True % of the Time
O Rh positive	Pitta or Pitta-Kapha dual	65%
O Rh negative	Pitta predominant	70%
A	Vāta predominant	80%
B	Kapha predominant	80%
AB	Vāta-Kapha dual	65%

Remember, blood in the Western sense includes rasa and rakta dhātus. A blood transfusion of the component called red blood cells, which is rakta dhātu, is required when a person has an extremely low blood count and is also necessary during a surgical procedure. Type A receives the blood from A. Type B should receive blood from type B. The universal donor is O and the universal recipient is AB. These four groups are important. It is simple to have your blood type checked in a lab. If by mistake blood of Type A is given to B or B to A, it is a mismatch. In addition, we must think about Rh positive and Rh negative. O Rh negative is highly pitta, and these people may develop peptic ulcer, ulcerative colitis and other pitta disorders. This group is likely to develop disorders of increased rañjaka pitta.

The Health of the Blood Vessels

Our blood vessels constantly change their diameters, depending upon our emotional states. In anger they dilate and there is increased blood flow. But in fear they constrict and cause decreased blood flow. Therefore, fear makes the person cold and anger makes the person hot. Alcohol dilates the blood vessels (stimulation) and increases the blood flow, because alcohol relaxes the muscles. That effect continues for six to eight hours. However, the next morning the blood vessels constrict and, because of the constriction, the brain receives insufficient oxygen and prāna, and the person feels drowsy (depressant). Anything that dilates the blood vessels is addictive, including caffeine. Many tranquilizers relax the musculature of the blood vessels but have an aftereffect of constriction.

Marijuana also dilates the blood vessels and relaxes the muscles, creating a tranquil state. However, drug induced tranquility is not true tranquility because it is a chemical effect that is responsible for the relaxation of muscles and relaxation of the muscular layer of the blood vessels, which is dilatation. But that has an aftereffect, which is constriction, and when the drug effect is over the blood vessels become more constricted and there is insufficient oxygen and nutrient supply, and therefore the person demands more of the drug. So drug induced tranquility is partial, temporary tranquility. It is just a chemical effect, and it has hazardous side effects.

Research has also found that meditation dilates blood vessels, relaxes muscles, and creates a tranquil state. If you meditate, your rakta dhātu moves silently and flows rhythmically. Blood vessels are dilated, muscles are relaxed, and you feel naturally tranquil. The more your breathing becomes quiet, the less oxygen your brain cells require. Following meditation, the dilated blood vessels and relaxed muscles do not have the aftereffect of constriction. The relaxation and dilation of the blood vessels remain until the person becomes stressed. In stress the blood vessels constrict and the person becomes rigid and tight. When the blood vessels relax, blood pressure is normalized. True tranquility, which comes through meditation, happens through the expansion of consciousness at the cellular level, tissue level and systemic level. Therefore, meditation is a form of stress reduction that improves the blood flow, brings more oxygen, and relaxes the muscles.

Psychedelic drugs suppress the thinking ability of the brain. The brain is made quiet, as opposed to being quiet. In drug-induced tranquility, chemical effects suppress all the thoughts, feelings, and emotions. Therefore a person feels some euphoria, a sense of well being, and it looks like real tranquility. But it is illusion. The true tranquility comes through meditation, where every thought, feeling, and emotion are completely understood, and in the process of understanding the thought, feeling, and emotion, there is total freedom. In that freedom, every thought, feeling, and emotion flower, and flowering of emotion is ending of it. Therefore, when emotions end by themselves, when thoughts end by themselves, then the brain becomes quiet, and that quietness is a natural, spontaneous, healthy tranquility.

So when someone takes a drug, his or her experience is an illusion. It is not a religious experience. It is not a spiritual experience. The chemical effects of the drug suppress the thoughts, feelings, and emotions. Therefore the brain is made quiet. It does expand consciousness, but that expansion is a limited, temporary affair. It looks like increased awareness, a spiritual experience, but it is not the same thing. It is like dim glimpses through a semi-transparent window at marvelously beautiful scenery. But when the window is opened, and there is no glass screen, there is a direct experience. The direct experience of the opened window is a spiritual experience compared to the dim glimpses of drug-induced tranquility.

The root cause of disease is not listening to the body. Intelligence is the flow of awareness, that tells us what we should and should not do. To purify the blood means to listen to the intelligence of the body. A sensitive body is the abode of God. With a sensitive body, life becomes a ceremony, because it is the action of awareness.

Māmsa Dhātu: the Muscle Tissue

The next dhātu is māmsa. The fully processed *sthāyi māmsa* is created from *asthāyi māmsa*, which is formed at the same time as sthāyi rakta. The transformation from āhāra rasa to sthāyi māmsa takes about 15 days.

Māmsa dhātu is the muscle tissue. The muscular system accounts for nearly half of the body weight. If a person weighs 120 pounds, nearly 60 pounds belong to māmsa dhātu. Muscles are derived from Earth and Water molecules, both of which are heavy. Fire molecules are also present in māmsa dhātu to a lesser degree. Ninety percent of māmsa dhātu is Earth and Water elements and 10 percent is the Fire element.

Muscle cells are specialized to undergo muscular contraction. As we have already studied, Ether is nuclear energy, Air is electrical energy, Fire is radiant energy, Water is chemical energy, and Earth is mechanical energy. When a muscle fiber contracts, the chemical energy of blood nutrients is converted into the mechanical energy of muscle movement. So for muscles to move, we need blood. The more movement of muscles, the more the requirements of the blood. When we exercise the blood flow increases, because muscles need blood, oxygen, and nutrients. So the Fire component of māmsa dhātu transforms the chemical energy of blood nutrients into the mechanical energy of muscle movement. An important function of māmsa dhātu is ambulatory movement and the movement of the joints during walking.

Māmsa dhātu is heavy, elastic, firm, dense, and bulky. It is derived from kapha dosha. Muscles give shape to the body. During an emergency, a muscle becomes rigid, contracted, and produces resistance against movement. Muscles can move fast. If you suddenly see that you are about to fall, the muscles contract, become rigid, and create resistance against forward movement. Like a moving vehicle, the body needs a brake, a control system. So māmsa dhātu has the capacity to create resistance against movement in order to stop the body. When standing on one leg, one group of muscles will contract and the opposite group will relax to maintain balance. Muscles bring skill in action, which is art. Handwriting, drawing a picture or even a straight line requires coordination. Art, whether it is dancing, walking on a rope, or climbing a mountain, needs coordination of the muscles. Coordination involves groups of muscles working together harmoniously in order to bring skillful action. Therefore, māmsa dhātu has the capacity to create coordination. This generates heat, another function of māmsa dhātu.

Māmsa dhātu also gives power, ambition, and courage. Along with the bones, it gives support to the person. Another function of māmsa dhātu is plastering or covering. Muscles provide protection by covering delicate organs and delicate parts of the body. They plaster the bones and joints and protect the nerves and blood vessels.

Māmsa dhātu is responsible for movement of bodily fluids—urine, sweat, lymph, and blood. The more the muscles move, the more the blood moves. The bladder muscles move the urine. The muscles under the skin promote sweating. There are subtle muscles at the root of the hair that contract, causing the hair to stand like a copper wire, creating goose bumps during an emergency. The muscles contract to keep you alert and awake.

Muscles are responsible for the personality and the appearance of the body. Well-developed muscles create a handsome body, like a Roman statue. When a muscle is stimulated, it contracts. Muscles express emotion. The facial muscles express joy, happiness, anger, or fear. A muscle can even become irritable and an irritable muscle is an angry muscle, a sore muscle.

Types of Muscles
Skeletal muscles (striated)— māmsa, kandara, snāyu
Smooth muscles (non-striated)— mrudu māmsa
Cardiac muscles—hrud māmsa

The tissue in the body that best resists gravity is the muscle tissue. Blood always moves downward with gravity, so rasa and rakta go with gravity, as does meda dhātu (adipose tissue). Anti-gravitation is levitation and levitation is the function of māmsa dhātu.

Types of Muscles and Their Functions

Muscle cells have different shapes. Some of them are spindle-shaped, some are fibers, some are long, flat fascia. The three basic classifications of muscles are skeletal (striated), smooth (non-striated), and cardiac. The skeletal muscles are called māmsa, *snāyu,* or *kandara;* the smooth muscles are known as *mrudu* māmsa (soft muscles), and the cardiac muscles are *hrud.* The smooth muscles and cardiac muscles are involuntary muscles and are not usually under our conscious control, whereas the skeletal muscles are under our conscious control.

Smooth muscles are non-striated and are more spindle-shaped. They are predominately present in the gastrointestinal tract, respiratory tract, urinary tract, and reproductive system. The muscles of the womb, vagina, and glans penis are smooth muscles. Smooth muscles also include the muscles of the gallbladder, urinary bladder, uterus, and diaphragm. They are controlled by vyāna vāyu and kledaka kapha, and their movements are regulated by the autonomic nervous system, as well as the central nervous system.

Cardiac muscles are specialized fibrous muscles. The fibers are hooked together to create a solid vessel, which is the heart. Cardiac muscles have the capacity to generate an electrical impulse that creates the pulsing action of the heart. Therefore, the heart functions somewhat like a battery. A sensitive galvanometer (electrocardiograph) can create a graphical record of the electrical impulse of the cardiac muscle (conductivity), which is a very specialized muscle that maintains life. When the heart stops, life stops. It is controlled by prāna vāyu and vyāna vāyu, along with avalambaka kapha.

The skeletal muscles are peripheral, striated muscles. These muscles are controlled by the cerebrospinal nerves and are under conscious motor control, while smooth and cardiac muscles are unconscious and are controlled by the autonomic nervous system. Skeletal muscles are controlled by prāna vāyu, apāna vāyu, vyāna vāyu, and tarpaka kapha. The skeletal muscles include the biceps, triceps, quadriceps, hamstrings, and gluteus maximus, in addition to the lingual muscles (the muscles of the tongue), the laryngeal muscles used to swallow, and the muscles of the pharynx.

In between two muscles there is a membranous structure called *māmsa dhara kalā*, which holds the muscles together and separates one muscle from another. This kalā is the fascia; this same kalā becomes muscle tendon. The connective tissue, fascia, goes beyond the end of the muscle and continues as a cord-like structure called muscle tendon, which is like a strong rope. This tendon is called kandara. The hamstring muscle is also called kandara. The kalā becomes thick in the muscle tendon because of tarpaka kapha and apāna vāyu.

Muscle fibers run parallel. One hair can easily be broken, but hundreds of hairs together are strong and difficult to break, because of strength in unity. In the same way, muscles have unity consciousness. They work as a unit. Muscle fibers are delicate, but thousands of muscle fibers run parallel and are quite powerful working in unity.

Each skeletal muscle fiber is connected to the end of a nerve. There is a gap between a nerve ending and a muscle fiber. That gap, that junction, is called the neuromuscular junction or synaptic cleft. There is abundant tarpaka kapha, prāna vāyu, and sādhaka pitta within this junction. Sādhaka pitta (the seat of emotions) exists as a neurotransmitter that stimulates the muscle to contract, while muscle tone is maintained by apāna vāyu and sādhaka pitta within the neuromuscular junction. The neuromuscular junction of the skeletal muscle is under the control of the reflex arc, which is vyāna vāyu, while tarpaka kapha maintains the nourishment of māmsa dhātu.

Tarpaka kapha exists throughout the body in every neuromuscular junction. In the brain, it is the fluid, the film. Tarpaka kapha is necessary for the transmission of each electrical impulse and it is the medium that carries the neurotransmitters. The same function exists in every muscle fiber junction point, because we have neurotransmitters all over the body. Therefore, tarpaka kapha functionally exists at every neuromuscular junction in the body.

By-products of Māmsa Dhātu
The superior by-products of māmsa dhātu are *tvacha* (the skin) and *vasā* (subcutaneous fat). Āyurveda says there are seven layers of the skin. The topmost layer is connected to rasa dhātu. The second layer of the skin is connected to rakta dhātu. The third layer, which is the subcutaneous tissue, is specifically connected to māmsa dhātu. Each subsequent layer is connected to the dhātus in sequence. However, we can also broadly group six layers (that is, all except the top layer) as the upadhātu of māmsa.

The inferior by-products of māmsa are nasal crust, earwax, sebaceous secretions, tartar on the teeth, and smegma.[16] These inferior by-products are called *khamala*. *Kha* means space; *mala* means impurity. Khamala is the nasal crust in the nose; the surface of the skin has sebaceous secretions and dandruff, which are khamala of the skin. These are impurities accumulated in the larger and smaller spaces. If māmsa dhātu agni is low, there is undue production of khamala. During ancient times rasa and rakta dhātus were measured in terms of añjali. But māmsa dhātu cannot be measured in these terms, because muscle changes. If you eat māmsa-nourishing food, such as meat and a high protein diet or even kapha-provoking food, it will add to māmsa dhātu. If you fast, within eight days your muscle mass decreases and you lose weight. There is a cleansing of māmsa dhātu in fasting and the muscle tissue reduces in size. Therefore, there is no generally agreed upon measurement of māmsa.

Māmsa sāra is present when māmsa dhātu is completely developed, with all its superfine qualities. Such a person has well developed cheeks, neck, shoulders, and a broad chest. The biceps and triceps appear healthy. The calf muscles and the muscles of the buttocks are well shaped.

The superfine qualities of healthy māmsa dhātu also include energy, power, strength, stamina, courage, confidence, determination, love, compassion, and forgiveness. A person with healthy māmsa dhātu makes money and has a strong sex drive. According to Āyurveda, longevity is due to strong, healthy muscles. Even during old age, a person can still have a good grip, strong muscle tone, and good muscle strength. Muscle tissue builds up weight slowly; five to ten pounds are a significant increase whereas meda dhātu (fat tissue) can put on 15 to 20 pounds more quickly. Māmsa works against gravity; meda is passive and yields to gravity. It is māmsa dhātu that nourishes meda dhātu, but without good rasa and rakta it is difficult to develop healthy māmsa.

By volume, if you consider equal amounts of muscle and fat, fat is less dense than muscle. Muscle is dense, firm, and bulky, while fat is malleable, spongy, and soft. Fat can float on water and muscle will sink to the bottom. If a person has a sedentary life, he or she may look heavier because of excess fat.

---

16. Smegma is a secretion of the sebaceous glands found under the labia minor about the glans clitoridis and under the male prepuce or foreskin of the penis.

When one exercises and loses weight, one loses fat and gains the firmness of muscle.

Disorders of Māmsa Dhātu

In *māmsa vruddhi*, when māmsa dhātu is increased by volume but reduced by quality, there may be enlarged, bulky muscles, or stiff muscles, undue enlargement of the lips, a large expanded nose, pendular breasts and a potbelly abdomen. The hips and the buttocks become enlarged and the body loses its proportion. There may be formation of muscle tumors, called myomas. The tongue becomes heavy and enlarged. The person may have repeated attacks of tonsillitis.

In a way māmsa dhātu is closely connected to the tonsils, because they regulate the immunity of māmsa dhātu. If the tonsils are removed, that function is taken over by the thymus. According to Āyurveda, the tonsil is a gland of immunity, called *gilayu*. Tonsils strengthen the immunity of smooth muscles—such as the stomach and pancreas. Tonsillitis may also affect the skeletal muscles, creating muscular rheumatism and arthritis. Chronic tonsillitis may cause myocarditis as a complication.

Increased māmsa may also lead to muscle hypertrophy, in which the muscle becomes enlarged. Myasthenia, a condition of muscular weakness, leads to swelling, water retention, and herniation, such as hiatal hernia. When a muscle becomes weak, it loses its tone and power. Tone is a sustained state of contraction. Because of lack of tone, the muscles have more space. Within that space, fluid retention creates swelling. One of the jobs of māmsa dhātu is to hold the joint and ligament in position. When the dhātu loses its tone, displacement or slipped disc may develop. All of these conditions are due to māmsa vruddhi, increased māmsa.

The opposite of māmsa vruddhi (increased māmsa) is *māmsa kshaya* (decreased māmsa dhātu). When māmsa dhātu is decreased, it can create muscle atrophy, muscle weakness, sunken cheeks and sunken eyes. The neck becomes thin and the bones are exposed. The ribs and vertebrae become visible. Because of māmsa kshaya, the temples, eyes and cheeks are sunken and the person has an emaciated appearance. The joints look big, because the muscles are wasted. The sacrum becomes prominent, the buttocks are withered and the breasts are thin. The person looks like a breathing skeleton.

I was traveling by train from Bombay to Pune. In the compartment there were many people. At a railway station a passenger entered. The moment people saw him, they ran away, saying, "Ghost, ghost, ghost." This man had extremely

> **Causes of Māmsa Disorders**
>
> Insufficient or excess protein consumption
> Heavy meats and dairy products
> Over or under eating
> Hydrophilous substances, such as yogurt, cheese, cucumber, watermelon, and sea salt
> Incompatible food combining
> Insufficient or excessive exercise (beyond one's capacity)
> Daytime sleeping
> Insufficient rest or sleep
> Physical trauma, such as an accident
> Emotional stress
> Liver disorders
> Tuberculosis
> Typhoid

debilitated muscles and he looked like a skeleton. That person came and sat near me. The moment I saw him I knew his condition was extreme māmsa kshaya, decreased māmsa. Even the expressions on his face were difficult to witness. He was full of grief and sadness, his hands were cold and he was extremely hungry. Although he constantly ate, all the food turned into charcoal. I said to him, "Come to our hospital and I will treat you." We performed pañchakarma, the Āyurvedic cleansing program, and gave him some muscle rejuvenating herbs.

About two years later I was teaching in an Āyurvedic clinic. A tall handsome man came up and hugged me. I said, "Who are you?" He said, "Do you remember, two years ago we were traveling from Bombay to Pune? I am that ghost man." He said, "I tried every medicine but only Āyurveda worked. Āyurveda has changed my life." He had been a living picture of extreme decreased māmsa dhātu. After treatment he became māmsa sāra, a handsome man. According to Āyurveda, damaged organs can be rejuvenated. The body can regenerate and it is quite possible for such an extreme condition to be healed.

Eating kapha-provoking food, such as cheese, yogurt, milk, meat, and heavy meals, causes increased māmsa dhātu. Insufficient exercise and sleeping during the daytime can also increase asthāyi māmsa dhātu. If you want to gain weight, eat four meals a day, sleep, and don't even wash the dishes. This increases asthāyi māmsa and meda. Working too hard, excessive physical activity, eating insufficient protein or insufficient kapha-nourishing food in general, causes decreased māmsa dhātu.

Certain diseases affect māmsa dhātu. The person described above, who looked like a ghost, once had typhoid, which caused his metabolism to become extremely hyperactive. After recovering from typhoid, he became quite skinny. Tuberculosis and cirrhosis of the liver can also affect māmsa. The liver transforms glucose into glycogen via bhūta agni and then stores the energy in māmsa dhātu. If the liver is weak, a person's māmsa dhātu is bound to be also weak. Trauma and accidents can also affect māmsa, as can neuromuscular disorders.

In diseases involving māmsa, there may be muscle twitching, spasms, rigidity, and stiffness, muscle aches and pains, or paralysis of the muscles. There may be involuntary movements of the muscles leading to convulsions, Bell's palsy (facial paralysis), quadriplegia, or paraplegia. Multiple sclerosis (demyelination of the nerve sheath, which is majjā dhātu) can also affect māmsa dhātu. MS creates progressive weakness and loss of muscle control leading to disability.

In cases of low māmsa dhātu agni, a person develops profuse accumulation of khamala—ear wax, nasal crust, or smegma. Increased earwax or smegma can be pre-cancerous. If a person develops these conditions after the age of 45, it may be an early sign of pancreatic cancer.

Table 16: Signs and Symptoms of Māmsa Disorders

Māmsa Vruddhi (*Increased Māmsa Dhātu*)	Māmsa Kshaya (*Decreased Māmsa Dhātu*)
Muscle hypertrophy Muscle flaccidity Undue growth of muscle, myomas, fibromas Fibrocystic changes in the breasts Uterine fibroids Enlarged lips, cheeks, tongue	Muscle atrophy, wasting Muscle rigidity Loss of muscle power Emaciation Fatigue Dislocation of joints TMJ disorders Craving for meat

For example, a 48 year old man came to me with only four symptoms—profuse earwax, repeated attacks of genital herpes, waking at night to pass urine, and difficulty swallowing food. I felt his pulse, which denoted vāta pushing pitta and pitta pushing kapha in the stomach. He also had an extremely low stomach pulse. I touched his belly and there was a hard lump. I said, "You must go for further testing. I suspect you have cancer of the pancreas." He told me he had just come from his medical doctor and nothing was found. I said to him that according to Āyurveda this was a serious condition. He went back to the doctor and an ultrasound showed cancer of the head of the pancreas.

The Role of Māmsa Dhātu in Emotional Well Being

The psychological manifestations of healthy māmsa dhātu are ambition, competition, confidence, courage, and determination. If the quality of māmsa dhātu is weak, these qualities are affected. The person loses confidence, power of determination, and complains of indecisiveness. Māmsa dhātu is connected to responsibility, especially the muscles of the shoulder, the trapezius. The person with weak māmsa dhātu feels like he carries the burden of the world on his shoulders.

Within the synaptic cleft, the neuromuscular junction, there are tarpaka kapha, sādhaka pitta, and prāna vāyu. Unresolved emotions or stress accumulate in the neuromuscular junctions in the form of unprocessed kapha molecules and, because of tension and stress, the muscles become stiff. This condition is called neuromuscular tension. Such stressed muscles are one of the causes of aging. When a muscle is stressed, the face and skin are wrinkled, because the skin is a by-product of māmsa dhātu.

To relieve this condition, bring conscious awareness to the groups of muscles. In meditation, bring awareness to the body and relax the muscles of the feet, calves, thighs, arms, belly, chest and even facial muscles. Opening the jaw slightly and touching the tip of the tongue to the palate behind the front teeth relaxes the muscles of the jaw. Relaxation of the muscles brings balance to tarpaka kapha, sādhaka pitta, and prāna vāyu in the neuromuscular junctions, leading to tranquility and relief of stress.

Māmsa dhātu is connected to the *marmāni*, the doors of relaxation and dynamic awareness. Marmāni are connected to the neuromuscular junctions. They are energy points, similar to acupuncture points, where Consciousness is most lively in expressing Itself. Pressing a marma point acts on receptors or neurotransmitters and brings relaxation to the muscle, and via the marma/muscle connection one can send a message to the heart, lungs, or pancreas. In this way, muscles are connected to the internal organs.

When a muscle is rigid, the flow of awareness is blocked. Emotions such as fear, anxiety, grief, sadness, and anger, in the form of neurotransmitters, become stuck in that muscle and create a neuromuscular block. In pañchakarma, application of oil to the skin goes into the deeper tissues, into māmsa dhātu, and begins releasing repressed emotions. Rubbing oil in the opposite direction of the lay of hair pushes the oil into the hair follicles, the sebaceous glands, the superficial fascia and deep fascia. The subtle quality of sesame oil helps to release those emotions by stimulating certain neurotransmitters in the central nervous system. Because of oil massage, those crystals of unresolved emotions become decrystallized and dissolve.

Meditation and Māmsa Dhātu

One of the primary functions of māmsa is *lepana*, plastering or holding. In meditation we hold, we have a grip on, awareness. This is *dhārana*, which also means holding. To have proper dhārana, we need healthy māmsa dhātu. The quality of healthy māmsa dhātu is a meditative mind. That quality of the meditative mind is love, compassion, and total relaxation. Meditation is love; meditation is awareness, and awareness is love. In love everything flowers, including grief, anger, and fear. Expression and suppression mean taking charge. That is a subtle trick that the mind plays upon itself. The moment you try to control life, then life loses its spontaneity.

When people use meditation solely for stress release, they frequently have problems with it. As they try to be quiet, many thoughts and feelings come to consciousness and they become disturbed. When there is a purpose behind meditation, the value of meditation is reduced. Purpose is expectation and expectation is desire. One should meditate with only the desire to meditate; that's it. Do not have expectation: "Yesterday, I meditated and I had a marvelous transcendental experience." To expect the same experience today reduces the value of today's meditation. Yesterday's experience may not happen and the person may become stressed. Then his or her expectation increases, creating boredom and they think they should try another technique.

Pitta people like structured meditation methods. But then we must go beyond structure. I think pitta people should do unstructured meditation. I do not know of a technique that does not make the mind mechanical, and a mechanical mind is a narrow and limited mind. Whenever following a system or a technique, don't get stuck with it or dependent on it. Use it, play with it, and then move on. The ultimate flowering of meditation should be spontaneous. Every action then becomes meditation. Eating food, drinking water, working, driving a car, ironing a shirt, and even washing dishes can be meditation. Then the entire life is meditation and stress has no place.

Meditation can help heal problems and there is nothing wrong in using meditation for healing purposes. However, do not use meditation only for that. Meditation has a higher purpose or flowering. I like to use the word flowering instead of purpose. A structured meditation, which is mechanical, creates a set pattern. When the brain works with a set pattern, it becomes senile. A healthy brain requires constant flow and movement, not rigidity.

The mind in meditation is a muscle in action with relaxation. If you walk two miles while looking at the beauty of the cloud and the mountain, and birds are singing, even in that action of walking there is relaxation and joy. So relaxation does not mean inaction. Action and inaction go together. And that is the highest spiritual function of māmsa dhātu.

If you meditate without expectation, then you begin loving without expectation. To love someone without expectation is the greatest love. That will happen only when your action becomes motiveless—not less motive, but motiveless. That one action for a fraction of a second, without motive, will bring transformation.

Meda Dhātu: the Fat Tissue

Now we go to the next dhātu, meda dhātu, or the fat tissue. Meda is adipose tissue, a loose connective tissue that includes fat, phospholipids, steroids such as cholesterol, and other types of lipids.

During the creation of processed muscle tissue, unprocessed fat molecules are also formed. The fatty tissue is watery and unctuous. It is slimy, soft, and has typical oily characteristics. Adipose tissue has a vital function in the cell. It participates in the formation of cell membranes, other structures of the cell, and also helps to nourish the cells. One of the functions of meda dhātu as adipose tissue is snehan (lubrication), which provides freedom of movement. Fats are used to build the cell and to store and supply energy for all cellular activity. Meda dhātu also gives groundedness.

In a way, fat acts as a fuel. When you exercise, your body needs some lubricating substance and that lubricant is provided through fat and cholesterol. Cholesterol has a function. It is necessary for lubrication of the tissue and for nourishment of the bones and cartilage, as well as the articular surfaces of the bones. Extremely low cholesterol, below 150, is one of the causes of cracking and popping of the joints, and may lead to degenerative arthritis and low libido.

Lipids include fats, oils, steroids, and other fatty substances. Cholesterol is a lipid from which steroids such as sex hormones are manufactured, and it is present in cell membranes throughout the body. There are two kinds of cholesterol, low density lipoprotein (LDL) and high density lipoprotein (HDL). Good cholesterol, the HDL, is thoroughly processed cholesterol. LDL is unprocessed cholesterol and has a tendency to deposit on the walls of the blood vessels and create plaque and arteriosclerotic changes. Ghee (clarified butter) in moderation enhances good cholesterol, or HDL. Total cholesterol count should be below 200 and numbers higher than this are associated with heart disease. However, there are other factors also involved in heart disease—triglycerides, stress, and blood sugar. I have seen a person with a cholesterol count of less than 200 have a heart attack. Cholesterol is not the only cause.

Fat molecules have similar properties to those of kapha dosha, and kapha is present in fat. According to Āyurveda, fat is predominantly Water and Earth. Fat has a tremendous capacity to store and yield energy into the system. Gram for gram, carbohydrates cannot give the same amount of energy. Fat molecules yield energy to the cell because they contain Water and Earth elements, which bring bulk and strength to the body. I am talking about fat in the correct proportion. I am not talking about fat that is in excess. An obese person has insufficient energy even to walk two blocks, because that excess fat is raw, unprocessed fat. I am talking about healthy, processed fat, which is necessary for the body. Overeating produces excess fat. If a person consumes too much food and his agni is not strong enough to digest it, the protein and carbohydrates can become fat. Conversely, when a person fasts, the adipose tissue loses fat droplets and shrinks. To find the amount of fat in the body, pinch the skin. A big pinch indicates there is much fat. A tiny pinch indicates little fat. Also look at the thickness of the skin. The thicker the skin, the more fat; the thinner the skin, the less the fat.

Meda dhātu is present beneath the skin as subcutaneous fat, the insulating material that maintains body temperature. It is closely connected to māmsa dhātu, whose upadhātu is subcutaneous fat. If meda is affected, then māmsa will gradually be affected as well, through its upadhātu.

In an obese person, the fire (enzymes) is pushed to the center because of the accumulation of fat under the skin. Therefore, a fatty person has a strong appetite. He or she may eat a full meal and again be hungry after three hours. Why? Because more agni (fire) is stored in the stomach and there is much less fire under the skin. Therefore, obese people have cold, clammy skin. In other words, the jāthara agni (gastric fire) is strong, but meda agni is low. If meda agni is low, fat metabolism is slow, which leads to excess accumulation of fat under the skin. Whatever that person eats is converted into fat. Even too much water will add to that adipose tissue, because fat is Earth and Water.

Fat is also present between two muscles, because the muscle fibers move and create friction. There is accumulation of fat on round organs, such as the kidneys, liver, spleen, heart, and diaphragm. Fat cells are also round. Behind the eyeball there is fat, because the eyes are the body's most active organs. They are constantly moving and need lubrication, and nature has provided fat to give them freedom of movement. If there is excess accumulation of fat behind the eyeball, the eyeball will protrude. This condition is present in hyperthyroidism. If there is high blood pressure, blood rushes to the brain and pushes kapha and meda behind the eyeball.

The omentum is an apron-like structure present as a fold under the stomach in the peritoneal cavity and this structure is rich in fat. It is the storehouse of meda dhātu. On the surface of the heart there is also fat. The heart is an active organ. To prevent friction between the parietal pericardium and the visceral pericardium there is a little fat. There is fat around the joints to protect them. Meda dhātu serves as a protective cushion for the joints. Under the skin, the fat acts as an insulator to maintain body temperature. Fat is a poor conductor of heat and holds heat within the body.

By-products of Meda Dhātu

In a healthy condition, meda dhātu takes 20 days to be formed. Again, there are two forms of meda dhātu—processed and unprocessed, sthāyi and asthāyi. Kledaka kapha is predominately present in meda dhātu. Meda dhātu gives energy and stamina, while the superfine molecules of meda bring love and compassion. According to Āyurveda, the upadhātu (superior by-product) of meda dhātu is snāyu, the flat muscles, sinews, tendons and ligaments. The mala of meda is *sveda* (sweat).

Two *añjali* is the ideal measurement of fat in the body, though the amount varies according to the size of body frame. It is difficult to know how the rishis made this measurement, because the number of fat cells changes depending upon diet, lifestyle, quality of food, and emotional states. According to Āyurveda, the dhātu that changes most slowly is meda. Meda and kapha are both slow. Eating kapha-provoking food will gradually create an increase in meda.

One thing is important. When the metabolism is normal, if you take your body weight before food and again after food, the weight should be about the same, even after a heavy meal. That indicates your jāthara agni is strong. If a person weighs more after consuming food, his agni is slow.

A person who receives love does not need much food. Food and love are interconnected. When you meet a loving, compassionate friend, your appetite is lessened, because you receive the higher food, love. The teachings of Āyurveda say that food is the food of the body and love is the food of the soul, consciousness. When a woman receives love, she looks beautiful and healthy. When she does not receive love, she tries to receive the missing love through food. Food becomes a substitute for love and over intake makes her obese. Obesity is a deeply rooted psychological problem, both in men and women. However, according to Āyurveda, fatty tissue is more feminine and women are more prone to accumulate fat.

A person who has superfine quality of meda dhātu, called meda sāra, has beautiful eyes, beautiful hair, and a melodious voice. A good singer is usually meda sāra. The skin is soft and shiny, the joints are flexible with no cracking or popping, and there is good endurance, energy, vitality, and longevity. Such a person rarely gets arthritis or osteoporosis.

Fat is necessary to nourish the glandular system—thyroid, parathyroid, adrenals, ovaries, and pituitary. Psychologically, meda dhātu is related to perception. The superfine molecules of meda dhātu help to retain healthy and blissful memories. The spiritual function of meda dhātu creates bliss molecules, such as endorphins.

Disorders of Meda Dhātu

According to Āyurveda, excess sugar, salt, sweets, and dairy products, a sedentary lifestyle, unresolved emotions, steroids, and typhoid are the main causes of meda disorders. After surgery, people may also put on extra weight such as in the case of a fracture of the leg and one is not able to be physically active. That person may become overweight.

In India, one cause of obesity is typhoid fever. Typhoid is a dangerous disease. It can create perforation of the intestine, leading to peritonitis (inflammation of abdominal membrane), endangering a person's life. Typhoid affects meda dhātu and, after having typhoid, a person often gains weight. Typhoid may affect metabolism in both directions. In pitta and vāta prakruti, it may create hypermetabolic activity, leading to malnourishment and emaciation. In kapha individuals, typhoid fever may slow metabolic activity and cause hypothyroid function, leading to obesity. In the United States, we rarely see a patient with typhoid, because the disease is under control. However, in Third World countries, many people still contract typhoid.

Meda dhātu is connected to the adrenals. Why does a person who takes steroids become overweight? According to Āyurveda, steroids are rich in Water and Earth molecules, which are similar to meda and kapha. Prolonged steroid therapy may induce anabolic activity by provoking kapha. This kapha will slow down bhūta agni in the liver and thyroid gland. Clinically, steroid toxicity manifests as a moon face, water retention, slow metabolism, and underactive thyroid function. Therefore, steroid toxicity is one of the causes of obesity.

Causes of Meda Disorders

Excess sugar, sweets, or simple carbohydrates
Excess salt or dairy products
Cold drinks
Regular consumption of meat
Oily or fried food
Lack of good quality fats in the diet
Incompatible food combining
Frequent emotional eating
Excess water
Stress and unresolved emotions
Sedentary lifestyle or daytime sleeping
Insufficient or excessive exercise (beyond one's capacity)
Alcohol, marijuana, tobacco, and other drugs
Steroids
Typhoid

Alcohol is also one of the causes of meda dhātu dushti. Alcohol is fermented sugar, which kindles jāthara agni. Alcoholics enjoy overeating and, because of the alcohol, the person puts on fat. Alcohol is metabolized in the liver and excess consumption of alcohol can create fatty changes in the liver, because alcohol is converted into sugar. The elements of sugar are Earth and Water, the same elements of meda. Alcohol leads to obesity, because it retains the elements of Earth and Water, due to low Earth and Water agni in bhūta agni. The molecules of these elements are unprocessed and stagnate in the adipose tissue. The result is fat. If there is only accumulation of fat on the liver, the liver appears round. With alcoholic cirrhotic changes, the liver becomes enlarged but feels sharp and hard on the surface, a clinical observation that can be confirmed through biopsy. With alcoholic changes, the person also develops prominent blood vessels on the nose.

What are the cardinal signs and symptoms that indicate fat metabolism is out of balance? When meda dhātu is increased because meda dhātu agni is low, the molecules of fat are not processed properly. This causes meda vruddhi, excess unprocessed meda dhātu. So adipose tissue retains more and more oil and water molecules, the skin becomes oily, and the person develops more tartar on the teeth. Increased meda can create lipomas (fatty tumors), gallstones, fatty stools, obesity, diabetes, and hypertension. It is also one of the causes of fibrocystic changes in the breasts.

Certain symptoms are an early sign of meda dhātu dushti and may lead to diabetes. Meda dhātu dushti, late-onset diabetes, and obesity go hand in hand, because all are metabolic disorders that involve kapha. An obese person will have plump cheeks, double chin, accumulation of fat in the mastic tissue and pendular breasts. There is also accumulation of fat under the skin on the rectus abdominus muscle. Sometimes it is difficult to palpate the abdominal muscles because of this accumulation of fat.

Before diabetes develops or obesity occurs, early signs of meda dushti appear. While passing the last drops of urine, a person gets goose bumps and a spasm develops (*vyāna dushti*). There is a craving for sugar, a typical foul smell under the armpits and breathlessness after walking. The teachings of Āyurveda say to watch for excess thirst and thick saliva, as well as over development of tartar on the teeth. Excessive tartar is caused by accumulation of unprocessed meda, and it is an early sign of diabetes and general meda vruddhi.

Such a person often develops steatorrhea (fatty diarrhea) and passes fat in the stool, so that the stool floats in the water. Floating stools can indicate no āma (undigested toxins) in the stool. However, they can also indicate there is excess fat coming into the bile and the liver is not properly processing the fat. Excess fat in the bile may create a tendency for gallstones. Before gallstones appear, a person develops a dull aching pain in the right hypochondriac area. Gallstones at the beginning stages of development are greasy and soft and cannot be seen on an x-ray. People do not understand the relationship between the pancreas and the choroid plexus in the brain. In the inferior horn of the lateral ventricle and in the roof of the third ventricle, there are a network of capillaries called the choroid plexus. There is also a choroid plexus in the roof of the fourth ventricle. Cerebrospinal fluid is secreted from the choroid plexus. The choroid plexus is called kloma in Sanskrit. The pancreas is also called kloma. If the pancreatic function becomes debilitated, the person becomes diabetic. Kapha type of diabetes is related to fat. So obesity and diabetes can go together. Diabetes and hypertension can also go together. Diabetes is not a single disease but a complex syndrome.

Table 17: Signs and Symptoms of Meda Disorders

Meda Vruddhi (*Increased Meda Dhātu*)	Meda Kshaya (*Decreased Meda Dhātu*)

Obesity
Lethargy
Pains in the joints
Breathlessness on exertion
Slow metabolism
Underactive thyroid
Profuse sweating
Lipomas (fatty tumors)
Hypertension (high blood
   pressure)
Gallstones
Low libido
Excess thirst and sweet taste in
   mouth
Diabetes
	Dry skin
	Cracking joints
	Emaciation
	Osteo (degenerative arthritis)
	Lumbago
	Overactive thyroid
	Osteoporosis (bone loss)
	Enlarged spleen

Excessive thirst is a common sign of meda dushti. But how much water should we drink? A healthy amount of water varies according to the person's diet, lifestyle, physical activity and prakruti, as well as the climatic conditions. A pitta person might require six to eight cups of water daily in summer, because there is so much heat in the body. A skinny vāta person may take less in humid conditions, but need to drink more than this in a dry climate. But a kapha individual who is 20 pounds overweight doesn't need much water. Four to five cups a day is usually enough.

People are told to drink more water to flush out the kidneys. However, when kidney energy is low, a person is not processing the water and the excess consumption is like beating a tired horse. That water will be retained in the connective tissues, leading to excess weight. Salt also retains water in the tissues. Nevertheless, some people drink 15 cups of water daily, which may flush the kidneys and cause loss of sodium and potassium. Because of the loss of sodium (salt), a person may develop muscle cramps and gas in the colon. In children, loss of potassium creates abdominal distention and gas, *apāna vāyu dushti*. These conditions are due to water toxicity, which changes the hydraulic pressure and affects osmosis.

The teachings of Āyurveda say that every person should have at least a moderate amount of fat in order to make the body round, firm and healthy. That amount of fat is measured as two añjali, approximately two pints. If there is too much fat, the veins are buried under the fatty tissue and it is difficult to find the vein. If the fat is insufficient, depleted fatty tissue creates a decrease of sweat or no sweat at all, even in a 90 degree temperature. The skin becomes dry and rough, and there is cracking of the joints.

In the process of nutrition of the tissues, if meda agni is intensely high, fat molecules are quickly utilized by the body. This can lead to meda kshaya, depleted meda dhātu. When a person is engaged in excessive physical activity but does not consume sufficient protein or lubricating substances, that person loses fat. Because of extreme loss of fatty tissue, a person's muscles become stiff and the joints begin to ache. This condition may even lead to osteoporosis or degenerative arthritic changes, as well as hair loss. The voice becomes hoarse, dry, and frog-like. Insomnia is also a problem. To have sound sleep requires some fat. Depleted fat also leads to menstrual irregularities. Emotionally, this imbalance creates insecurity, fear, and anxiety. Extremely debilitated meda dhātu, or meda kshaya, manifests as spontaneous fractures due to the bones being unable to bear the body's weight.

Āyurveda considers beauty to result from good health. In Western culture, being slim is fundamental to the concept of beauty. Women jog, work out, and eat a limited diet to try to be slim. However they then show signs and symptoms of depleted fatty tissue, such as cracking of the joints, arthritic changes, and constipation.

Say you have decided to maintain normal fat, which is two añjali. How can we determine two añjali of fat? The quality of the pulse reveals this information. If the meda dhātu pulse at the fifth level is vāta, fat is depleted. If the pulse shows pitta, the woman has excess pitta in the fat that may create gallstones or multiple boils. Multiple boils can also indicate diabetes. If the meda pulse shows kapha, it can indicate lipomas, gallstones, or fibrocystic changes in the breasts. However, if the meda pulse has no doshic spike, it means meda dhātu is healthy.

When fat is depleted and the person craves meat and cheese, that person should eat those foods. If an obese person craves cheese, that craving is emotional, psychological. There is a great difference between the need of the body and a psychological craving. The mind creates emotional cravings. A person with excess kapha symptoms and craving for cheese should not eat it. Cheese will increase fat and make the bile thick. It will slow down metabolism.

Ghee is the best. Ghee in moderation does not increase total cholesterol and it helps to build good cholesterol (HDL). But if total cholesterol is high, beyond 230, don't eat ghee. If cholesterol is borderline, you can eat ghee. But how much ghee should one eat? One teaspoon per meal is enough. For three meals each day, one should not take more than three teaspoons. If you take two or three tablespoons of ghee daily, your cholesterol may rise, because your agni may not be strong enough to burn that much fat. It may also add to your triglyceride level.

Cholesterol is transformed into testosterone in the liver. For that reason, when the liver is weak, a person's testosterone may be low. According to Āyurveda, bitter ghee (tikta ghrita) helps balance HDL and improves the processing of cholesterol into testosterone. However, tikta ghrita and all bitter substances will reduce the production of sperm.

Both increased cholesterol and high triglycerides (fat) make the blood thick. When the viscosity of the blood is high, then blood pressure becomes high. Obesity and hypertension go together. That does not mean every person who is hypertensive is obese, but every person who is obese is likely to be hypertensive. Each organ in the human body has its own ojas, tejas, and prāna to perform its normal physiological function. When either tejas or ojas is depleted in the liver, that organ may not process fat and carbohydrates, leading to hyperlipidemia and increased triglycerides. The blood in these individuals flows with resistance, causing hypertension.

According to Āyurveda, the liver is the most important organ involved in the transformation and processing of fats and lipids. I have seen many people with a cholesterol reading of 230 or 240, and triglycerides also beyond normal level, because their liver function is below normal. These people often have a history of jaundice or mononucleosis.

A man with high blood pressure came to see me. His systolic pressure was 140 and diastolic was 90. A diastolic of 90 indicates hypertension. He had a history of mononucleosis and hepatitis, and his liver was not properly processing cholesterol. I gave him kutki, an Āyurvedic herb that is a good liver cleanser, and his blood pressure and cholesterol returned to normal.

As we have already studied, within the synaptic cleft, or neuromuscular junction, there is an important neurotransmitter that Āyurveda calls tarpaka kapha, an acetylcholine-type substance. Acetylcholine brings relaxation and tranquility. According to Āyurveda, tarpaka kapha is essential in bringing that action. Molecules of tarpaka kapha help yield the molecules of bliss. Certain endorphins are secreted into the nervous system and a person experiences joy and happiness.

But exactly the opposite happens if the molecules of meda dhātu are of inferior quality. Inferior meda molecules inhibit the secretion of serotonin and other substances, which can lead to depression. Depression and obesity go together. Some obese people feel more depressed during the winter, because of clouds in the sky and lack of sunlight. According to Āyurveda, the presence of sunlight stimulates sādhaka pitta and a person becomes happy. Lack of sunlight creates depression, and winter depression (Seasonal Affective Disorder—SAD) is common when meda dhātu dushti is present.

It is possible to have decreased meda in one part of the body and increased meda in another part at the same time. For example, when prāna vāyu is hyperactive and apāna vāyu is hypoactive, a woman may be obese in the thighs but at the same time have emaciated breasts. In this case, hyperactive prāna is not allowing the fat molecules to stay in the upper part of the body, creating a lack of meda there. Displacement occurs because of weak prāna or weak apāna; the fatty cells are pushed into the upper or lower part of the body respectively.

Obesity is divided into central obesity, where the belly is big; truncated obesity, where the breasts and belly are big; and peripheral obesity, where the extremities are big. These conditions are due to displacement of meda molecules in a particular direction, depending upon the person's lifestyle and emotions. If a person has deep seated grief and sadness in the lungs, which are vāta emotions, there will be less chance for the meda molecules to stay there. They will be pushed down. So such a person may have chubby thighs. This condition is not increase or decrease, but rather displacement of fat molecules.

Meda dushti is created when meda dhātu is qualitatively deranged. With meda dushti a person may develop an enlarged spleen, constant low backache, or perhaps difficulty putting on weight. The spleen becomes enlarged because meda agni is low, which affects the agni of the spleen. When there is meda dhātu dushti and the spleen is enlarged, the liver also tends to be enlarged. Fatty degeneration of the liver indicates that the liver cells cannot metabolize fat molecules, and unmetabolized fat molecules accumulate in the liver. When there is enlargement of the liver due to fatty degeneration, the liver feels long and soft when palpated. If the enlarged liver has a sharp, hard, and irregular border, it may be malignant, which denotes a tridoshic disorder.

A clinical examination of the liver reveals these changes. When the liver is hard, painful, tender, and swollen, it could be the result of hepatitis. In cirrhotic changes, the liver shrinks and becomes hard. Cirrhosis means death of the liver cells. We can live without the spleen but we cannot live without the liver. Surgical transplantation of the liver is risky. If you are vāta and you receive a pitta or kapha person's liver, your body will not accept it. So there is a high rate of mortality with a liver transplant. To make your body accept a foreign liver is difficult and particularly depends upon the prakruti paradigm.

The lumbosacral joint needs a little pad of fat as a cushion. If that cushion is gone, which can happen when someone has depleted meda, the joint becomes weak and the person develops low backache. In obese people with a large abdomen, the angle between the lumbar and the sacrum becomes too straight. So obese people also complain of low backache. Obese people frequently develop arthritis of the ankles and knees, because those joints are vulnerable when carrying the extra weight of the body. A weight reduction program can help pain in the joints.

Some sleep disorders are associated with meda dhātu. Some people feel sleepy while walking or driving a car. Others sleep during the day. Their metabolism is slow and, because of slow metabolism, agni is low. Because of low agni, sādhaka pitta does not maintain awareness. Taking *trikatu chūrna* (ginger, black pepper, long pepper) with honey can correct this type of sleep disorder. Another complication of meda dhātu dushti is the deposition of fat on the blood vessels that may create arteriosclerosis or atheroma.

Ideal weight depends upon height and exercise. On clinical grounds, ideal weight is connected to the size of the muscles and bones and the amount of fat. If you are a physically active, muscular person of average height and weigh 150 pounds, the weight is due to physical activity. Some people have strong bones, are tall and also have high weight. That is not obesity. Obesity is connected to the weight of the fat, not the muscle.

Therefore, ideal weight depends on the balanced quality and quantity of the tissues. If you have strong muscles and strong bones and your weight is high, that is acceptable. But if the weight is high and the muscles are flabby, that is obesity and it is a problem. If a person who regularly lifts weights is overweight, the weight may be due to increased māmsa dhātu. Māmsa dhātu governs one-third of our body weight and that weight is acceptable. The teachings of Āyurveda do not give a fixed figure for ideal weight. It varies from person to person.

Awareness and Meda

Āyurveda, which is a spiritual science of healing, says that within your DNA molecules you carry the memory of your parents' illnesses. If your father had diabetes, tuberculosis or rheumatoid arthritis, your cells carry the memory of those illnesses. Even obesity can become a genetic factor. In certain families, the grandfather was obese, the father was obese, and the son is also obese. Or the grandmother was obese, the mother was obese, and the daughter, even at age 16, is obese. The desire is created to eat the same kind of fat-producing food. This desire is recorded in the adipose tissue as a biochemical phenomenon. Your thought is a biochemical vehicle, and that vehicle is an important instrument through which you can communicate with your cells. The entire body is a body of awareness. If you stretch out your arm and hold it, you can feel that prāna is moving, awareness is moving. If you hold it for a couple of minutes, you begin to feel tingling and numbness. Tingling and numbness indicate there is inadequate flow of prāna. That is one of the signs that meda molecules are blocking the flow of prāna. If your prāna is strong, you can hold your hand out for a couple of minutes without feeling tingling and numbness. Then when you slowly move your hand down, you feel awareness moving with your hand. This feeling is quite subtle. An obese person can sit in a cross-legged posture for only five minutes before his legs go to sleep, because the weight of adipose tissue blocks the flow of awareness.

When you sit quietly, bring more awareness to the toes and move the toes in awareness. Then bring awareness to the ankle and move the ankle in awareness. Bring more awareness to the knee and move the knee with awareness. Breathe into it. Slowly raise your awareness to the hip area and bring action with awareness to those muscles.

This is the art of visualization. You visualize your own body and begin communicating with the cells with your internal perception and intention. A Vedic sūtra says, if you have right intention, you will create right attention. And right attention will bring right awareness. The inner flow of awareness becomes the pathway of the inner pharmacy. This awareness will erase the memory of your cells that are carrying the memory of obesity. Then your cravings for sugar, candy, cookie, and chocolate will come to an end.

Food is a need of the body but food can be a focus of temptation. Some people are so insecure they use food as a drug to satisfy their insecurity, fear, and anxiety. So eat with awareness every time you put a lump of food in the mouth and chew. Feel the food go into the esophagus and into the stomach after you swallow. When you bring more awareness to the stomach, you will not overeat. People eat too much because of temptation, inattention, and lack of awareness.

The teachings of Āyurveda say to divide the capacity of the stomach into three parts—one part food, one part water, and one part air. But some people eat to full capacity, leaving no space for air or water. That is emotional eating. Such an emotional habit comes from toxic connective tissue. The connective tissue is the seat of the subconscious mind and the subconscious mind is your own creation. There is no clear line of demarcation between the conscious and subconscious. The subconscious can become conscious. Your conscious mind is a door into the subconscious mind. If you increase the radius of the dimension of your conscious mind, then your subconscious will become conscious. With this expansion of consciousness, you will be able to see your childhood traumas, which are responsible for incorrect eating.

If you observe carefully, the inferior quality of meda dhātu retains hurt, grief, and sadness. However, the superfine quality of meda dhātu can retain the bliss of awareness.

Asthi Dhātu: the Bone Tissue

The next dhātu is asthi, the bone tissue, which is the densest tissue in the body. According to Āyurveda, asthi dhātu is predominately made up of Earth, Air, and Water. Earth is about 80 percent, Air about 15 percent, and Water, found in the periosteum, around five percent. Due to the Air molecules, bones are porous. Because asthi dhātu is composed primarily of the Earth element, the intracellular matrix of asthi dhātu is rich in iron, copper, zinc, other minerals, and mineral salts.

Asthi dhātu provides internal support. It gives shape to the head, face, thorax, limbs, and nose. It protects delicate vital organs—the brain, eyes, ears, tongue, heart, and lungs. The pelvic bones protect the ovaries, fallopian tubes, uterus, colon and prostate gland.

Asthi dhātu creates cranial, thoracic, and pelvic cavities and one of the functions of this dhātu is to confine the cavities, like a wall. If there is no wall, there is no room. The walls of a house create confined space. In the same way, the walls of the skull create the confined space of the cranial cavity, the rib cage creates the thoracic cavity, and the pelvic bones create the pelvic cavity. Bones serve as attachments for the muscles. The muscles need support and for that reason all muscles are attached to the bones by ligaments.

Asthi dhātu also acts as an excretory tissue. The unwanted molecules of toxic heavy metals, such as arsenic, mercury, and lead are retained in asthi dhātu, and the body tries to eliminate them in the nails and hair. In hair analysis, some people show excessive amounts of these metals, which come from the bone. Indirectly, asthi dhātu maintains water electrolyte balance through the molecules of calcium, magnesium, sodium, and potassium.

This dhātu also conducts sound waves that aid in hearing. We hear through both air conduction and bone conduction. All ambulatory movement, locomotion, is governed by asthi dhātu through the joints. Another important function relating to the bones is the formation of red blood cells through the bone marrow. However bone marrow is majjā dhātu, which we will discuss in the next section.

Meda dhātu nourishes asthi dhātu. Immature asthi dhātu, called asthāyi asthi dhātu, is formed at the same time as sthāyi meda dhātu, and this unprocessed dhātu is transformed into processed asthi dhātu by asthi agni, the fire component of asthi dhātu. This transformation takes place through a fine membrane called the periosteum.

The bone, asthi dhātu, is composed of compact cells. Inside is the bone marrow. The outer covering is the periosteum, which is called *asthi dhara kalā*. As we discussed earlier, kalā is a membranous structure. Purisha dhara kalā in the colon absorbs minerals and directs them to the periosteum (asthi dhara kalā). Asthi dhara kalā is rich in lymphoid tissue, specialized plasma. Within the periosteum, there is unprocessed asthi dhātu and there is agni, which transforms the unprocessed asthi into processed asthi. Part of the unprocessed asthi dhātu is *taruna asthi* (cartilage), a specialized form of asthāyi asthi dhātu. The full transformation of asthāyi asthi into sthāyi asthi requires 25 days. Therefore, if there is a fracture of a bone, it takes a minimum of 25 days to heal.

By-products of Asthi Dhātu

In the process of this transformation, some by-products are formed. These are teeth, nails, and hair, and the immature majjā dhātu (the next dhātu). *Danta* (teeth) is the upadhātu (superior by-product); *kesha* (hair) and *nakha* (nails) are mala (inferior by-products). There are no nerve endings (majjā dhātu) in the nails and hair, and for that reason they do not have sensation of pain. However, majjā dhātu is present at the root of the hair and nail; if you pull the nail or hair, it will cause pain. If you cut the hair or clip the nail, there is no pain. Thank God! Otherwise, there would be pain with each hair cut.

The hairs of the secondary sexual characteristics (pubic hair, moustache, and axillary hairs) are the superfine products of asthi dhātu in relation to shukra and ārtava, the reproductive tissue. They are specialized hairs and are not directly functionally connected to asthi dhātu. However, the superfine part of asthi dhātu (asthi sāra) is utilized by processed shukra or ārtava dhātu to form these hairs from the time of puberty. In young children, the shukra/ārtava dhātu is not yet mature, so a young girl or boy before puberty has no pubic or axillary hair.

By looking at the nails, we can understand the condition of asthi dhātu. If asthi dhātu is brittle, the nails are brittle. If asthi dhātu is strong, the nails are strong. In certain cultures, the nails are thin and brittle because of diet and certain environmental conditions. Some people get a fungus growth in their nails, which may be due to external or internal causes. For example, fungal infection is common in damp, humid weather.

The teachings of Āyurveda convey that asthi dhātu is a crystallization of rasa, rakta, māmsa, and meda dhātus. People

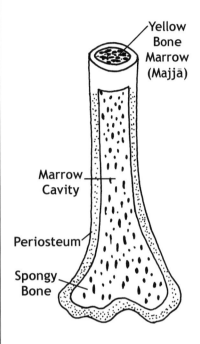

Asthi Dhātu

Yellow Bone Marrow (Majjā)

Marrow Cavity

Periosteum

Spongy Bone

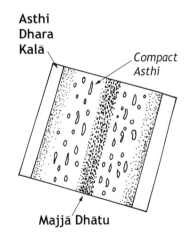

Asthi Dhara Kalā

Compact Asthi

Majjā Dhātu

with a kapha prakruti will have better asthi dhātu, because the Earth and Water components that mostly comprise asthi dhātu are predominately present in the kapha person. If you compare the x-ray of a femur of a kapha person, a pitta person, and a vāta person, the large femur belongs to the kapha person, the medium femur to the pitta person and the tiny femur to the vāta person. I was taught to identify the prakruti of a person by looking at an x-ray of his or her femur.

Asthi agni, in conjunction with thyroid and parathyroid hormones, maintains calcium metabolism. The thyroid gland secretes a hormone called calcitonin that controls calcium blood levels. Over activity of the thyroid stimulates more and more calcitonin. That dysfunction reduces blood calcium levels. Calcium is needed for blood formation and for the clotting function of blood. If a person's blood does not clot properly, that person is probably lacking calcium. Natural coagulation needs adequate calcium in the blood.

Exactly the opposite happens when the thyroid gland is underactive. Then there is a low level of calcitonin, which raises calcium levels in the blood. Calcium is needed for the conduction of impulses to the muscles and for maintaining muscle tone and relaxation. There are many forms of calcium. Calcium citrate is highly absorbable and quick acting. Calcium carbonate has slow, sustained action. Calcium gluconate is good for helping the muscles relax. Āyurveda says to treat the thyroid gland. *Shilājit*, a mineral resin, particularly helps to bring its function back to normal.

Excess vāta or pitta can lead to hyperthyroidism, with increased metabolism and loss of weight. When kapha is aggravated, kapha molecules can diminish the agni of the thyroid, leading to hypothyroidism. A person with kapha prakruti has large bones. But in kapha vikruti (disorder) when kapha inhibits the function of the thyroid gland, calcium metabolism is affected. Hypothyroidism slows metabolism and many obese people have underactive thyroid function.

The parathyroid gland secretes a hormone that stimulates osteoclasts to break down the bone tissue and release calcium salts into the blood. If a person has an overactive parathyroid, that person has increased urination, excess thirst, and may even develop osteoporotic changes. The bones lose calcium and the person can get spontaneous fractures, kidney stones, or gallstones. Underactive parathyroid is extremely rare.

According to Āyurveda, asthi dhātu is a crystallization of consciousness. Within the interstitial cellular matrix of asthi dhātu, we carry seeds of past lives. We have lived before. We came here because we were somewhere else. Coming here from somewhere is what we call birth. We are here and we go somewhere else. Going somewhere, by dropping this mortal frame, is called death. Therefore, death is the cause of birth and birth is the cause of death. There is no birth without death and there is no death without birth. Within our bones, we carry the seeds of the desires of our past lives.

Though bone tissue appears to be a hard, compact, supportive mass, it is a living tissue that is sensitive to emotions and feelings. Little changes can create a shift of consciousness. In craniosacral work, a slight shift in the plates of the skull can release emotions and widen the field of consciousness, which is one of the healing factors in this treatment.

Vedic philosophy says that minerals deposit in the periosteum, which is the mother of bone tissue. The periosteum contains thick concentrated calcium, magnesium, iron and other minerals necessary for bone formation. Bone tissue is a rigid, hard, firm connective tissue and, within that tissue, we carry unresolved, crystallized emotions. Desires, emotions, and unresolved hurts are accumulated within the matrix of asthi dhātu. These emotions can affect the function of the parathyroid and thyroid glands as well as formation of bone tissue. Severe bone disorders can indicate a great deal of unresolved and unexpressed emotions.

An asthi sāra person has strong bones, good height, strong teeth and thick, strong nails. This person has great endurance, strength, vitality and stamina. A man is as old as his bones, so an asthi sāra person has a long life. Asthi sāra people are also forgiving, hardworking, and honest.

Disorders of Asthi Dhātu

What are the causes of asthi dhātu dushti? One cause is lack of minerals—calcium, magnesium, zinc, and certain trace minerals necessary for bone health. Nail biting is caused by a deficiency of zinc and calcium, although anxiety, insecurity, and nervousness can also lead to nail biting. Thyroid and parathyroid dysfunction, as well as physical and psychological trauma, may also cause asthi dhātu dushti.

When asthi dhātu is decreased, it is called asthi kshaya. One of the causes of decreased asthi dhātu is increased asthi agni. The increased metabolism burns the calcium, magnesium, and other mineral salts. White spots develop on the fingernails, the fingernails become brittle and they get ridges and creases. Brittle nails indicate asthi dhātu deficiency. These people may

---

Causes of Asthi Disorders

Poor diet – especially excessive vāta provoking foods, such as dry foods, beans, and leftovers

Lack of minerals

Insufficient or excess protein consumption

Poor posture

Overly vigorous or excessive exercise (beyond one's capacity)

Irregular intense exercise that provokes vāta, such as mountain climbing or running

Physical trauma, such as an accident

Psychological factors, such as trauma, loneliness, insecurity, lack of support

Thyroid and parathyroid disorders

Menopause

Hormone replacement therapy

---

also have many cavities in the teeth. Teeth become brittle and fractures of the crowns may occur. If there is a deep pocket of infection within the gums, the teeth become sensitive to cold because of vāta. But when pitta is present and creates inflammation, the teeth become sensitive to hot drinks, indicating the nerve is involved.

According to Āyurveda, delayed teething in children is caused by decreased asthi dhātu. The bones become fragile. The mala (inferior by-product) of asthi dhātu is hair, so a person with asthi kshaya may begin losing hair, caused by high pitta in asthi, or the hair may become brittle and dry or kinky, due to vāta. Hair loss can be related to a deficiency of calcium, magnesium, and zinc, or to excess salt consumption, which can provoke pitta in asthi dhātu. Both these causes can result in decreased asthi dhātu.

It is interesting to note that hair loss can also be connected to pituitary dysfunction. If the agni of shukra dhātu is high, which burns shukra dhātu, a person can start losing facial or pubic hair. This loss is connected to hormonal dysfunction of the pituitary, and is not asthi dushti. In addition, it may be connected to the lack of male or female hormones. When a young woman has hair around the nipple, she has difficulty conceiving. According to Āyurveda, hair around the nipple means the woman's body is rich in testosterone, a male hormone. These women may develop endometriosis.

During menopause, asthi agni becomes hyperactive because the body produces less estrogen. When less estrogen is present, asthi agni becomes overactive in an effort to compensate for that lack of estrogen and the agni it contains. The result can be osteoporosis. Eating a vāta provoking diet will worsen osteoporotic changes. According to Āyurveda, a woman should take natural herbal estrogen that is present in shatāvarī and other herbal remedies. Shatāvarī is effective in preventing osteoporosis during menopausal age. However, if you give a woman synthetic estrogen, her menstruation can return, or she may develop pitta symptoms, because estrogen is pitta provoking. In addition, there is the possibility of cancer. It is more balancing to use natural herbal estrogen, which is present in shatāvarī, guduchi, and aloe vera, as these all decrease pitta.

Table 18: Signs and Symptoms of Asthi Disorders

Asthi Vruddhi (*Increased Asthi Dhātu*)	Asthi Kshaya (*Decreased Asthi Dhātu*)
Bony protuberances, spurs	Hair loss
Osteomas (bone tumors)	Rough, dry, brittle, crooked nails
Calcification	Osteoporosis (bone loss)
Lordosis (abnormal convex curve of lumbar spine)	Osteo (degenerative) arthritis
Kyphosis (hunchback)	Rheumatoid arthritis
Bone fusion	Arthralgia (joint pain)
Extra teeth	Spontaneous fractures
Excessive hair growth	Shortened height
Scoliosis and spinal misalignment	Scoliosis and spinal misalignment

Decreased asthi dhātu can also create degenerative arthritis, as well as receding gums. Some people brush their teeth as if they were brushing the toilet. That is hurtful to the gums and may result in receding gums and bone loss in the jaw. On an emotional level, when asthi dhātu is depleted, a person is insecure, lonely, nervous, and ungrounded.

When asthi dhātu is increased (asthi vruddhi), there are often thyroid and parathyroid dysfunctions. There is more deposition of calcium on the bone, creating spurs. There may even be deposition of calcium in the soft tissue, such as the lungs or other organs. A person may get an extra tooth or a wisdom tooth may become twisted. Each tooth is connected to a different organ. For example, the wisdom teeth are connected to the heart and the canines are connected to the liver and eyes.

The teachings of Āyurveda say that toothpaste should be astringent and bitter. If sweet toothpaste is used, the saliva will become thick and will be rich in calcium, leading to the development of tartar on the teeth. Āyurvedic toothpaste is bitter and astringent. It cleans the pockets between the teeth and makes the saliva thin.

After brushing the teeth, before going to bed, place 10 drops of tea tree oil in a small cup of water and swish. Tea tree oil is astringent and bitter. It kills bacteria and is a good antiseptic. It also strengthens the gums. Neem is also a good choice. Brushing the teeth with neem toothpaste will make the saliva thin and the tartar will disappear with no receding gums. Triphala tea is also good for swishing or gargling when brushing the teeth.

Relationship of Teeth, Dhatus, and Organs

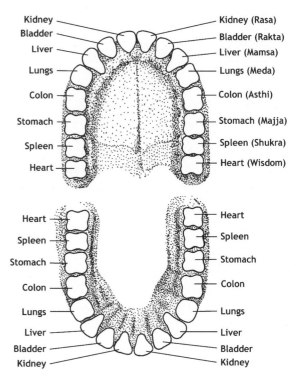

Kidney — Kidney (Rasa)
Bladder — Bladder (Rakta)
Liver — Liver (Mamsa)
Lungs — Lungs (Meda)
Colon — Colon (Asthi)
Stomach — Stomach (Majja)
Spleen — Spleen (Shukra)
Heart — Heart (Wisdom)

Heart — Heart
Spleen — Spleen
Stomach — Stomach
Colon — Colon
Lungs — Lungs
Liver — Liver
Bladder — Bladder
Kidney — Kidney

Alum, salt, and baking soda are good to remove dead bacteria. Alum is antiseptic and soda is alkaline. They make the teeth shiny. However, sometimes soda erodes the gums and creates inflammation. Once every 15 days, put a little baking soda on your toothbrush and gently brush the teeth. Salt is strong and will irritate the gums and create gingivitis. Use salt rarely.

Consuming excess *kaphagenic* food, such as wheat and dairy products, increases asthi. Some people have the habit of taking minerals and vitamins every day. It is usually unnecessary, and sometimes difficult to know how much to take. If you take excess vitamin C, it may increase pitta. Excess intake of calcium may create arteriosclerosis and increase the possibility of a heart attack, because calcium is responsible for clotting the blood. A person with varicose veins, caused by clotted blood, should not take too much calcium, because excess calcium may deposit on the clot.

When asthi dhātu is increased, there will be deposition of calcium on the muscle tendons, one of the causes of myofibrosis. In myofibrositis, muscle fibers become inflamed, irritated and the person develops aches and pains. This condition may look like muscular rheumatism. Increased asthi dhātu can also create bony tumors (osteomas) and misalignment of the spine (scoliotic changes). The majority of people have a little misalignment of the spine because of the way they walk. Misalignment of the spine may be present both in increased and decreased asthi dhātu.

Some people grind their teeth, which may indicate deep-seated anger and fear. That action is asthi dhātu dushti. Sometimes children grind due to worms. In adults, worms can create wet dreams, dreams of sex. The female worms hatch eggs around the perineum, which creates a peculiar itching sensation and, in deep sleep, the itching becomes pleasurable. For grinding teeth, chew half a teaspoon of uncooked basmati rice before going to bed. Then brush the teeth and hold a mouthful of warm sesame oil for five minutes and swish. Spit it out and go to bed. Leave a little oil in the mouth. Grinding of the teeth in deep sleep disappears. There are several Āyurvedic herbs that will help rid the body of worms.

Majjā Dhātu: the Nerve Tissue and Bone Marrow

Majjā dhātu is the sixth tissue. The word *pūrana* means "to fill space" and a major function of this dhātu is to fill the spaces of the innermost tissue of the body, the bones. Majjā dhātu includes both the nerve tissue and the bone marrow. Bone marrow is a soft jelly-like tissue within the cavity of the bone. Every bone has a little foramen, a small hole, through which the nerves and blood vessels enter the bone tissue. Therefore, the bone tissue has a sense of pain, pressure, and position of the joint. Whenever your joint is flexed or extended, you know its position because of majjā dhātu.

There are two kinds of bone marrow, red and yellow. Red bone marrow is found in the spongy bone and is rich in pitta and its function is to produce red blood cells and hemoglobin. As the person becomes older, a part of the red bone marrow becomes yellow. Yellow bone marrow is found is the medullary canal of long bones and consists primarily of fat cells and connective tissue. It does not produce red blood cells; it just stays in the cavity to support the bone. Unresolved emotions that are stuck in the matrix of bone marrow can alter the property of the marrow. Radiation also affects the bone marrow. Some broad-spectrum antibiotics, such as tetracycline and chloramphenicol, depress the bone marrow and create blood dysplasia, or dysfunction of the red bone marrow.

Majjā dhātu also has an important function of communication. It is present in the brain, hypothalamus, spinal cord, and in all interspinal nerves and cranial nerves, including subcutaneous nerves. Learn the 12 cranial nerves: olfactory, optic, oculomotor, trochlear, trigeminal, abducens, facial, acoustic (vestibulocochlear), glossopharyngeal, vagus, accessory and hypoglossal. Some of these are sensory, some are motor, and some are mixed nerves. The sensory stimulus is carried to the brain. The energy that carries the sensory stimulus is prāna and that which carries the motor response is apāna.

Majjā and the Prenatal Development Stage

As we considered earlier, the agni of asthi transforms immature asthi into mature asthi. In that transformation, asthi agni also creates immature majjā dhātu. The nerve tissue is well protected by bones. The flat bones of the skull provide the cavity for the brain, called the cranial cavity. When a child is born, the pulsation of the cerebral artery can be felt at the anterior fontanel. The anterior fontanel gives space for the brain to grow. If a child is born without an anterior fontanel, there will not be sufficient space for the brain to grow and that child may become mentally or physically retarded.

There are two fontanels. In Sanskrit, the anterior fontanel is called *brahmā randhra*. Randhra means opening. The posterior fontanel is called *shiva randhra*. Mystic anatomy says that consciousness enters the fetus through the anterior fontanel and consciousness leaves the body of a *yogi* at death through the posterior fontanel, leading to the liberation of the yogi. But an ordinary person's consciousness leaves through the other nine gates (2 ears, 2 eyes, 2 nostrils, mouth, anus, and penis or vagina), so the soul is caught in the cycle of birth and death. One can become liberated and realized while living in the body through meditation and yogic practice. The brain is a vital organ that is created by individual consciousness. The kundalinī shakti, which is electromagnetic energy, or neuro-electricity, is present in the brain of the fetus. For that reason, the fetus is in ecstasy, in samādhi.

Physiologically, all 72,000 nādis (channels) have their root in the navel. Through the belly button the baby's kundalinī and the mother's kundalinī are connected. At the belly button is the celiac plexus, or celiac ganglion, which governs the contraction of the diaphragm. But in the womb the baby breathes through the mother's lungs and that breath o consciousness is breathing without air. This is a mystica expression. Science tries to explain this process mechanically while Āyurveda tries to explain it spiritually. The brahmā randhra (anterior fontanel) and the shiva randhra (the posterior fontanel) are under the control of prāna. As long as prāna within the brain is pulsating, there is no need for the lungs to open for air, because the baby is breathing through the mother's lungs in the womb. The baby's digestion also happens through mother's digestion.

The womb is a most blissful state of unconsciousness. Modern psychologists say that every person is seeking the womb of bliss. The child cries because it has lost the song of bliss. You know pain because you have already experienced bliss. Without the experience of bliss, there is no experience of pain. Bliss is not the mere absence of pain, but is a most positive state of existence. This state of bliss is present in the mother's womb.

The child in the mother's womb is in a passive, blissful state. There are no phone calls, no bank accounts, and no responsibilities. Sometimes the child sucks its thumb. Sometimes the child kicks. At that moment, the anterior fontanel is open. There is subtle communication between the mother's heart and the baby's heart. The baby expresses its feelings and emotions through the mother's emotions. A woman has two hearts during pregnancy—her own heart and the baby's.

When does consciousness enter? Some people say that consciousness enters with the first breath. No, that is not the fact. Consciousness enters the ovum right at the time of fertilization, and the fertilized ovum is a conscious living tissue. The moment the sperm enters the ovum, it creates a subtle dynamic space of consciousness. That space is called non-ākāshic space, which is the *bindu* of consciousness, pulsating and throbbing without breath. In the fertilized ovum, jīva, the individual consciousness, is isolated from Brahmā, the universal consciousness. *Nādam* (the soundless sound), bindu (pulsating consciousness), and kalā (membranous structure) are all present in the zygote. It is not a dead tissue growing in the womb.

The cell division into two, four, sixteen cells, is accomplished by prāna vāyu. Thus the shape of the body is formed by prāna vāyu. Kapha helps to nourish each cell and pitta brings transformation of the immature cell into the mature cell, within the core of the zygote. This mitotic division of the fertilized ovum leads to the growth of the fetus.

The body is objective material consciousness and the mind is subjective material consciousness. Body and mind are one. When consciousness is operating with kundalinī shakti within the crown chakra of the fetus, we are conscious only in a blissful way. We are not conscious of life. We are only conscious subjectively. But the moment a child takes its first breath, objective consciousness enters. At the time of delivery, the mother pushes down the body of the child, helping the dilation of the cervix and contraction of the uterus. When the three Ps— passenger, pressure and passage—are in perfect order, the child comes out through the tiny canal of the birth passage. During the delivery, stress causes the baby's kundalinī to push down into the mūlādhāra (root) chakra. There, apāna vāyu is activated for the first time and it stimulates prāna vāyu. Then contraction of the diaphragm takes place, the lungs open and the baby breathes. At this moment of the first breath, the baby has forgotten the sound of bliss.

The moment you are born physically, you are separated from your mother's neuro-electricity. As long as the umbilical cord is pulsating, ojas is moving from the mother to the baby. The experienced obstetrician feels the pulse of the umbilical cord, and when the pulsation is diminished, he places forceps on each side and cuts in between. If the umbilical cord is cut before the slowing of pulsation, the child may not receive adequate ojas from the mother and that child may become sick. What is ojas? Ojas is the sap of the seven dhātus. It is the vital force that governs immunity. We will discuss ojas in detail in the next chapter.

At the time of delivery, a baby passes from a blissful state to a physical state. When kundalinī moves from the crown chakra along the spinal cord and hits the solar plexus and the celiac ganglion, then the diaphragm works, the lungs open, the first breath enters, and the child cries. At that first breath, the baby's kundalinī is pushed down into the pelvic cavity. So downward movement of kundalinī separates the individual consciousness (jīva) from higher consciousness. However, the upward movement of kundalinī helps the union of jīva with higher consciousness. The moment the child cries, at that moment, the blissful state of subjective awareness is gone and the physical state of objective awareness is born. We forget the blissful state in the mother's womb. We are only physically conscious and when we dream we are subconsciously conscious.

Many times a baby is still one with the blissful state, as well as with unfinished emotions of a past life. Sometimes a baby smiles in a deep sleep. Charaka says a baby is still experiencing subjective, subconscious, past life experiences. The Western world does not believe in past lives and rebirth, but it is necessary as far as majjā dhātu is concerned. Past life subconscious experiences center in the hypothalamus. There is a respiratory center in the hypothalamus, but it is dormant in the fetus. The first breath activates that center. Similarly, there is a memory center, but the memory center in the fetus is active only for past lives. Present life memories are not yet there. For the physiological functions of majjā dhātu, these past life subconscious memories create a bed for new centers to be developed.

The Functions of Majjā Dhātu

Sthāyi majjā dhātu is formed from asthāyi majjā dhātu via majjā agni. Majjā agni is composed of enzymes, amino acids, and neurotransmitters necessary for the nourishment and metabolism of nerve cells.

In general, the main function of majjā dhātu is communication. Because of majjā dhātu we have collective experience and the physical awareness of "This is my finger; this is my hand." Majjā dhātu brings all the organs together through conscious awareness. Through the motor nerves, majjā dhātu responds to stimuli. Through the sensory nerves, majjā dhātu carries the stimuli from the periphery to the center of the brain.

We have five senses—seeing, hearing, smelling, touching, and tasting. These five senses are carried by majjā dhātu from the peripheral organs to the center, where each sensation is interpreted. So, both sensory stimuli and motor response are carried by majjā dhātu. This dhātu is also responsible for the voluntary actions of the skeletal muscles and for the involuntary actions of smooth muscles. The cardiac muscle and the muscles of the gastrointestinal tract are governed by majjā dhātu via prāna.

The function of majjā dhātu depends upon sādhaka pitta, which is present in the gray matter of the brain tissue. The gray matter regulates the temperature of nerves and neurons. Within the cerebral cortex, which is rich in gray matter, the interpretation of sensory perception takes place. When you look at an object, the image that is formed on the retina is inverted. That image is carried as an optical sensation to the occipital cortex. Sādhaka pitta in the occipital cortex digests, absorbs, and assimilates that image and brings understanding.

Understanding is subtle neurological digestion and a process of assimilation. It is governed by majjā agni. Every experience and sensation carried to the brain is unprocessed and unmetabolized. In the brain, these unmetabolized sensations are processed and transformed into understanding.

Modern thought says that consciousness is the outcome of bodily existence. However, consciousness exists prior to a physical existence. Therefore, Consciousness Itself is the phenomenon that gives rise to the thought process we call neurotransmitter production, or stimulus response. Scientists do not want to accept Purusha (Pure Consciousness), which is the source of insight. They say there is some area of the brain that gives insight. But insight is not a thought process. It is just a "happening."

We create neurological images and psychological images. You have been looking at your wife for the last 10 to 15 years. You have a psychological image of her. That image is an experience recorded within the matrix of majjā dhātu on the sensitive film of tarpaka kapha. On that sensitive film, every good, bad, and ugly experience is recorded. This image-making machinery is present within majjā dhātu, the nerve tissue. The total number of images that you gather creates your own image. Your teacher has judged you, your father has judged you, and you have judged yourself. That judgment is conclusion and that conclusion is confusion. The moment you look at your wife based upon past experiences and past images, you will never understand her as she is now. This happens because within the matrix of majjā dhātu, we carry images that condition our experience. Thus, our perception becomes polluted by past images and that may be the reason why we do not see the truth.

The core of majjā dhātu is to create a feeling of "I am." We all carry an ego. Our ego is our culture, education, and background. What we have accumulated over the last 10,000 years remains within the matrix of our nerve cells. If we minutely observe, majjā dhātu is a material thing. Thought expresses as a material process (neurotransmitter secretion) that needs a medium in which to flow. That medium is majjā dhātu. The ego is another material process within thought, and the ego "creates" the thinker. In actuality, thought is a thinker and there is no separation between thought and thinker. We create a center and around that center, thinking is active. That center is the ego. In a sense, the ego is a bundle of material processes stuck within majjā dhātu, and the core of majjā dhātu is the crystallized, material process of the ego. Thought is a material process. Within that process, time as another material process begins, because thought needs time. Thought creates pathways within the neuron and thought shapes the brain. Intense thoughts of anger, fear, or grief can damage the pathways.

So because of majjā dhātu, you are you and I am I, she is she, and he is he. Majjā dhātu creates self-identity. If you do not have your own identity, that is agony. If you have identity, your majjā dhātu functions happily and strongly. When a teenager does not have identity it is difficult, because there is no psychological recognition. That is the way society functions. If you are recognized as an expert, people come to you. If you are not recognized, you are nobody. One of the functions of majjā dhātu, through recognition, through identity, is to nourish the ego. All these functions are governed by sādhaka pitta in majjā dhātu.

Anything that has form is bound by time and space and is therefore limited. Bliss has no form. In essence, you have no form. When Buddha's disciple went to Buddha, Buddha told him, "Bring your original face." So the man went and shaved his face. "No, not this face, your original face." The man said, "This is my original face. This is what I have." Buddha said, "This face is a false face. This is a mask." When you go home, you change your mask. When you go to the office, in front of the boss, you change your mask. So this face is unreal. It is a projection of your emotions, ideas, feelings, and sensations. This face is just a pseudo face.

The light of awareness is your true face. You face everything through awareness. Awareness that carries things from the last 10,000 years is your true original face. If you look at your own picture when you were a child, you were so different. When you became an adult, you had to change your face. It is all superficial and has nothing to do with your true face. The process of changing the face is not the real face; it is a phase of the face.

So, majjā dhātu, as the nerve tissue, has important functions. When majjā dhātu is absolutely healthy, there is clear perception, right understanding, and right comprehension. A majjā sāra person is bright, brilliant, intelligent, and has attractive eyes, because the eyes are related to majjā dhātu. But if there is too much āma in majjā dhātu, or if majjā dhātu is raw, unprocessed, then there is misunderstanding, misconception, confusion, delusion, and even hallucination. All these are unhealthy states of majjā dhātu.

Majjā dhātu is responsible for the tactile sensations of touch, pain, and temperature. It has the capacity to experience pressure and deep sensitivity. In this way, we understand touch, pain, temperature, pressure, and stereognosis (three-dimensional experience).

Awareness and Majjā Dhātu

When you are in a totally blissful state, you are not conscious of it. In real awareness, you are not aware that you are aware. The moment you are aware that you are aware, your awareness is gone. The moment you are conscious of joy, something goes out of it. When joy becomes the object of perception, only the ashes of joy remain. In a way, the meditative state is not a conscious act. Conscious meditation unfolds the unconscious state. Whatever we do as conscious meditation is still an act of will, an act of desire, the ego.

In a state of beauty, when you see a marvelous sunset or an extraordinary light behind a cloud, at that moment, you are in a blissful state. The beauty is not in the sunset. It is within you. But the sunset has the ability to unfold the beauty within you. Not everyone sees the sunset as beautiful. If you are in a sad mood, you cannot see the beauty of the sunset, because the perception of beauty is within you. A flower, the beautiful face of a woman, the marvelous face of a child; at that moment of beauty there is no observer. There is only pure awareness. There is no objective experience of beauty, but there is a total presence of beauty, without subjective or objective division.

The subjective comes when you identify. The root meaning of the word "identify" is "to consider as identical, to equate." So, it is based on a repetition of a previous experience. Then, through the process of identification, the subjective comes into being, and you say, "Oh, I saw a beautiful sunset. I hope I will see the same sunset tomorrow." Hope means desire, and then the beauty becomes desire.

Your objective experience is limited, because the objective is limited. Though your objective experience is vast, still it has boundaries. Bliss is a total, innermost subjective experience. Objective consciousness is absent. The moment you are aware that you are aware, then that awareness becomes the subject, the observer. When you are aware that you are happy, it is pleasure. In joy, there is more pleasure, but joy is not pleasure. Joy is a totally subjective feeling, because joy is your true nature. When joy is over, then you have the memory of that joy, and the remembrance of that joy is pleasure. Therefore, the root cause of all desire is the memory of joy. You can invite pleasure, but you cannot invite joy. Unfortunately, joy becomes sensory and many times, we think pleasure is joy. Joy and pleasure are not the same.

Awareness is our true nature, but our awareness is not total. It is fragmented and we are only aware of a fragment. When you are in pain, you are aware of the pain and the rest of your body is forgotten. The pain becomes an emergency. Meditation goes into the center of awareness. You come to the source of awareness and there is tremendous joy, bliss, beauty, and ecstasy. That is called samādhi. In samādhi you are not aware physically. Objective, physical awareness is totally absorbed into the subjective presence, into pure existence. You forget the presence of the body. In a deep sleep, you also forget the body, but deep sleep is not samādhi or meditation. Meditation transcends sleep into pure awareness.

The world is objective experience and samādhi is subjective experience. Modern science wants to prove everything objectively. But the teachings of Āyurveda say objectivity is limited. How can you read an individual based upon an objective barometer? Objectivity will give only a guideline. Both objectivity and subjectivity are necessary for understanding. There is a space where objectivity and subjectivity meet. That meeting point is called perception. Perception is awareness of where subjectivity merges with objectivity.

Majjā dhātu also gives a sense of vibration. If there is an earthquake, you know it is an earthquake because majjā dhātu transmits the sense of vibration. This dhātu in animals such as birds, dogs, and cats is quite sensitive. They know before an earthquake happens, because their majjā is more sensitive than ours.

Majjā dhātu is present from the brain to the surface of the skin. On the skin, there are contact receptors that convey messages, in conjunction with neurotransmitters. All neurotransmitters are sādhaka pitta and tarpaka kapha. Tarpaka kapha is the actual material that is necessary for building the neuron, the nerve cell. The nerve cell has a myelin sheath and that sheath is formed by tarpaka kapha. From one neuron to another neuron, an impulse is transmitted without losing the intensity of the impulse. On the contrary, the impulse is amplified within the synaptic space. The synaptic space is called *chidākāsh*. *Ākāsh* means space and *chid* means awareness. So within the space between two neurons are certain neurotransmitters. Neurotransmitters are necessary for carrying the impulse from one neuron to another neuron.

The autonomic nervous system, which is one part of majjā dhātu, is closely connected to the subconscious mind. The sensory and motor systems, another part of majjā dhātu, are under voluntary control and connected to the conscious mind. However, the ventricles of the brain are beyond conscious and subconscious.

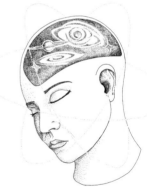

The inner space is one with the outer space.

The space within the cavity of the brain is synonymous with the vast outer space. When you enter that inner space through visualization, through awareness, you can feel that the inner space is one with the outer space. Then you literally begin to lose your physical consciousness and enter into subjective expansion. That is profound meditation.

The space of the spinal column opens into the fourth ventricle and continues into the third ventricle. Within the roof of both the fourth and the third ventricles, and the inferior horn of the lateral ventricle, are the choroid plexuses, from which cerebrospinal fluid is secreted. The horn of the lateral ventricle is called Ganga, the celestial river. There is a Ganga in India and there is a Ganga in your brain, which secretes sacred water, the cerebrospinal fluid. Majjā dhātu is surrounded by cerebrospinal fluid, which nourishes and protects the neurons. This fluid keeps the spinal meninges well lubricated so that they can absorb shocks from outside.

We use only one-tenth of our brain at a time. Meditation brings to use the unused part of the brain. But meditation should not be mechanical; it should be unstructured. To bring discipline you need structured meditation. To bring focus and attention you need structured meditation. Use structure for a short time and then go into pure unstructured meditation, because truth is unstructured. Ultimate reality is not a man-made, structural calculation. It is great order, and that order is virtue, which has a mathematical order.

Extrasensory perception is awareness beyond the sensory tract. In between you and me, there is a pranic current, a srotas. Just by looking at you, I can read your thoughts. Physically you are separate from me and I am separate from you, but we are connected by photons, by light particles. In the same way, extrasensory perception occurs when your awareness is functioning on the molecules of the lights that are within you and without you.

When you enter into the passive state of awareness, you suddenly pick up somebody's thought. That is called extrasensory perception. You can even communicate with trees and animals. ESP is the superfine function of majjā dhātu. There is even a global majjā connected to the global plasma, which is called cosmic *soma*. Extrasensory perception is possible when there is moment-to-moment awareness without choice. Choice is desire. Desire makes you choose, and choosers are the losers. This is important. Once you choose, you lose. There are times to choose and times not to choose. If you go to buy a refrigerator, you must choose. If you go to buy a shirt, you must choose. Judgment is choice and in these situations, choice is necessary.

However, if we bring judgment to our psychological fields, our relationships become difficult. We start measuring our wives, our husbands, our girlfriends or boyfriends, and these measurements are expectations. When expectations are not satisfied, relationships become frustrating. We expect them to be perfect. This kind of choice brings confusion. Here judgment is not necessary. Where to choose and where not to choose is intelligence. We must have right understanding, right judgment, but where? In the scientific and technological fields, we need choice, we need judgment. But in the psychological field, in daily relationships, it is harmful to judge or criticize.

The Chakra System. The chakra system comes under majjā dhātu and is also connected to the endocrine system. For example, *sahasrāra* is related to the pineal gland; *ājñā* to the pituitary; *vishuddha* to the thyroid and parathyroid; *anāhata* to

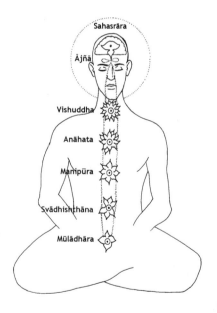

Sahasrāra

Ājñā

Vishuddha

Anāhata

Maṇipūra

Svādhishthāna

Mūlādhāra

the thymus; manipūra to the pancreas; *svādhishthāna* to the adrenals; *mūlādhāra* to the gonads. The chakra system is explained in detail in the section on Mano Vaha Srotas in chapter six, beginning on page 195.

By-products of Majjā Dhātu

The upadhātu (superior by-product) of majjā dhātu is *ashru* (lacrimation or tears). The mala (inferior by-product) of majjā dhātu are *akshi sneha* (oily secretions from eyes) and *vit sneha* (epithelial and mucous secretions that help discharge the bowel). Scanty lacrimal secretions in the eyes indicates inferior majjā dhātu. There are two tear glands in the eyes, located just above each eye. Small apertures, called the nasal lacrimal ducts, open from the eyes into the nose; therefore, whenever tears come into the eyes, they also go into the nose. That is why you blow your nose when you cry. The initial function of tears is to lubricate the eyeball and keep the cornea clean. The cornea cannot be exposed to the air. The moment the cornea becomes dry, we begin shedding tears. Blinking cleanses the eyes.

Where tears fall from the eyes, reveals whether they are of vāta, pitta or kapha origin. The tears of kapha are the tears of joy and happiness and they are sweet to the taste. They are scanty and they come from the outer corner of the eye. Tears of anger are hot and sour; they fall from the center of the eyelid and are related to pitta. Tears of frustration and intense grief are bitter and astringent to the taste, related to vāta, and fall from the inner corners of the eyes. (see illustration on page 64) Though tears come from the eyes, we never pay attention to whether they are tears of love, anger, frustration, or grief and sadness, but Āyurveda does.

Majjā dhātu tries to discharge emotions in the form of tears, so tears are liquefied crystals of emotions. Most of the time, we do not express our tears, our grief, sadness, and emotions. The moment you suppress your tears, a choking sensation occurs and an aching feeling in the throat chakra arises. Suppression of grief and sadness affects the pituitary and thyroid glands, leading to hypothyroidism due to kapha, hyperthyroidism due to pitta, or irregular thyroid function due to vāta. There is an emotional factor in the functional disorders of the endocrine glands.

Dreams

One of the important functions of majjā dhātu is to create dreams. Dreams are a discharge of the nerve cells, the drainage of incomplete thoughts, actions, and feelings. Many times thoughts come during our daily activities, but we are not completely aware of them. Any thought without total awareness

---

Vāta Dreams

Falling, being attacked, being pursued, doing something, sex, frozen with fright, death of loved one, being locked up, flying, snakes, autumn, fulfillment.

Pitta Dreams

Schooling, teaching, studying, sex, arriving too late, eating, fire, failing an examination, killing someone, being inappropriately dressed, being nude in public, summer, problem solving.

Kapha Dreams

Swimming, finding money, eating candy, sex, doing the same thing again and again slowly, arriving too late, seeing self as dead, snow, spring, winter, satisfy unconscious needs.

is an incomplete thought. The brain cells pick up that incomplete thought, and because incomplete thoughts stay in the brain cells, our brain has to complete these thoughts to restore order. One of the functions of majjā dhātu is to drain or complete our incomplete actions. In that way, dreams are necessary. In a dream, you finish unfinished business and the brain is able to restore order.

According to Āyurveda, dreams are classified as vāta, pitta or kapha. Vāta dreams are active, pitta dreams are fiery, and kapha dreams are romantic. Classify the dreams, then treat the dosha and you will see good results. Let us not separate the body from the mind, because body and mind are one. In a dream, the subconscious mind comes up. Many times, if you study the dreams, you will know the subconscious cause of a disease. Make a record of your dreams and try to analyze them as vāta, pitta or kapha. Do it for one month. Within that time you will discover the pattern of your dreams and how your majjā dhātu is functioning in your life and relationships.

Areas of the Brain with Their Functions

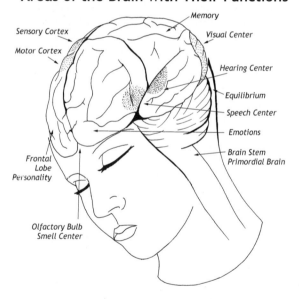

Sensory Cortex
Motor Cortex
Memory
Visual Center
Hearing Center
Equilibrium
Speech Center
Emotions
Brain Stem
Primordial Brain
Frontal Lobe Personality
Olfactory Bulb Smell Center

Disorders of Majjā Dhātu

In the material on the other dhātus, we talked in terms of increase, decrease, and dushti (disorder). The table "Signs and Symptoms of Majjā Disorders" on page 167 lists the signs and symptoms of increased and decreased majjā dhātu, but the text talks more in terms of vāta, pitta, and kapha affecting majjā dhātu. The signs and symptoms can be classified either in terms of the qualitative changes caused by each dosha, or in terms of quantitative changes, which are vruddhi and kshaya. Kapha is responsible for increased majjā dhātu, while either vāta or pitta may be responsible for decreased majjā dhātu. Dushti can be mono-doshic, dual-doshic or tri-doshic caused by the provocation of the bodily doshas—vāta, pitta, and kapha.

As we have seen, majjā dhātu is the seat of the conscious and subconscious mind. The frontal lobe of the brain governs the emotional brain. There are superior and inferior frontal areas and right side and left side. According to Āyurveda, the superior area governs vāta, the middle governs pitta, and the inferior governs kapha.

Anxiety, fear, and nervousness are located more in the vāta area. Anger, judgment, and criticism are in the pitta area. Attachment, greed, and possessiveness are found in the kapha area. How did the ancient rishis discover this? I do not know. They had no modern equipment but they did have great insight.

Vāta. If vāta becomes hyperactive in majjā dhātu, it creates certain signs and symptoms that later become neurological problems. Due to the aggravation of vāta in the nervous system, a person may become anguished and anxious. There may be nervousness, causeless fear, or fear of the unknown. In other individuals, there may be insomnia. Physically, a person may have tingling and numbness, muscle twitching, nervous twitching of the eyelids, or cold hands and feet.

Increased vāta in majjā can mean the perception becomes shaky and unclear, which may lead to dizziness. If prāna vāyu is affected, an upper motor neuron type of lesion may develop, leading to increased rigidity in the muscles. The muscles become rigid because of increased muscle tone, hypertonia. On the other hand, if apāna is affected, which creates a lower motor neuron type of lesion, the person has exactly the opposite effect—hypotonia, which is flaccidity. So, both rigidity and flaccidity are symptoms of vāta involvement.

One of the functions of majjā dhātu is to maintain the coordination of groups of muscles, thereby maintaining equilibrium and the center of gravity. Because of coordination, we can put food in our mouths, button our shirts, and perform many skillful actions. Ask a person to draw a straight line. If the line is zigzag, it means coordination is affected. Lack of coordination is also a vāta symptom. In addition, the reflexes become exaggerated. If you observe a Parkinson's patient, the knees, ankles, hips, and elbows are flexed and he walks like a

---

Causes of Majjā Disorders

Poor diet - especially excessive vāta provoking foods, such as dry foods, beans, and leftovers

Incompatible food combining

Physical trauma, such as a bone fracture

Hectic lifestyle and emotional stress

Conflict

Unresolved deep emotions

Extreme climatic conditions

Lack of sleep

Spiritual possession (energy field affliction)

High fever

Bacterial or viral infection

Cerebral concussion, compression, or contusion

Heavy metal toxicity

Radiation exposure

Alcohol, marijuana, tobacco, and other drugs

Any doshic disturbance that overstimulates or otherwise affects the nervous system

---

statue. It is difficult for him to stop, unless some chair or table stops him.

When vāta affects majjā dhātu, especially in the frontal area of the brain, a person may develop schizophrenia. In vāta type of schizophrenia a person is anxious, anguished, and hyperactive. He or she also has hallucinations, especially auditory or olfactory.

Disturbance of prāna is another factor in majjā dhātu dushti. If the gastrointestinal tract is clogged with āma (toxins), the person may have nightmares. Eating a late dinner may also cause nightmares, because the heavy food in the stomach blocks the flow of prāna. So, nightmares are due to blocked prāna in majjā dhātu.

Rapid eye movement (REM) is an extremely high vāta condition. When a person in sleep has rapid eye movement, it indicates dreaming. Every thought and emotion moves the eyeballs and the eyeballs can be very active. In meditation, keep the eyeballs still. When you keep the eyeballs still, your thinking becomes slow. So there is a connection between the speed of thinking and the speed of eyeball movement. REM is associated with anxiety, stress, nervousness, and insecurity, as well as with dreaming.

Observe the movement of the eye. If a person moves his eyes to the right when he talks, that means he is talking from intuition. If he moves his eyes to the left, it means he is engaging in intellectual or manipulative talk. Oscillating movement means the person is uncertain about what he is saying. Do not take seriously the person who moves his eyes, because he does not know what he is talking about.

Eye movements are motor actions. In addition, they are subconscious actions of your thoughts, feelings, and emotions. When you are looking into someone's eyes while he is talking and the person avoids looking at you, he is telling a story that is not true. Eyes are the windows of the soul. Very few people look directly into someone's eyes, especially in the West. To look into someone's eyes is scary, as if one were entering into the person's private space. But in India we look directly into the eyes. It is cultural.

Pitta. When pitta is affecting majjā dhātu, a person may develop polyneuritis, which is common in diabetes, with burning hands and feet. I have observed that if the grandmother or grandfather is diabetic, this condition may occur in the granddaughter or grandson. They may not develop diabetes but they may have polyneuritis, a pitta disorder.

Recently I saw a young woman, who came with the complaint of burning hands and feet, all polyneuritis symptoms. Her grandmother was diabetic. She went to a neurologist who recommended B_{12} shots, but they did not help. She had extremely high pitta. I gave her shatāvarī, guduchi, and *brahmī*, which reduced her pitta and successfully treated her symptoms. Sometimes if you treat the dosha, the symptoms simply disappear. Try to look at the problem with simplicity.

Excess pitta may create inflammation of the nerve endings. Neuralgia is pain along the track of a nerve. Trigeminal neuralgia is common in extremely high pitta/vāta people. Sciatica is also pain along the track of the sciatic nerve. So radiating or migrating pain along the track of a nerve means pitta is moving around the nerve. This condition happens frequently when majjā dhātu is affected by pitta dosha.

At the neuromuscular junction, pitta accumulates and waits for a situation in which to manifest. A person may suddenly get shingles (herpes zoster), which is a pitta condition. Herbs to help this condition include *gulwel sattva*, to pacify pitta, and *kāma dudha*, to reduce inflammation. Long-standing, lingering pitta in majjā dhātu attracts the virus of herpes zoster and a person develops that inflammatory change and burning pain along the track of a nerve. If the herpes moves along the nerve passage of certain subcutaneous nerves in the scalp, it may affect the optic nerve.

Herpes simplex is localized inflammation and stagnated pitta in the nerve ending. If a person has repeated attacks of herpes simplex, it affects the immunity of majjā dhātu. There is general immunity and localized immunity. A person with repeated herpes may have a history of mononucleosis, chronic fatigue syndrome, Epstein Barr virus, or may even develop AIDS, all of which are pitta. AIDS begins with pitta. We are looking at these modern labels with a different perspective. Please understand the significance of this. Sometimes these serious disorders can be greatly improved simply by treating pitta.

Pitta disorders of majjā dhātu are serious. In some people, extremely high rakta dhātu may affect majjā dhātu and create cerebral hemorrhage or cerebrovascular accident (CVA). A patient can die from a cerebral hemorrhage. If a patient is unconscious, look for a pinpoint pupil that does not react to light. That is serious and the patient's life is in danger. Pitta conditions of majjā dhātu can create extremely high risk factors. Hypertension, cerebral hemorrhage, cerebrovascular accident, cerebral embolism, and stroke paralysis begin in pitta and end in vāta.

A patient came to see me with sickle cell anemia, in which the red blood cells disintegrate and look like the sickle of a farmer. The condition is the result of extremely high pitta in the bone marrow. It is a genetic immunological disorder. We gave him tikta ghrita with *abhrak bhasma*. Within three months, his red blood cells regained their normal shape. In sickle cell anemia the red blood cells are disintegrated or deformed because of excess pitta in the red bone marrow, which is responsible for erythrogenesis. Abhrak bhasma acts on majjā dhātu (bone marrow) and on pitta.

Certain disorders, such as trigeminal neuralgia, begin with pitta and end in vāta. Stroke paralysis also begins as pitta, then manifests as vāta. Another example is demyelination, as seen in multiple sclerosis, which is excess pitta that burns the myelin sheath. As a result, the patient has more vāta symptoms—rigidity, difficulty walking, and muscle wasting. The person develops tiredness, tingling and numbness, and muscle fatigue due to sensitivity to extremes of both heat and cold. These are signs and symptoms of both vāta and pitta.

Āyurveda's language is the language of the tridosha—vāta, pitta, and kapha. Do not label a condition as trigeminal neuralgia, Parkinson's disease or herpes zoster. These are Western terms. We have to look at it in a simpler way—which dosha is out of balance, which dhātu is affected, which organ or system is involved, and which quality of the dosha is out of balance. Take the entire history, family and personal, and you will understand which dosha is involved. Āyurveda gives an approach of simplicity and treatment should be plain and simple.

Kapha. Excess kapha in majjā dhātu may create thickening of the nerves, which is a serious condition. A man came to see me with a thickening of the nerves of the skin and shiny skin. He had lost his eyebrows. I said, "This is the beginning of leprosy." Even today, there are cases of leprosy in this country. There are two types—tubercular and non-tubercular. The tubercular type is found in those who are resistant to the disease-causing bacteria; the other type is seen in those with little resistance. Kapha in majjā dhātu is serious business. When a patient of leprosy gets an ulcer, it does not heal. Even if a cigarette burns his finger, he does not feel it because there is a loss of sensation of pain. Vāta, pitta, and kapha, these three doshas together can create space-occupying tumors in the brain. Majjā dhātu is a deep connective tissue and disorders of majjā dhātu are quite complicated and difficult to cure.

Table 19: Signs and Symptoms of Majjā Disorders

Majjā Vruddhi (*Increased Majjā Dhātu*)	Majjā Kshaya (*Decreased Majjā Dhātu*)

Pineal and pituitary tumors
Neurofibromatosis (tumors on
   peripheral nerves)
Heaviness of eyes
General heaviness and
   sluggishness
Excess sleep
Hydrocephalus (accumulation of
   fluid in ventricles of brain)
	Osteoporosis (bone loss)
	Anemia
	Osteo- and rheumatoid arthritis
	Sexual debility
	Insomnia
	Neurological problems
	MS, Parkinson's
	Stroke paralysis
	Epilepsy
	Attention Deficit Disorder (ADD)
	Lack of understanding
	Poor communication

People do not know what to eat, when to eat, and how to eat. We must teach them Āyurvedic principles. A patient of mine came back to see me after some time. She said, "Dr. Lad, I came to you thinking that I would get some pill but I received philosophy instead. And amazingly, it works! I am dancing and happy." I asked her what her problem was. She said, "I had the beginning of a central cataract and the doctor says it is gone. I am so pleased. You saved me from an operation." Her diet was kapha provoking and she was a kapha woman. There were many kapha molecules in the lens of her eyes and she was developing cataracts. I told her to follow a kapha soothing diet and to squeeze the juice of one organically grown pomegranate seed into the eye. It burns for a while but then it feels soothing. That drop of pomegranate juice in the eye helped remove the kapha molecules within the tissues of the lens. Pomegranate is astringent and removes kapha. She now has clear vision. Even her doctor was surprised and asked, "What have you done?" She said, "Philosophy."

Āyurveda is a system of individual healing that treats the whole person. Modern medicine analyzes statistical observations and considers that which is common amongst a hundred people as the normal value or state. Based upon that normal value, modern medicine tries to judge every individual. However, Āyurvedic medicine says that normality varies from person to person, because every individual is a unique phenomenon.

Everything is waiting to catch your perception. But if you do not pay attention to something, that something does not exist for you. In awareness, there is no concentration. Concentration involves narrowing the mind. In concentration, you create a wall of resistance. The more you concentrate the more you become exhausted and lose energy. Although meditation begins with concentration, it is pure, all-inclusive attention and awareness. In awareness, you look at a chair, at the clouds, at the beautiful sky, or the lovely mountains. Nothing is rejected and everything is welcome. In that way, you receive tremendous energy. You simply jump into the inner abyss. In meditation, there is no concentration. You enter a dimension beyond perception. Perception is directed attention and, in meditation, there is no direction; you become vast like an ocean. When you become established in this state then even while driving a car, there is awareness. When painting a picture there is awareness. Your whole energy is painting the picture through your hand. Then your whole life becomes meditation. Eating food and walking with a friend become meditation. There is total action, which is freedom.

Mysticism is the perfume of life. Without mysticism, life becomes mechanical and a mechanical life is a boring life. Mystery and beauty go together. Life is a mystery; it is not a puzzle. A puzzle can be solved and understood. Then once you understand the puzzle, the puzzle is no more a puzzle. Birth, death, the breath and heartbeat are all mysteries. Mystery means to enter into the unknown. Those people who do not feel comfortable with mystery feel fear of the unknown.

We must not separate the body from the mind. Superfine molecules of majjā dhātu have the capacity to become aware moment to moment, enter into meditation, and go into ecstasy, causing mutation and transformation of the brain cells. The transformation of majjā dhātu is the transformation of the human being. If one looks at majjā dhātu only as nerve tissue, it becomes rigid and mechanical. One must see the energy aspects of majjā dhātu. Then it becomes complete.

Shukra and Ārtava Dhātus: Male and Female Reproductive Tissues

Shukra dhātu is the male reproductive tissue and *ārtava* is the female reproductive tissue. *Prajanana* means producing, generating, bringing forth and procreating. Both male and female reproductive tissues are specialized to produce a new life and their vital function is the continuation of the human species.

The pure substance of existence is the soul, ātman. You existed before your physical birth. You were born as a collection of a few atoms. Remember, before your birth the atoms of your body already existed. Whether you were born with a silver spoon, a golden spoon, or a plastic spoon in your mouth was your choice. You chose your parents according to karmic influence.

Jāyati means to be born. You begin to grow, *parināmati*. *Vardhati* means to grow to maturity. Then, as part of physical experience, we must finally die, *mriyati*. As psychological experience, we do not die when the body dies. Moreover, as spiritual experience, as pure ātman, we are beyond birth and death.

> Asti means existence.
> Jāyati means to take birth.
> Parināmati means to begin to grow.
> Vardhati means to grow to maturity.
> Mriyati means death.
> This is the flow of life.

Birth and death are the wheel of time in which we are all caught. Liberation means to go beyond the wheel of time, the cycle of birth and death. The body is objective experience and the mind is subjective experience. The soul is the otherness. In other words, the soul is pure consciousness, pure awareness, pure existence, pure presence.

One of the vital functions of the reproductive tissue is to create offspring. I like to call a sperm a subtle atomic cell. It is the male seed that is created in special organs called testicles. The ovum, the female egg, is created in the ovary.

In the formation of tissues, sthāyi rasa is formed within five days from āhāra rasa, which is formed within 12 hours after the ingestion of nutrients. Then in 10 days, sthāyi rakta is formed; in 15 days, māmsa; in 20 days, meda; in 25 days, asthi; and in 30 days, majjā. And it takes approximately 35 days after the ingestion of nutrients for sthāyi shukra or ārtava to be formed.

By-products of Shukra and Ārtava Dhātus

The upadhātu of shukra and ārtava is ojas. Ojas is produced during the nutrition of all the dhātus, but it is the by-product of shukra/ārtava dhātu in particular. This ojas goes to the heart and nourishes para ojas. Some people say there is no mala for shukra/ārtava dhātu, whilst others say that secondary sexual characteristics (pubic and axillary hair) are the mala.

Shukra Dhātu

Within the pouch of the scrotum, there are two testes. Before descending in the ninth month, they hang near the kidneys in the body of the male fetus. The testicles begin descending because of apāna vāyu, which is a downward pull that brings the testicles down through the inguinal canal into the scrotum.

When a male baby is born, the doctors and nurses check to see if the testicles are descended. If the scrotum is empty, the doctors are concerned. Within the first few days, the testicles must descend. Chronic undescended testicles may be one of the causes of sterility in a man. Abdominal temperature is high and under this high temperature, the testicles do not produce sperm. In order to produce sperm within the cavity of the scrotum, we need a temperature of .5 degrees lower than the visceral temperature. Therefore, nature has provided a small pouch between the thighs. If a man wears tight underwear and his testicles get heated by the temperature of the thighs, he may become sterile. Optimal temperature is needed in order to produce sperm.

The teachings of Āyurveda describe a number of interesting factors about the sperm. A sperm has a head, neck, body, and tail. Prāna, the life force, is present in the sperm. Apāna vāyu and vyāna vāyu are also present. Actually, the sperm has all 20 attributes, five elements, three doshas—vāta, pitta, kapha—and in microform has all seven dhātus, the seven tissues. There is also a mind and a presence of soul in the sperm—soul in the sense of pure consciousness. The sperm is the atomic cell of life. It is not a dead thing but is alive and vital. In addition, a sperm has the three qualities—sattva, rajas, and tamas—and contains ojas, tejas, and prāna.

In Sanskrit, the sperm is called shukra. The word shukra means white. The rishis have described shukra as liquid, unctuous, jelly-like, cool, with the smell of honey, and a sweet taste. Shukra is like ghee and ghee enhances production of semen.

The testicles contain seminiferous tubules, the epididymis and the spermatic cord. Within the wall of the seminiferous tubule is a kala, a membranous structure, called *shukra dhara kalā*. From here, the sperm are created. Agni is present there, consisting of enzymes, amino acids, and hormones.

Shukra dhara kalā becomes active at the age of puberty. Because of the maturation of its content, it produces male hormones that are responsible for the manifestation of secondary sexual characteristics, such as development of the beard and moustache, axillary hair and pubic hair.

Shukra dhātu is present throughout the body. There are seven layers of the skin, each with a name and a measurement. The deepest layer of the skin is connected to shukra dhara kalā. When someone touches you with great love, the touch creates a desire for sexual union. Shukra dhara kalā is also present in the

Shukra Dhātu

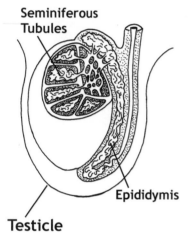

Seminiferous Tubules

Epididymis

Testicle

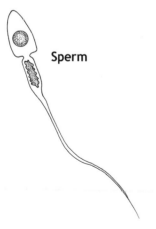

Sperm

eyes. Seeing a beautiful man or woman stimulates the desire for sex. Even smell is stimulating. Dogs have a highly developed sense of smell and, when a female dog is in season, the male dog senses that fact just by smell.

In the human body, every cell is a sex cell and sex governs the polarity of life. Sex is love, creativity, a dynamic life force, and it is present in you. Those who fight with sex do not understand the beauty of life. Celibacy is a great thing. You go beyond sex. But, some people, under the name of celibacy, suppress sex and become angry and violent.

So, sex is present all over the body. However, here we will concentrate on the seminiferous tubule, which is part of shukra dhara kalā. Shukra dhara kalā is rich in ojas. When immature sperm are formed, they are carried into the epididymis, and they stay there for 35 days. The epididymis is a pouch on the top and back of a testicle where newly born sperm are brought and stored to become mature. If you observe celibacy for 35 days, imagine how much strength and vitality you receive.

There is a mind and a consciousness in each sperm. When sperm become mature, they develop ojas. Ojas, located in the epididymis, sends electricity to the heart. Therefore, the heart is also a seat of ojas. A blow to the epididymis can kill a man, because it stops the heart. That is why striking someone's genitals is forbidden in martial arts.

The epididymis is the mother of sperm. The mature sperm pass from the epididymis through the spermatic cord into the prostate, another powerful gland, which secretes prostatic fluid. When sperm mix with prostatic fluid, it is called semen. Sperm need a medium in which to flow. Through the prostatic fluid, the sperm swim rapidly and pass through the urethra into the genital organ. When the sperm in the epididymis become mature, they create an incredible desire for making love. They send electromagnetic energy to the penis and the penis becomes erect.

When a man ejaculates, many millions of sperm are released. Only one is needed to fertilize an egg. If there are no spermicidal chemicals present in the vagina, sperm can stay alive there for up to seven days.

The coiled tubes of the epididymis are about six meters long (20 feet). Within that long tubule, new sperm are born every moment. When a sperm dies, it becomes bodily protein. A sperm is rich in fluid, protein, zinc, and also mercury. For that reason, in Vedic philosophy mercury is called the semen of Shiva.

Mercury is a most important metal. In Indian alchemy, mercury protects semen. It helps the maturation of sperm and gives vitality. Sperm is transformed into neuro-electricity so that a person receives intelligence. For that reason, if you observe celibacy for one month, your brain is charged with supreme intelligence. A person engaging in sex 10 times in a week depletes his body fluids, throws away his energy, reduces his memory, intelligence, and ability to concentrate.

Ārtava Dhātu

Shukra is cool and active, so it is predominantly kapha in structure, but moved by vāta. Ārtava, the female egg, is hot and passive, so it is more pitta. The orgasmic fluid secreted during intercourse by a woman is called female shukra, but the female reproductive system itself is ārtava dhātu.

The female egg contains prāna, apāna, vyāna, the 20 attributes, five elements, three doshas, and seven dhātus from the mother. The egg also contains the three universal qualities—sattva, rajas, and tamas. Additionally, there a mind and a presence of soul in the egg, in the sense of pure consciousness. The 20 attributes refer to those gunas we studied in chapter two. They are connected to the Western concept of biochemical synthesis of the main amino acids. All these ingredients are already present in microform in both male and female seeds. Without a female egg, the sperm cannot create new life. Without sperm, the female egg cannot create new life. Therefore, life is a creation, a union, between male and female energy.

Female eggs are formed in the ovaries. Cells called *ārtava dhara kalā* are present in the ovary. Agni is present in the kalā and that agni helps the creation of egg cells. The ojas of the female is also present within ārtava dhara kalā, along with tejas and prāna.

During ovulation, some women have pain, because apāna vāyu, ojas, tejas, and prāna, which are necessary for ovulation, become disturbed. If tejas is intense, the woman develops hot flashes, the nipples become sensitive, and there is tenderness in the breasts. If there is raw ojas within ārtava dhara kalā, the woman becomes emotional during ovulation. She retains water. The breasts become enlarged and tender. She becomes drowsy and craves sweets because of imbalanced kapha. If apāna vāta is provoked during ovulation, the woman develops low backache and muscle cramps. She has constipation, insomnia, anxiety, insecurity, nervousness, and fear of the unknown.

The ovaries are the primary organs of the female reproductive system. They serve a two-fold purpose: at maturity, they produce the ova (eggs) and also the hormones, estrogen and progesterone.

The ovaries are smooth and firm, similar to almonds in both shape and size. Located in the pelvic cavity, they are attached to the uterus at one end and float just below the ends of the fallopian tubes at the other. The ovaries mature in the fourth month of fetal development. There are approximately 400,000 follicles present in the ovaries at birth. However, less than 400 eventually mature into an egg during the reproductive period of a woman's life.

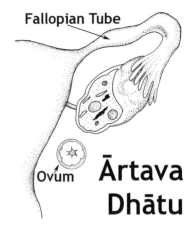

Fallopian Tube

Ovum

Ārtava Dhātu

The cortex of the ovaries consists of follicles at primary, growing, and mature stages of development. At ovulation, which normally occurs every 28 days, a mature egg ruptures from one of the follicles and is then drawn into one of the fallopian tubes. The fallopian tubes drape over the ovaries in tiny, finger-like structures called fimbriae. The fimbriae move in a wave-like manner and initiate a peristalsis that pushes the egg down the tube to the opening into the uterus. The uterus, a hollow, pear-shaped organ, holds and nourishes the fertilized ovum from implantation of the blastocyte until birth.

The mature ovum waits within the fallopian tube to meet the sperm. If the sperm doesn't arrive within five to seven days, the ovum dies. The dead ovum is discharged during menstruation. So menstruation is a funeral, a cry for dead ova. Again, a new endometrium is formed.

However, if the egg is fertilized, cell division begins. It reaches the two-cell stage within 36 hours and splits into four cells within 48 hours of fertilization. Cellular development continues and implantation in the lining of the uterus takes place at about seven or eight days after fertilization.

The other major function of the ovaries is to produce the female sex hormones, estrogen and progesterone. This process also begins at puberty. While the ovarian follicle is maturing in preparation for the rupture of the ovum (egg) from the follicle, it is secreting estrogen. Once the ovum has left the follicle, the corpus luteum, a small yellow endocrine structure, develops within the follicle and begins to secrete progesterone as well as estrogen. Estrogen is responsible for estrus and the development and maintenance of secondary sex characteristics. Progesterone is responsible for preparation of the uterus for pregnancy, the development of the placenta after implantation and the development of the mammary glands.

Causes of Shukra and Ārtava Disorders

Incompatible food combining
Having intercourse at midday or midnight, dawn or dusk
Retention of ejaculation
Over indulgence in sexual activity
Having several orgasms during one night
Having sex during the menses
Intense sex while under the influence of intoxicants
Violent or exotic sex in the wrong position
Use of chemical spermicides
Physical or surgical trauma, such as surgical intervention in the lower pelvic floor
Gonorrhea, syphilis, or herpes
Genetic predisposition to reproductive disorders
Following tantric sexual practices without proper guidance
Emotional stress and worry

The male and female reproductive organs have similar properties and functions. The only differences are that the sperm is alkaline and the vagina is acid; the sperm is cool and the ovum is hot; the sperm is active and the ovum is passive. In the higher state, Purusha is passive and Prakruti is active. What is active in the higher consciousness becomes passive in the lower atomic life. The harmony of creation continues to move.

Disorders of Shukra/Ārtava Dhātus

What are the causes of shukra dhātu dushti and ārtava dhātu dushti? The primary causes are sex at an inappropriate time and excessive sexual activity. An acceptable frequency of sexual activity varies from person to person, and season to season. However, Āyurveda says that sexual fluids take 35 days to be replenished, so it is important not to overdo sexual activity if ojas is to be preserved. The texts say that around once per month is the limit for a vāta person in autumn, whilst once a day can be good for a kapha person in winter. Sexual energy is sacred, and if people have sex for the sake of pleasure, or to satisfy a desire, they lose ojas. However, when two people truly love each other and, within that loving relationship, they make love with awareness, they can transform ojas into profound bliss.

Table 20: Signs and Symptoms of Shukra and Ārtava Disorders

Shukra/Ārtava Vruddhi (*Increased Shukra/Ārtava Dhātu*)	**Shukra/Ārtava Kshaya** (*Decreased Shukra/Ārtava Dhātu*)
Preoccupation with sex Increased desire for sex **Shukra only:** Excess semen flow with increased prostatic secretion but low sperm content Premature ejaculation Prostatic calculi **Ārtava only:** Premature orgasm Sterility Multiple cystic ovary	Low libido Sterility Pain during coitus Fear of sex **Shukra only:** Oligospermia (low sperm count) Impotence (failure to achieve or maintain erection sufficient to maintain penetration and coitus) **Ārtava only:** Primary sterility No ovulation

Conclusion

Sex is a profound energy. If you do not understand the value of sex, your life will be incomplete. There is a great deal of misunderstanding about sex in the West. Sex organs are connected to the root chakra, where kundalinī shakti is located. In other words, when kundalinī is stuck in the root chakra, a person becomes crazy for sex. If kundalinī moves downward, the person will masturbate and deplete his ojas. But when kundalinī moves upward, one can go beyond sex and sex can be transformed into samādhi. If you transform sex into pure love, you will become enlightened.

Remember, in sex you are experiencing *mithuna*. Mithuna is a better word than sex. The word sex is overused and misused in today's world. Mithuna means male and female energy merging together. We have a right brain, the female brain, and a left brain, the male brain. When the right brain is active, a person writes poetry, is interested in religion, and is filled with love and compassion. When the left brain is active, the person becomes analytical, logical, mathematical, calculating, ambitious, and competitive. The left brain is male energy and the right brain is female energy.

When your right nostril is active, you breathe better through the right nostril and the left hemisphere of your brain is active. You become more judgmental, critical, analytical, mathematical, and scientific. When your left nostril is breathing, you are filled with love and compassion and poetry flows through you. Right brain and left brain merge together in the limbic area, where there is a sex center, the primordial brain. Sex does not take place in the sex center, but it arises through the merging of the right and left hemispheres. At that moment of merging, there is a craving to meet the opposite partner.

Sex energy stimulates the pituitary gland, the pituitary gland stimulates the gonads, and sex hormones are produced—in the woman more estrogen, in the man more testosterone. As that energy develops, the heart beats faster. Even the thought of sex makes the heart beat increase, because of vyāna vāyu, prāna vāyu, and ojas. Then the breath becomes rapid; when you are in the midst of sex energy, you can breathe like a bull. Sex energy descends down to the organs. Then there is an awakening of the genital organs and an incredible craving to meet the partner. This happens in a fraction of a second.

There are descending tracts and ascending tracts passing through the spinal cord. Therefore, profound higher love energy descends down into the root chakra and becomes sexual desire.

Sex is the highest form of the lowest energy and samādhi is the highest form of the highest energy. Samādhi is a state of perfect bliss, tranquility, and joy. A person who has gone beyond the sex center can attain samādhi. If your sex center is blocked, twisted, or under stress, you can never attain samādhi. You have to do the homework first, to clean the kundalinī shakti which is stuck in the root chakra. *Tantra*, *yantra*, mantra, *mudrā*, and meditation are profound ways through which you can transform sex into a supreme state of awareness. These are sacred secret teachings that are taught only to the chosen authentic yogic student.

Many of our problems are rooted in sexual energy—male and female. Many classic psychological problems stem from imbalances of sexual energy. Most problems in relationships are connected to the root chakra and associated with shukra or ārtava dhātu.

6

Srotāmsi
The Bodily Channels and Systems

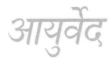

Introduction

We have examined the three biological organizations: vāta, pitta, and kapha. These doshas move from one part of the body to another along channels—both physical and energetic—called *srotāmsi*.[17] A srotas is like a river. The beginning of a river is small. This small beginning is joined by others and becomes a stream; the stream becomes a flow and the flow becomes an even larger current. It moves and meets many other rivers, becoming bigger and bigger. Finally, the river meets the ocean.

Similarly, in the human body there are many small srotāmsi and they come together to create a larger *srotas*. The largest srotas is called maha srotas, which is the gastrointestinal tract. Maha means large. Synonyms for srotas are *mārga* (passage), *nādi* (channel), and *patha* (path). The English word path comes from the Sanskrit word patha. Other Sanskrit words for specific srotas include *dhaminī* (arteries) and *sirā* (veins).

In the human body, a single cell under a powerful microscope reveals that it has porosities, which can also be

---

17. Srotas is singular and srotāmsi is plural.

called srotāmsi. Through these porosities, oxygen enters the cell carbon dioxide comes out, sodium ions go in, and potassium ions go out. These ions are electrically charged particles.

The body has many forms of srotāmsi. Capillaries are srotāmsi. The blood and nutrients, along with the plasma, mix in the capillary and come to the cell. Carbon dioxide from the cell passes into the capillary. In this way, gaseous exchange takes place within the capillary. The body itself is porous; even the skin has small openings. Near each hair there is a little duct called the sebaceous duct. These ducts form a channel called *sveda vaha srotas,* the channel that carries sweat.

A srotas is a passage, path, road, or highway. In addition to the gastrointestinal tract, other main highways include the respiratory, cardiovascular, auditory, nasal, and optic tracts. In ancient times, the rishis observed the human body as made up of billions and billions of srotāmsi. Organs are made of srotāmsi. An organ is organized systematically to perform certain functions, which are governed by the structure of the organ. The chakra system is also composed of srotāmsi. The central canal of the spinal cord is a srotas connected to the billions of srotāmsi all over the body. There is a srotas for each sensation. The srotas for hearing is the auditory pathway; for touch, the tactile pathway; for vision, the optic pathway; for taste, the gustatory pathway; and for smell, the olfactory pathway.

Each srotas has a *sroto mūla* (root), a *sroto mārga* (passage), and a *sroto mukha* (mouth or opening). For example, in the urinary system the kidney is the sroto mūla; the two ureters, the urethra and the bladder form the sroto mārga and the urethra opening is the sroto mukha. See "Srotāmsi, the Systems and Channels of the Body" on page 288 for detailed information on each srotas.

As seen from the table, the srotāmsi are: anna, the food carrying channel; prāna, the channel carrying prāna (the life force); ambu/udaka, the water channel; rasa, the plasma channel; rakta, the blood channel; māmsa, the muscle; meda the fat; asthi, the bones; majjā, the bone marrow and nerve tissue; shukra/ārtava, the reproductive tissue; purisha, the feces mūtra, the urine; sveda, the sweat; and mano vaha srotas, the srotas which carries the mind. There are three srotāmsi to receive—prāna, water, and food; seven srotāmsi to nourish and maintain the body—rasa, rakta, māmsa, meda, asthi, majjā and shukra/ārtava; and three to eliminate—urine, feces, sweat.

The other channels are stanya vaha srotas and rajah vaha srotas, which have structural confluence with ārtava vaha srotas but different functions—lactation and menses, respectively. However we will regard them as being part of ārtava. Stanya and rajah are also functionally related to rasa dhātu, as they are both upadhātus of rasa, but they are not regarded as part of rasa vaha srotas.

Srotāmsi	Channel
Anna Vaha Srotas	Food
Prāna Vaha Srotas	Prāna
Ambu or Udaka Vaha Srotas	Water
Rasa Vaha Srotas	Plasma
Rakta Vaha Srotas	Blood
Māmsa Vaha Srotas	Muscle
Meda Vaha Srotas	Fat
Asthi Vaha Srotas	Bones
Majjā Vaha Srotas	Marrow, Nerve Tissue
Shukra Vaha Srotas	Male Reproduction
Ārtava Vaha Srotas	Female Reproduction
Rajah Vaha Srotas	Menses
Stanya Vaha Srotas	Lactation
Purisha Vaha Srotas	Feces
Mūtra Vaha Srotas	Urine
Sveda Vaha Srotas	Sweat
Mano Vaha Srotas	Mind

The concept of srotas is both structural and functional. For example, dhātu srotāmsi are made up of the dhātus and are more structural, while mala srotāmsi are more functional. In some cases, the srotas itself, the flowing channel, is not obvious, as in the case of muscle, fat, bone, or even the reproductive system. We do not see the actual channels, but the ancient texts say they exist.

Even the mind has a srotas, called mano vaha srotas, and every thought or emotion has a micro-srotas within mano vaha srotas. If a person has intense fear, the mano vaha srotas is charged with fear and that eventually becomes disease. Mano vaha srotas is both structural and functional.

Sroto Dushti

All srotāmsi are made of dhātus and dhātus are nourished by srotāmsi. A defective space (*khavaigunya*) will primarily affect the dhātu or srotas, depending upon whether it is within the structure of the dhātu or a functional defect. Often it affects both. When a srotas is flowing normally, it is in a state of health. Disease begins if the srotas becomes imbalanced. Disease is often classified as inflammatory (which is pitta), infectious (pitta), congestive (kapha), anabolic (kapha), or catabolic/degenerative (vāta). However, we can also categorize disease according to four types of imbalance in a srotas.

Overflow of a srotas is one disease condition. The srotas begins flowing too much, as in the case of diarrhea, which is abnormal. The opposite of diarrhea is constipation, which is an example of stagnation. The feces do not move. Stagnation also includes varicose veins, blood clots, and tumors. The thickening of srotas, as in arteriosclerosis or enlarged lymph nodes, is also stagnation. Dilation means too much expansion or enlargement. The srotas can undergo a radical change and create a tumor, which is a localized dilation. If someone has varicose veins, the vein is dilated, as well as stagnated.

Table 21: Four Types of Sroto Dushti

Atipravrutti	Excess Flow, Overflow	Diarrhea, vomiting
Sanga	Stagnation, Accumulation	Constipation, blood clots, lymphatic congestion
Sirā Granthi	Dilation, Growth, Swelling	Tumors, diverticulosis
Vimārga Gamanam	False Passage	Bleeding gums, bleeding into lungs, pleurisy, fistula, perforation

Sometimes the content of a srotas goes the wrong way. This is called false passage. For example, edema or swelling results when plasma leaks from the blood vessels into the interstitial tissues. Other symptoms of false passage are bleeding gums or hematoma, in which the blood vessel is ruptured and blood accumulates under the skin. False passage also includes perforation, such as an ulcer.

When a srotas is affected, health is affected. Good health and balanced srotāmsi go together. For instance, when mūtra vaha srotas is filled with excessive fluid, the person wakes up at night to pass urine. If there is stagnation, a person may not pass urine for three or four days, which is a disease condition. Thickening of the srotas—such as thickened blood vessels walls or hardening of the liver—is also a disease condition, as is any dilation or tumor.

The four modes of sroto dushti (disorders of the channels) can be observed in our daily lives. The Āyurvedic student should pay attention to these various manifestations of sroto dushti. Diet, lifestyle, and emotional factors that provoke the dosha can affect a dhātu and disturb the normal function of a srotas.

Each dosha and doshic subtype has its own srotas. There is also a central channel from the crown chakra that is connected to the higher consciousness, which is an invisible srotas. In between you and me, there is also a srotas. Relationship is a srotas. When you give and take, when you understand, share your thoughts, feelings, and love, that is a srotas. When there is overflow or stagnation of srotas in relationship, both the relationship and the health will be affected.

Happiness is called *sukha*. Khā means space (ākāsha), *su* means healthy, clean. Where clean, healthy srotāmsi are present, one is in a state of sukha. The opposite of happiness is *duhkha*. *Du* means disturbed. If a person has deep-seated grief and sadness, he is not healthy, because there is duhkha and his srotāmsi are clogged with unhappiness, grief, and sadness. When there is fear, let it go. Keep channels free of fear. Do not let them stagnate or become suppressed. A suppressed srotas will create anxiety, insecurity, nervousness, and unhappiness. If the emotions do not flow properly, they stagnate and disturb the srotas. Therefore, diet, lifestyle, relationships, and emotions that provoke vāta, pitta, and kapha are bound to disturb the function of srotāmsi.

The Channels to Receive: Food, Prāna, Water

Anna Vaha Srotas: The Channel of Food

The first three channels—*anna vaha srotas*, *prāna vaha srotas*, and *ambu vaha srotas*—receive energy from the

Anna Vaha Srotas

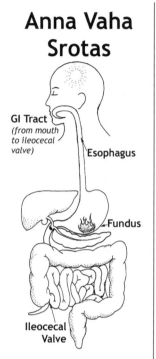

GI Tract
(from mouth to ileocecal valve)

Esophagus

Fundus

Ileocecal Valve

outside—water, food, and air. These channels are connected to outer energy. Prāna vāyu, udāna vāyu, and apāna vāyu are all connected to these three srotāmsi.

The first channel, the channel carrying food, is called anna vaha srotas. The mūla (root) is the esophagus and greater curvature of the stomach (fundus). The mārga (passage) is the gastrointestinal tract from the lips to the ileocecal valve at the juncture of the small and large intestines. The mukha (mouth or opening) is the ileocecal valve. Anna vaha srotas contains bodhaka kapha, kledaka kapha, prāna vāyu, udāna vāyu, apāna vāyu, samāna vāyu, and pāchaka pitta, in addition to the subtypes of vāta listed above.

Anna means food, vaha means to carry, and srotas means channel. This srotas starts with the mouth, lips, and tongue and then moves down to the laryngopharyngeal area. The larynx leads to the lungs and the pharynx leads to the esophagus, stomach, duodenum, jejunum, and ileum, and on to the ileocecal valve.

The tongue is the organ of taste, the teeth are responsible for mastication, and the esophagus carries the food into the stomach. They are all responsible for mechanical digestion. Digestion in the stomach is governed by kledaka kapha, pāchaka pitta, prāna vāyu, and jāthara agni. The liver is also important in the digestive process. We have discussed in the Agni chapter how the bhūta agni in the liver is necessary to transform food into living cells. Digestion in the duodenum is governed by rañjaka pitta, pāchaka pitta, samāna vāyu, and kloma agni (pancreatic juices). Samāna vāyu continues to predominate to the ileocecal valve. When the foodstuff comes into the ileocecal valve, apāna vāyu takes over in the astringent stage of digestion.

Usually, six or more hours are required for the digestion of a meal. There are six tastes (sweet, sour, salty, pungent, bitter, astringent), and each taste relates to a one-hour stage of the digestive process. Each taste nourishes rasa dhātu during its respective stage of digestion, resulting in rasa dhātu containing all six tastes.

The state of anna vaha srotas can be examined on the tongue. If the tongue is heavily coated in the back, that indicates āma in the colon. Indentations around the margins of the tongue show lack of absorption of minerals. If the central part of the tongue is coated, there are toxins in the gastrointestinal tract.

The lips, teeth, tongue, esophagus, stomach, duodenum, jejunum, ileum, ileocecal valve, liver, and spleen all need to be examined in the context of clinical evaluation. But here we are learning theory and philosophy.

Prāna Vaha Srotas: The Respiratory Channel

Prāna vaha srotas is the life-carrying srotas, the respiratory channel. The mūla (root) of prāna vaha srotas is the left chamber of the heart, which receives oxygenated blood from the lungs, and the maha srotas, the entire gastrointestinal tract. The mārga (passage) is the respiratory tract and the bronchial tree, including the alveoli. The mukha (opening) is the nose. The important organs in this vital air channel start with the nose, the nasal pharynx, the larynx, trachea, bronchi, bronchioles, and alveoli.

Prāna is located in the hypothalamus of the brain. Inhalation is governed by prāna. The intercostal muscles widen, the diaphragm descends, the air from outside rushes into the trachea, bronchi, bronchioles, and alveoli. Exhalation is udāna. Udāna vāyu pushes out the unwanted waste gases accumulated in the alveoli.

Carbon dioxide is necessary for the stimulation of respiration. However, carbon monoxide is quite toxic. Improper combustion in a fireplace, car, or someone's body can yield carbon monoxide, whereas carbon dioxide is complete combustion. If there is incomplete combustion of gases in your home, the accumulated carbon monoxide will affect your hypothalamus, stimulate your deep sleep center, and kill you. Carbon monoxide has no smell and is very dangerous. On the other hand, carbon dioxide stimulates the respiratory center.

There is agni in prāna vaha srotas, which maintains the lumen of the alveoli. Avalambaka kapha, prāna vāyu, udāna vāyu, and vyāna vāyu are present in the heart and lungs. Sādhaka pitta is in the heart and brain. All of these have functional integrity. Sādhaka pitta in the brain processes information and words into knowledge. Sādhaka pitta in the heart processes thoughts into feelings and emotions.

The transformation of food into energy and energy into vitality is governed by the digestive tract as well as prāna vaha srotas, the respiratory tract. In a way, you are blowing on the fire in the stomach by breathing. Because of respiration, the oxygen goes into the alveoli, mixing with the blood and becoming oxyhemoglobin. This is carried to the different tissues, organs, systems, and cells. All cells, tissues, organs, and systems breathe through the lungs. The lungs are not breathing for themselves but are breathing for all cells in the body.

Prāna Vaha Srotas

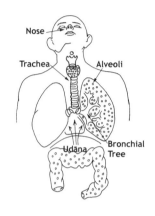

Prāna vaha srotas is also connected to the colon. In the Chinese system of healing, the lung meridian is connected to the colon meridian. If the colon is clogged, the lungs will not function properly. The lungs and colon are connected, because apāna vāyu in the colon, udāna vāyu in the lungs, and samāna vāyu in the intestines have functional integrity. Whenever the colon is clogged, the person develops bad breath. Cleansing the colon with basti (medicated enema) will improve breathing. Modern anatomy says there is no relationship between the lungs and colon. But functionally there is a relationship. During exhalation, apāna vāyu pushes udāna vāyu upwards. In that sense, the colon is functionally connected to the lungs and heart. Inhalation is prāna vāyu and exhalation is called apāna in yoga terminology. However, Āyurveda distinguishes udāna vāyu, which moves upwards and outwards, from apāna vāyu, which moves downwards and outwards. So exhalation is udāna vāyu in Āyurvedic terminology.

Ambu Vaha Srotas: The Channel for Water

Ambu vaha srotas is also called udaka vaha srotas. Ambu and udaka both refer to water. Ambu is also a name given to the deity Lakshmī. Ambu vaha srotas includes cerebrospinal fluid, salivation, gastric mucosal secretions, and the secretions of the pancreas. As there is a channel for food, the gastrointestinal tract, so there is a special channel for water called ambu vaha srotas. It is connected to the plasma (rasa dhātu), a liquid, watery tissue. There are subtle capillaries that are connected to the lymphatic system, blood vessels, and the mucosal membrane on the tongue, lips, and gastrointestinal tract. Around the gastrointestinal tract, there are blood vessels that constantly absorb water. Whenever water is lacking, salivation is stimulated.

The mūla (root) of ambu vaha srotas is kloma (the pancreas), *tālu* (the soft palate), and the choroid plexuses in the brain. The mārga (passage) is the gastrointestinal mucous membrane. The mukha (opening) is *vrukkau* (the kidneys or kidney glomeruli), *jihva* (tongue), and *roma kupa* (sweat glands).

The pancreas is called kloma in Sanskrit. The function of the pancreas is to digest the water component of sugar, the sweet taste. Sweet has Earth and Water elements, and the Water component is assimilated by the pancreas. In other words, the pancreas regulates blood sugar.

The choroid plexuses in the brain are related to kloma. They are venous plexuses that secrete cerebrospinal fluid, which enters the subarachnoid space and travels along the spinal

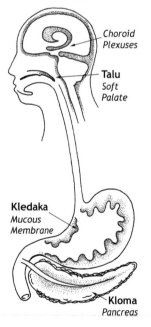

Ambu Vaha Srotas

Choroid Plexuses

Talu
Soft Palate

Kledaka
Mucous Membrane

Kloma
Pancreas

column. The entire brain is well protected by cerebrospinal fluid. This is all ambu vaha srotas. The kidneys and adrenals also play a secondary role in this srotas.

When the tip of your tongue touches the palate behind your front teeth, you are relaxing the choroid plexus. That action creates a uniform flow of cerebrospinal fluid along with the release of bliss molecules. Your entire body has molecules of bliss. That is a beautiful function of the cerebrospinal fluid. When you take your tongue off the roof of the mouth, then your lower chakras are activated which can lead to aggression or competition. When your tongue touches the roof of the mouth, your higher chakras are activated, balancing the flow of energy and unfolding a meditative quality in the mind.

Other important functions of ambu vaha srotas are to create lacrimal, nasal, and salivary secretions. Ambu vaha srotas is also connected to sveda vaha srotas, the channel of sweat, and mūtra vaha srotas, the urinary channel. Whenever you drink lots of water, you pass more urine or sweat, because that excess water cannot stay in the body. So mūtra and sveda are outlets of ambu vaha srotas.

There is agni in ambu vaha srotas. Whatever water you take in needs to be processed and digested. That digested water enters the plasma cells (rasa dhātu). If the agni of ambu vaha srotas is low, then unprocessed water accumulates in the interstitial cells and this leads to edema and swelling.

The Channels to Nourish and Maintain the Body: The Dhātu Srotāmsi

The function of the first three srotāmsi—anna vaha srotas, prāna vaha srotas, and ambu vaha srotas—is to receive food, prāna, and water from outer sources. We will now consider the seven dhātu channels that maintain the functions of the various bodily tissues.

Rasa Vaha Srotas: The Channel for Plasma

The first dhātu channel is the channel carrying rasa, called *rasa vaha srotas*. The mūla (root) is the right chamber of the heart and the ten great vessels. (see Appendix page 294) The mārga (passage) is the venous and lymphatic systems. The mukha (opening or mouth) is the arteriole-venous junction in the capillaries. Veins carry deoxygenated blood to the right chamber of the heart. Then from the right chamber the blood goes to the lungs for oxygenation. All oxygenated blood goes to the left chamber of the heart through the arteries. The left

Rasa Vaha Srotas

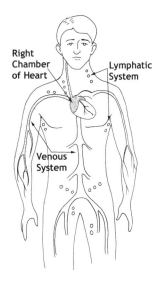

Right Chamber of Heart

Lymphatic System

Venous System

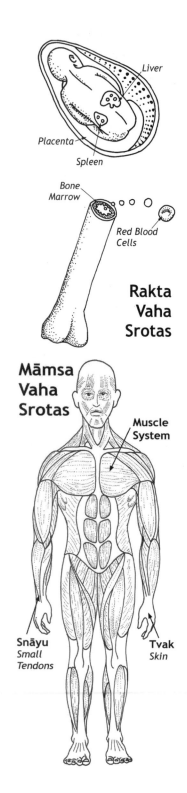

Rakta Vaha Srotas

Māmsa Vaha Srotas

Liver

Placenta

Spleen

Bone Marrow

Red Blood Cells

Muscle System

Snāyu Small Tendons

Tvak Skin

chamber of the heart is connected to prāna vaha srotas and the right chamber is connected to rasa vaha srotas.

Rasa vaha srotas is made up of rasa dhātu so it includes plasma, serum, the cardiovascular system and the lymphatic system. The doshic subtypes associated with this srotas are kledaka kapha, bodhaka kapha, avalambaka kapha, tarpaka kapha, prāna vāyu, vyāna vāyu, and sādhaka pitta.

Rakta Vaha Srotas: The Channel for Blood

The second dhātu channel is *rakta vaha srotas*, the channel carrying blood. The mūla (root) is the liver and spleen. The mārga (passage) is the arterial circulatory system. The mukha (opening or mouth) is the arterial-venous junction. Rakta vaha srotas includes the red blood cells, the heart, liver, spleen, bone marrow, and arteries. In the body of the fetus, the blood is formed through the liver and the spleen. The moment the child takes its first breath, the function of the liver and the spleen changes and the production of red blood cells becomes the function of the bone marrow. Doshic subtypes related to rakta are kledaka kapha, avalambaka kapha, prāna vāyu, vyāna vāyu, and rañjaka pitta.

Māmsa Vaha Srotas: The Channel for Muscle

The channel carrying nutrients for the muscle tissue is called *māmsa vaha srotas*. The mūla (root) is *snāyu* (in this case the superficial fascia and small tendons) and *tvak* (the six layers of the skin), plus the embryological mesoderm. The mārga (passage) is the entire muscle system. The mukha (opening or mouth) is the pores of the skin.

The epidermis of the skin is related to rasa dhātu, the dermis is rakta dhātu, and the third layer of the skin is particularly related to māmsa dhātu. When the skin is massaged, the muscles relax. So there is some functional integrity of these skin layers with māmsa. For that reason, the skin, fascia, tendons and ligaments are connected to the channel for the muscle tissue. The doshic subtypes related to māmsa vaha srotas are kledaka kapha, avalambaka kapha, prāna vāyu, apāna vāyu, vyāna vāyu, and rañjaka pitta.

Meda Vaha Srotas: The Channel for Fat

The channel carrying nutrients for the fat tissue is called *meda vaha srotas*. The mūla (root) is the omentum and adrenals. The mārga (passage) is the subcutaneous fat tissue. The mukha (opening or mouth) is the sweat glands. (see illustration page 192) Sweat is a by-product of meda and is also included in this srotas. The doshic subtypes associated with meda vaha srotas are kledaka kapha and avalambaka kapha.

This srotas is connected to and rooted in the adrenals and kidneys. (see illustration page 191) The adrenal cortex regulates fat metabolism. All anabolic steroids increase fat in the body. Adrenocorticotropic hormone (ACTH) secreted from the anterior pituitary gland and the hormones secreted from the adrenal cortex have functional integrity. A person who suffers from nervousness and insecurity goes on eating and eating, which stresses the adrenals. Fat metabolism changes and the result can be either obesity (excessive meda) or inadequate meda dhātu.

Meda vaha srotas is also associated with and rooted in the omentum, an extension of the abdominal lining (peritoneum) that drapes over the stomach and intestines like an apron where fat accumulates. Whenever examining meda vaha srotas, be sure to evaluate the omentum as well as the adrenals. If the tone of the abdominal muscle is diminished and the muscle is flabby, the person will appear obese. Fat also accumulates on the lower back, hips, thighs, and buttocks.

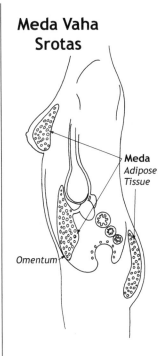

Meda Vaha Srotas

Meda *Adipose Tissue*

Omentum

Asthi Vaha Srotas: The Channel for Bone

The channel carrying nutrition for the bone tissue is called *asthi vaha srotas*. The mūla (root) is the pelvic girdle and sacrum. The mārga (passage) is the skeletal system. The mukha (opening or mouth) is the nails and hair. This srotas is connected to the bones and joints.

In examining asthi vaha srotas, examine the nails and the hair, because they are waste products of the bones and the mukha of this srotas. If bones become brittle, the nails become brittle. If bones become fragile, the hair and nails become fragile and the person loses hair. The doshic subtypes corresponding to this srotas include kledaka kapha, avalambaka kapha, shleshaka kapha, prāna vāyu, apāna vāyu, and rañjaka pitta.

Asthi vaha srotas is affected by not enough exercise or by excessive exercise such as heavy weight lifting and intense, irregular, and improper physical activities such as jogging, jumping, mountain climbing, hiking, skiing, or physical trauma. Vāta provoking food, such as black beans, pinto beans, adzuki beans and raw vegetables in addition to leftover food will also affect this srotas. Menopause can also contribute to its imbalance. On an emotional level, loneliness, lack of support, and insecurity will affect asthi vaha srotas. Because bones are porous and need the pull of gravity, astronauts in space lose bone tissue. Bones contain Earth and Air. Earth helps build bone and being in space makes the bones fragile.

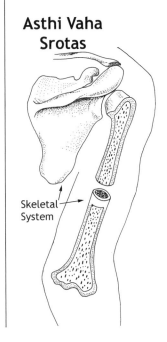

Asthi Vaha Srotas

Skeletal System

Majja Vaha Srotas

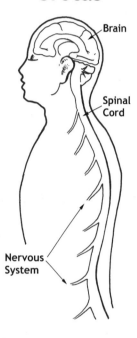

Brain

Spinal Cord

Nervous System

Ārtava Vaha Srotas

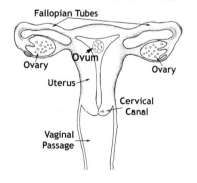

Fallopian Tubes

Ovary

Ovum

Ovary

Uterus

Cervical Canal

Vaginal Passage

Majjā Vaha Srotas: The Channel for the Nerves and Bone Marrow

The channel carrying nutrients for the bone marrow and nerve tissue is called *majjā vaha srotas*. The mūla (root) is the brain, spinal cord, joints, and the junctions between dhātus. The mārga (passage) is the central, sympathetic, and parasympathetic nervous systems. The mukha (opening or mouth) is the synaptic space. This srotas includes cavities of the bone, such as the auditory cavity and the spinal column. It is also connected to the emotions and to lacrimation, which is present in the eye orbit. Therefore, there are tears of fear, anxiety, nervousness, anger, and frustration.

Rañjaka pitta is mainly present in the liver and the spleen. However, after a child is born, rañjaka agni is present in the bone marrow, while majjā dhātu as nerve tissue is connected to sādhaka pitta for comprehension. Apāna vāyu and vyāna vāyu are present in the bones. The channel carrying bone marrow contains kledaka kapha, avalambaka kapha, prāna vāyu, vyāna vāyu, sādhaka pitta, and rañjaka pitta.

Majjā vaha srotas also includes the nervous system, brain, spinal cord, and sensory and motor nerves. Their major function is to bring communication and to maintain the flow of intelligence and coordination. The governing doshic subtypes in majjā vaha srotas as nerve tissue are prāna vāyu, sādhaka pitta, and tarpaka kapha.

Shukra/Ārtava Vaha Srotas: The Channel for Reproductive Tissue

The channel carrying nutrients for the male reproductive tissue, the sperm, is called *shukra vaha srotas*. The mūla (root) is the testicles and the nipples. The mārga (passage) includes the vas deferens, epididymis, prostate, urethra, and urinogenital tract. The mukha (opening or mouth) is the urethral opening. Apāna vāyu is connected to this srotas. (see illustration on page 52 and page 170) The channel carrying nutrients for the female reproductive tissue, the ova, is called *ārtava vaha srotas*. The mūla is the ovaries and areola of the nipples. The mārga includes the fallopian tubes, uterus, cervical canal, and *yoni* (vaginal passage). The mukha is *yoni oshtha* (the labia).

The channel carrying sperm contains kledaka kapha, avalambaka kapha, prāna vāyu, apāna vāyu, and ojas. The channel carrying ova contains more heat, more tejas, because the ova are hotter than the sperm. The by-products of rasa dhātu—stanya and rajah (lactation and menstruation)—are functionally related to ārtava vaha srotas. Reproduction and pleasure are functions of both shukra and ārtava vaha srotas

Drinking a cup of hot milk at night immediately nourishes shukra in men and stanya in women through rasa dhātu agni.

Rajah Vaha Srotas: The Channel for Menstruation

Rajah vaha srotas and ārtava vaha srotas have structural confluence, but their functions and fields of action are different. The fields of action for ārtava vaha srotas are primarily the ovaries, fallopian tubes, and the fundus of the uterus. Rajah vaha srotas is more connected to the fundus of the uterus, endometrium, cervical canal, and the vaginal passage. The function of rajah vaha srotas is to clear away the unfertilized ovum and prepare the uterus for the next cycle. If fertilization does not occur, the endometrium begins to shed and bleed, leading to menstrual flow. Rajah vaha srotas matures at puberty and, when fertilization does not take place, it is responsible for menstruation. Rajah itself is a by-product of rasa dhātu. After each menses, it creates a new endometrial lining. The old endometrial lining, along with the dead ova, are washed away by rajah vaha srotas.

Stanya Vaha Srotas: The Channel for Lactation

Stanya vaha srotas, the channel carrying nutrients of lactating tissue, is present in both breasts. There are different lactiferous (lactation) glands (the mūla, root), which are connected via the lactiferous ducts (the mārga, passage) to the nipple (mukha, opening or mouth) like a honeycomb. Along with ārtava vaha srotas, this srotas becomes mature at the time of puberty, when the girl develops secondary sexual characteristics, such as pubic hair, axillary hair, and development of the breasts. However, this srotas becomes active only after the delivery of a child. When the fetus is growing, stanya vaha srotas is growing. Within a couple of days after delivery, lactation begins.

Kledaka kapha, avalambaka kapha, vyāna vāyu, prāna vāyu, and udāna vāyu are related to this srotas. Their job is to create lactation. Lactation (stanya) and menstruation (rajah) are both by-products of rasa dhātu. When a mother is lactating, she does not menstruate and when she stops lactating, she begins menstruating.

Channels of Elimination: Feces, Urine, Sweat

Purisha Vaha Srotas: The Channel for Feces

The channel carrying feces is *purisha vaha srotas*. The mūla (root) is the cecum, rectum, and sigmoid colon. The mārga (passage) is the large intestine. The mukha (opening or mouth) is the anal orifice. The channel of feces contains kledaka kapha, pāchaka pitta, rañjaka pitta, and apāna vāyu. Purisha vaha

Stanya Vaha Srotas

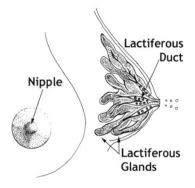

Nipple

Lactiferous Duct

Lactiferous Glands

Purisha Vaha Srotas

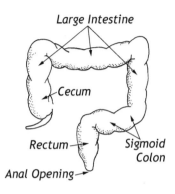

Large Intestine

Cecum

Rectum

Anal Opening

Sigmoid Colon

srotas is also called *mala vaha srotas*. Both purisha and mala mean feces, vaha means carrier, srotas means channel.[18]

As we have seen, the digestive tract opens through the ileocecal valve into the cecum. The cecum is the second stomach where food rests for awhile. The appendix opens off the cecum and secretes certain chemical enzymes to maintain the flora of the cecum and to destroy unwanted bacteria. Hence, the appendix is called the abdominal tonsil. It has its own protective function. The appendix secretes enzymes that are necessary for the digestion of legumes (beans etc.) and grains. If you do not have an appendix, go easy on beans, because gases form more easily.

Purisha vaha srotas includes the cecum, ascending colon, transverse colon, descending colon, sigmoid colon, and rectum. Apāna vāyu governs the activities of purisha vaha srotas, which accumulates the end products of digestion, or unessential foodstuffs, called *kitta* in Sanskrit. Kitta also means feces.

When the rectum is full of feces, apāna vāyu sends a message to the brain, the brain sends a message to the autonomic nervous system and mass peristalsis starts from the ileocecal valve, creating pressure to push out the feces. The feces are thrown out in the morning or in the evening, depending upon lifestyle, the quality of food eaten, and the way food is chewed.

There are some lucky people who wake up in the early morning to the call of evacuation. Some unfortunate people have to have an enema just to move the stool. Some partly fortunate and partly unfortunate people have to smoke a cigarette, drink coffee, or eat a meal before they can have a bowel movement. One should have a bowel movement before the sun rises. Constipation creates āma and affects the mind, leading to negative thinking.

Why don't people have regular bowel movements? First, they do not exercise. Exercise is necessary for the elimination of feces. We must bring discipline into our lives. Discipline is most important and brings energy and positive thinking. People develop constipation because their diet habits are irregular. Some days they eat breakfast and some days they do not. Some days they eat less, some days they eat too much. They also eat at the wrong time. Today in America, lunch often means a business lunch. Constipation is also due to not eating sufficient

18. Please note that Purusha and purisha are different. Purusha means higher consciousness and purisha means feces.

roughage. People eat bleached flour, white bread, and no whole grains. Eating whole grains, sprouts, and greens help the colon to move.

Āyurvedic literature speaks a great deal about the examination of the stool. Just examine whether the stool is well formed or whether it is like whipped cheese with no form, indicating poor assimilation. If a person is passing undigested food, his digestion is poor. Undigested food makes the stool heavy.

You may ask if floating stools are good or bad. A healthy stool without toxicity (āma) floats and that is good. A stool with toxins (āma) sinks to the bottom. That is not healthy. If there is severe āma, it sticks to the bottom. However, undigested fat in the stool also makes it float and that is not healthy either. The heaviness of the feces depends upon the quality of the food and the toxins present in the stool.

Generally, in vegetarian people the stools are light, whereas if a person eats meat, the feces will be heavy and sink. Both āma and undigested food are heavy, so the stool becomes heavy and sinks. However, undigested food can also undergo fermentation and the gases formed can make a stool light so that it floats. Floating of the stool and sinking of the stool are connected to the quality of the food and the quality of digestion and of agni (digestive fire).

Mūtra Vaha Srotas: The Channel for Urine

The next srotas is *mūtra vaha srotas*. The mūla (root) is the kidneys. The mārga (passage) is the ureters, urethra, and bladder. The mukha (opening or mouth) is the opening of the urethra. The channel carrying urine, or mūtra, involves kledaka kapha, avalambaka kapha, apāna vāyu, and rañjaka pitta. When someone with diabetes eats sugar, kledaka kapha sends the sugar to the kidneys.

Water consumption is regulated by the kidneys. Excess water is excreted through the urine, a liquid waste filtered through the kidneys. There is a connection of the colon mucous membrane to the kidneys. Excess liquid from the colon is absorbed through the colon mucous membrane and excreted in the urine.

The color of the urine changes according to water intake and the type of food eaten. For example, beets will create red urine. Vitamin C, folic acid, and the B vitamins accumulate rañjaka pitta, which is yellow in color, and so these substances color the urine yellow. In liver disorders, such as jaundice or hepatitis A with icterus (jaundice), the urine is dark yellow in

Mūtra Vaha Srotas

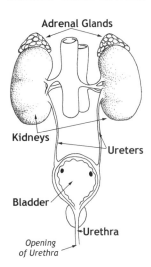

Adrenal Glands

Kidneys

Ureters

Bladder

Urethra

Opening
of Urethra

color. When blood passes through the urine because of trauma, the urine becomes red. Body wastes from the plasma are also excreted through the kidneys.

Sveda Vaha Srotas: The Channel for Sweat

The channel carrying sweat is called *sveda vaha srotas*. The mūla (root) is the sweat glands. The mārga (passage) is the sweat ducts. The mukha (opening or mouth) is the pores of the skin and the opening of the sweat glands under the skin. This channel is closely related to meda dhātu (the fatty tissue), the sebaceous glands, and the skin. Whenever examining sveda vaha srotas, be sure to also examine the sweat glands, fat, sebaceous glands, and the texture of the skin. The subtypes present are kledaka kapha, pāchaka pitta, rañjaka pitta, bhrājaka pitta, and vyāna vāyu.

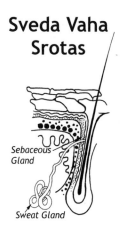

Sveda Vaha Srotas

Sebaceous Gland

Sweat Gland

There is skin all over the body and on the skin there are small hairs. Near the root of the hair, there is a small hole that is connected to a small sweat gland. Sweat is a by-product of meda dhātu and it helps to remove impurities from the plasma.

Bhrājaka pitta under the skin maintains the proper temperature of the skin by producing sweat. If the body is too hot, the person sweats and that cools the body down. If it is too cold, the sweat glands constrict and the body temperature is maintained. Sweat is a liquid, oily substance that keeps the skin soft and moist. It also strengthens the hair roots.

There is a connection between sweat and urine. If a person urinates in excess, then he or she sweats less. If someone sweats excessively, there is less urination. The same thing happens in regard to the seasons. People sweat a lot in summer and therefore do not pass much urine. In the winter season, they sweat less and urinate more. Sweat indirectly regulates water electrolyte balance and blood pressure. Too much sweating reduces blood pressure. No sweating increases blood pressure. If a person with low blood pressure sweats excessively, he or she may pass out, because of a drop in blood pressure.

Sveda vaha srotas is affected by exposure to the sun, working in hot temperatures, and eating sugar and salt beyond one's requirement. Alcohol and hot, spicy food also affect sveda vaha srotas. Sweat is connected to anger. If a person has repressed anger, hate, and envy, his sveda is affected by pitta. If a person has deep-seated fear, anxiety, and insecurity, his sveda is affected by vāta, and becomes constricted. Anger creates hot sweat, whereas fear creates cold sweat, or else the person does not sweat and gets dry skin. Daily application of oil all over the body keeps sveda vaha srotas balanced and relieves anger, fear, and anxiety. When you take a warm shower after this application of oil, your skin, kidneys, and colon are nourished.

Mano Vaha Srotas: The Channel of the Mind

Mano vaha srotas, the channel of the mind, is a complex srotas. The mūla (root) is the heart (cardiac plexus) and the ten important sensory pathways. These are five bilateral pairs, one pair for each of the five senses. The mārga (passage) is the entire body. The mukha (opening or mouth) are the sense organs (ears, skin, eyes, tongue, and nose) and the marmāni, energy or acupressure points.

According to Āyurveda, there is *vibhu* mind, which is the universal mind, and there is *anu* mind, the individual mind. In India, five thousand years ago, the rishis discovered that there is a universal unified field of the mind. Modern Western psychologists also believe there is a universal mind. There is mind in everything, living and non-living, organic and inorganic. However, the state of consciousness differs for various things. For example, the mind of a rock is as if in a deep coma. Rocks have feelings and expressions and, if one is aware, one can sometimes sense that a rock feels happy, sad, or perhaps frightened or angry. However, one must have an open mind to perceive these emotions. It is beneficial to develop one's intuition, the mystic aspect of the mind.

States of Mind

The teachings of Āyurveda describe five different categories of a person's state of mind. The first type is called *mūdha*. Mūdha means idiotic or mad mind, a mind that is deluded or hallucinates. This type of mind is rigid in outlook and opinions. The second type is *kshipta*. Kshipta means an active mind. Like a butterfly that flies from flower to flower, this type of mind flits from idea to idea. When prāna becomes agitated, the mind becomes kshipta, hyperactive. Such a mind is like a free bird flying high in the sky of imagination.

The third type is *vikshipta*. Vikshipta is partly active and partly inactive. It is evidenced by a lack of clarity and focus. One moment this kind of mind is heavy and slow and the next moment it is active. The fourth type is *ekagra*. Ekagra means one-pointed or focused mind. It is the mind that solves a problem, reads a book, or probes deeply into a subject. The last type of mind is *mukta*, completely free and liberated. A mukta mind is attentive, aware, and liberated. Such a mind is blissful. A person who is enlightened is called *mukta ānanda*. Such a person is in a blissful state and every moment is a moment of meditation. Each person is born to become mukta. It does not

matter how much money is in one's bank account. It does no
matter how many university degrees one has. It is al
meaningless without a mukta state of the mind. To attain the
mukta mind is the ultimate goal of human life.

Some people may have a problem trying to distinguish
between mūdha and mukta. How do we tell whether we are
experiencing cosmic consciousness or are simply mad; seeing
the angels or just hallucinating? To the mūdha mind, mukta is
mūdha. There is a clear-cut distinction between mūdha mind,
the mad mind, and the mukta mind, the liberated mind. Who
understands the liberated mind? Only a liberated person.
According to worldly views, it appears that mūdha and mukta
are the same. But mukta mind is for liberation and mūdha mind
is used for sex, power, prestige, and position in society. Mūdha
has inferior goals and mukta has profound and superior goals.
Mukta mind is described more extensively in the section on
Universal mind, but first we must understand the functions and
properties of the individual mind.

Manifestations of the Mind

Mano vaha srotas has different manifestations. The
crystallization of the mind is the body. The mind is subjective
experience; the body is objective experience and the materia
world is objective experience. Because of the differen
frequencies of images, experiences, thoughts, and emotions, the
mind manifests into different layers or *koshas*. Kosha also means
sheath.

The most basic sheath of the mind is called the *annamaya
kosha*, the sheath of food, and is equated with the physica
body. Anna means food and the physical body needs food
water, and air. Maya means "made of." Outward from this
kosha is the electromagnetic field of the body. It is called
prānamaya kosha, the sheath of prāna or vital essence. It is also
known as the etheric body. This electromagnetic field is six
centimeters away from the skin. As one moves away from the
surface of the skin, this field becomes fainter and fainter and,
after two feet, it merges into universal space. Approximately one
foot six inches away from the body begins the *manomaya
kosha*. It is one of several layers directly related to the mind,
called the mental body. Manomaya kosha is related to manas,
the sensory and emotional mind. The term astral body is
generally given to a combination of the prāna kosha and the
mano kosha, which together relate to the emotional nature of a
person. Approximately two feet away from the body is the
kosha of *jñāna*, the sheath of knowledge. This sheath is often
incorporated into the next (*vijñāna*) kosha. Three feet away

from the physical skin is *vijñānamaya kosha*, the sheath of the intellect, buddhi. This is usually termed the causal body. And about three-and-a-half feet away from the body is *ānandamaya kosha*, the kosha of bliss or bliss body.

These koshas—anna to ānanda—are vibrations of the mind and the mind operates in them through a central canal. This central canal runs from the center of the head to three-and-a-half-feet above the crown, where a person is connected to the universal mind. At that point, there is a meeting of the universal mind and the individual mind. A line passing from that center goes through the spinal cord to the tip of the tailbone, extending out below the body. Along this central line, from the tip of the tailbone to the crown, is the chakra system, which is also included in the srotas of mind.

The Koshas (Sheaths) of the Body

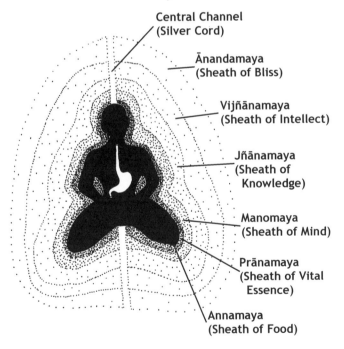

Central Channel (Silver Cord)

Ānandamaya (Sheath of Bliss)

Vijñānamaya (Sheath of Intellect)

Jñānamaya (Sheath of Knowledge)

Manomaya (Sheath of Mind)

Prānamaya (Sheath of Vital Essence)

Annamaya (Sheath of Food)

Chakras, Koshas, and the Mind
The fundamental chakra system consists of seven energy centers aligned along the spinal column. These energy centers, sometimes called wheels of light, are non-physical links between body, mind, and spirit. Each of the seven major chakras acts as a repository of information and experience about the individual.

The root chakra holds every experience related to the person's survival and position, the second carries information about procreation and prestige, and the third contains experiences that raise issues of control and ambition, which is power. The fourth is the seat of "me," the seat of love. However, this love in the heart chakra is not sexual love. It is a profound, emotional, compassionate love. The throat chakra is the power of communication and expression. The sixth chakra, the third eye, is where alpha meets omega. The sixth and seventh, the third eye and the crown chakra, are places of bliss.

Table 22: The Chakras and the Koshas

Chakra Name	Related Kosha	Function
Mūlādhāra (Root chakra)	Annamaya	Survival, Groundedness
Svādhishthāna (Second chakra)	Prānamaya	Procreation, Self-identity, Self-esteem
Manipūra (Third chakra)	Manomaya	Ambition, Achievement, Power, Control
Anāhata (Fourth chakra)	Jñānamaya	Love, Immunity
Vishuddha (Fifth chakra)	Vijñānamaya	Communication, Will
Ājñā (Sixth chakra)	Ānandamaya	Alpha meets Omega, which is intuition
Sahasrāra (Seventh chakra)	Beyond the koshas	Self Realization, Bliss

Each chakra is connected to a kosha: The first chakra is connected to the annamaya kosha, the food sheath, relating to survival; the second to prānamaya kosha, and to self identity; the third to manomaya kosha, relating to ambition; the heart chakra relates to *jñānamaya kosha*, to the "me" and emotional love; the throat chakra to vijñānamaya kosha, relating to communication; and the sixth chakra to ānandamaya kosha, to the third eye and bliss. The crown chakra is beyond the koshas of the mind.

The channels of the mind are connected to the autonomic nervous system in the body, which is also related to the chakra system. In addition, the chakra system is connected to the endocrine system: the root chakra to the gonads or ovaries; the second chakra to the adrenals; the third to the pancreas; the fourth to the thymus; the fifth or throat chakra to the thyroid and parathyroid; the sixth or third eye to the pituitary; and the crown chakra to the pineal.

Perception, Awareness, and the Mind

Pure awareness and consciousness, when reduced to sensation, perception, and thought, become the mental faculties. The mind comprises two main components. Manas is the sensory mind, which includes perception, thinking, and emotion. Buddhi is the intellect. Buddhi includes the faculties of *dhī* (cognition), *dhruti* (retention), and *smruti* (memory). The mind is a movement of prāna, which is necessary to create perception, the product of the mind. There is a mind in every cell, the cellular mind, and a center of awareness is also present in each cell. The flow of awareness from one cell to another is intelligence and that flow of intelligence is called prāna. At what level does the universal mind become the individual mind? It is the buddhi or individual intellect that performs the process of recognition. The moment buddhi recognizes an object, the universal mind becomes the personal, individual mind.

In pure awareness, there is attention, but the flow of attention takes place through the mind. The mind causes the attention to flow in a particular direction and that direction is called perception. When manas touches the object of perception and perceives the quality of that object of perception—its color, shape, and form—these attributes are carried by manas into the inner faculty of buddhi, intellect, where recognition takes place. Buddhi is subtler than manas.

The mind is absolutely necessary in order to experience anything. Experience means to go through, to become that. The moment you eat sugar you become one with the sugar and experience the sweet taste. The moment you eat cayenne pepper, your mind becomes cayenne pepper—hot, sharp, penetrating, and burning—and you have that same experience. Your mind becomes one with the object of perception, whether it is olfactory, gustatory, optical, auditory, or the tactile perceptions of touch, pain, and temperature. Therefore, to know is to become. We need experience because experience is the food of knowledge—little experience, little knowledge; more experience, more knowledge. Therefore, experience nourishes knowledge and knowledge is experience. There is no knowledge without experience, there is no experience without the mind, and there is no mind without the movement of attention.

In a classic story, there was a beautiful house and the master went away for a vacation, telling the servant to take care of the house. Within a few weeks, the servant became the master of the house, as if the master did not exist. Exactly the same thing happens with us. In our bodies the mind rules, as if the master is absent. When the master is absent, then the mind creates madness and unfocused activity. The moment the master returns, the mind becomes focused, the mind is mukta. You are the perceiver of the mind, because you are pure soul. However, you are in the prison of identification. You identify with the body even though the body is not you. You are not the hand, you are the mover of the hand. In the same way, you are not the mind, you are the mover of the mind, the master of the mind. Unfortunately, it is often the case that the servant becomes the master and the master becomes the servant.

Individual Mind and Universal Mind

The individual mind is constantly thinking, inquiring, and investigating. Manas experiences through the senses. Emotions, feelings, sensations, and thinking are the normal functions of manas. Based upon conclusions of the buddhi, manas creates a goal. A goal is a desire for becoming somebody, so a goal is the product of desire. If it is a positive desire, the goal is positive. If it is a negative desire, the goal is inferior or neurotic.

The mind also has the capacity for conclusion and judgment. These are functions of the buddhi. The mind gathers experience into a faculty of the mind called smruti (memory), the mother of knowledge, where we store experience and knowledge. Then, based upon stored knowledge, we create an image about the self or others. This image nourishes ego, which is nothing but image.

The mind is a material process within consciousness. Anything that can be recognized is a material process. If we say that consciousness is a container, then the mind is the content. Similarly, we can see the mind as a container and thoughts, feelings, and emotions as the content. The senses are agents of the mind. The senses do not have consciousness themselves, but the mind yields knowledge from the interaction of the senses.

The particular mind is a mind that is always judging, evaluating, recognizing. The moment this particular mind drops its measurement, its process of judgment, then it is vibhu, the Universal Mind. The Universal Mind is the common ground of existence, the Ground Mind. The Ground or Universal Mind further evolves into passive awareness, which is Purusha. But the moment the Universal Mind judges, it becomes the particular mind, and this particular mind suffers through its process of recognition and judgment.

Can the Universal Mind perceive? Vedānta says, yes, the Universal Mind perceives and the particular mind also perceives.

The difference between the perception is that the Universal Mind is non-judgmental and unconditional, whereas the particular mind has judgment. As long as we are in the particular mind, we are in division and darkness. Within this darkness and division, there is much suffering.

One can listen to the statement that there is no darkness or division. Hearing that statement from an enlightened person brings some clarity and helps to dispel my darkness. When such a person speaks, one can hear in the darkness. The statement that there is no division helps me wipe out my darkness. A tiny beam of light begins to penetrate. That is what a mantra does. A mantra is a word coming from the heart of a wise person. This person says, "There is no division." That statement helps to wipe away the center of darkness. It is a glimpse of the light. Then I have to meditate upon it and the spark becomes a wave. Then this particular mind is no longer a particular mind. It becomes universal and the light is glimpsed. The moment the glimpse becomes a constant phenomenon, the person is enlightened. We have glimpses of enlightenment, just a flash of light. When there is flash after flash after flash, it becomes constant. The light becomes broader and more encompassing. It begins to pulsate in our very being.

Our concept of light is as the opposite of darkness. Still this is a division—darkness and light. However, light hugs both darkness and light. We think in terms of dualism, but it is both things simultaneously. Twilight is neither darkness nor light. In twilight, one sees the form of a human being, but can't identify the person, which means there is no recognition. The moment you recognize, you belong to the division.

Sānkhya says that mind is *tanmātric*. This world is also tanmātric. When I look at an object, this particular mind senses its tanmātrās (objects of the senses) and takes the tanmātrās of that object's appearance and brings them back to Purusha. In the Sānkhya system, the tanmātrās are the "atoms" of the elements and activate the senses when prāna goes out to engage them. The mind goes and touches an object in the form of tanmātrās, through the action of prāna. Through that conjunction there is exchange of tanmātrās. The flow of prāna carries the tanmātrās to the senses, to manas, to buddhi, to ahamkāra, and eventually to Purusha.

You exist here, but at the same time you exist in non-existence. I smell a flower and I walk away to try to smell the flower from a greater distance. I can smell the flower from a certain distance, but if I walk one more step, I enter into the non-existent field of the flower. As long as I can smell the flower,

I am in touch with the existential *gandha* (smell) *tanmātrā* of that flower. The moment I walk further away, I enter into the non-existential gandha tanmātrā of the flower. When the particular mind's gandha tanmātrā meets with the flower's gandha tanmātrā, that meeting changes the tanmātrā of both. The observer influences the object and the object also influences the observer. The individual's tanmātrās create certain pathways, located in the individual mind.

Mano vaha srotas is also connected to the Universal Mind. Insight is the meeting point of the individual mind with the Universal Mind. The Universal Mind doesn't need to learn. It is vast, pure knowledge—Mahad, Supreme Intelligence. But the individual mind needs to go through much practice to develop that communion with the Universal Mind. If the individual mind operates without judgment, recognition or division, then the individual mind becomes the Universal Mind.

Mind in the Lower Three Chakras

When the mind is working through the root chakra, the mind will work for survival, food, and position. When the mind is working through the second chakra, it is concerned with self-identity and procreation. When the mind is operating though the third chakra, its concerns are ambition, power, control, competition, and achievement.

These three chakras are the lower chakras. They belong to the animal nature. Animals need food, sleep, and sex, and we also need food, sleep, and sex. In the root chakra there is sex manifesting as the highest form of the lowest energy. Every animal has self-identity and also has power, ambition, and control. There is an alpha monkey who controls the other monkeys and even with fish, one fish leads and the other fish follow. The leader and follower relationship is animal nature. As long as we need a leader to lead our country, we belong to animal nature. As long as we are looking for a leader, our consciousness belongs to the third chakra of power and control.

From mūlādhāra to sahasrāra is a journey of the mind. In mūlādhāra, the first chakra, we work day and night to pay the bills for survival. Many people simply work for that and die. Others may come from the second chakra and work not only for survival but also for self-identity. In the third chakra a person becomes a leader, who nevertheless is still in animal nature.

Heart Chakra: Bridge to Higher Consciousness

Pure human consciousness is the heart chakra, the bridge between the lower three and the higher three chakras. Love is in the heart chakra but this love has nothing to do with sex. When you are charged with love energy and your mind is working through the root chakra, you will end up with sex. If you are filled with love energy and your mind is working in the second chakra, you will work for self-identity. If you are filled with love and your consciousness or mind is working through the third chakra, you will have ambition and desire to achieve.

Love in the heart chakra is beyond sex. It is pure love for humanity and devotion, or bhakti. In the heart chakra, the heart center, there is a small window. If you meditate at the heart chakra and open that window, you will see light within. There is a little staircase to climb from the heart to the throat chakra. When you enter the heart chakra and go to the throat chakra, you gain the art of communication, the power of speech and expression. When the heart chakra is open, you listen to the music of life and dance with inner music. When you sit for meditation and your heart chakra is open, your body automatically starts swaying. Then you can listen to the sound of one hand clapping. When your heart chakra is open, you can read other people's minds, because the heart chakra is a bridge between the inner world and the outer world. This is an important chakra. The pure "me" is located here. Jīva (the "me") is seated in svādhishthāna, but moves into the heart to feel and think. It moves into the vishuddha chakra to communicate with others.

The Mind and the Higher Three Chakras
When your consciousness is working at the throat chakra, whatever you speak is true. You will touch the hearts of people through your throat chakra and your words will be filled with love and compassion. When your female energy is awake and your throat chakra is open, you become a singer. When your male energy is open, you become an orator.

When consciousness is operating through the third eye, the male and the female merge and cross the center line of the body. The third eye is the place where alpha meets omega. The third eye is an important springboard from which one can jump into the inner abyss. But this is not jumping as into a swimming pool, which is a descending action. Jumping into the inner abyss is an ascending action. One uses the third eye as a springboard to jump upward. Pranic energy from the toes rises to the third eye, where prāna meets with tejas and tejas uses ojas to expand consciousness. Then a person's entire body can become numb. This numbness is not a neurological symptom but is called *vairāgya*, which means true prosperity.

In your inner abyss, you become light to yourself. There you can see the golden egg and the head of kundalinī shakti, the cobra. On the head of the cobra, there is a beautiful blue pearl, the pearl of spiritual wisdom. The shining light of this pearl does not need a wick, nor does it need fuel. It is the flame of life, light, and love. It is a smokeless flame, bright, brilliant, and luminous, and it gives light within and without.

States of Awareness

The ending of the mind happens in the crown chakra. Your daily operating mind must be understood. To look at your mind means to observe your thinking; to observe what you are sensing; to be completely aware of your feelings and emotions, of your goals, your conclusions, your experiences, your image, and your tiny ego. Then you become aware of the watcher and the watched. That is witnessing, pure awareness. All your idiosyncrasies, questions, and even your mind disappear. As long as you are questioning and inquiring, you are not in the highest state of bliss.

It is good to inquire and investigate. However, if you spend your entire life inquiring and investigating, you will never reach the ultimate purpose of life. Some pitta people spend their lives inquiring—changing gurus, mantras and relationships—and they end up with confusion and lack of clarity. Still they inquire. They burn their ojas with excessively high tejas, which can lead to mental imbalance and fanaticism. This is not to say that one should not inquire. Make inquiries. At some point, it is time to stop inquiring and jump into the faculty that is inquiring, which is the inquirer. Then the mind ends and one enters into bliss. Such a mind in the blissful state is called vibhu, universal.

The Universality of Mind

We all have separate bodies, separate thoughts and separate emotions, but thinking as a whole is universal. Mind is not personal but is universal. Unfortunately, we identify ourselves with mind. Therefore, my mind becomes separate from your mind. This division between mind and mind is the division between human and human, between one religion and another, between one nation and other nations. Linguistic division, racial division, national division, and economic division are based on the dividing mind. Division is the root cause of confusion, conflict, and war in this world.

We are the world and the world is us. There is conflict and fear in us, therefore there is conflict and fear in the world. The world is a screen where we project our pictures. If we change and project love and peace, the world will change. People try to change the world without changing themselves. Only when we change will the world change. When we are full of love and compassion, loving and compassionate people will come to us and our world will become different.

Disorders of Mano Vaha Srotas

Greed, anger, envy, pride, self-importance, ambition, competition, and comparison all adversely affect mano vaha srotas. People become dishonest with their feelings and emotions and carry a mask on their faces. This is a cause of psychological problems, when we are not honest people. The moment we realize our minds are deceiving us, that very realization brings a radical change.

If we do not look at ourselves as we are, if we look through someone else's eyes, we will never know ourselves. Self-knowledge is not like learning chemistry or biology. Learning about ourselves requires watching the total movement of our consciousness at every moment. This action is real meditation and it demands awareness, sacrifice, and discipline. Discipline means to learn, not to imitate. Imitation is a lie. Discipline is the first step in dealing with a psychological problem. The second stage is to bring clarity in your relationships, both living and non-living. Your relationships with your mother, father, wife or husband, children, brother, sister, and friends, as well as your relationship with your own thoughts, feelings, emotions, and goals, must all be absolutely clear. That clarity is the greatest discipline.

This is the beginning of mano sāra. Sāra means essence. A mano sāra person is a person whose mind is healthy and sane. He is capable of looking at himself without judgment, criticism, and without listening to others. When your mind is sāra, pure and healthy, it is in meditation. Such a mind has clarity and clarity breeds compassion for all. Wherever such a mind goes, there is samādhi.

A mano sāra person may not be intelligent. He or she may not have a degree from a prestigious university or be a highly skillful person. However someone who is mano sāra is a person whose mind is sane, healthy, compassionate, spiritual, and meditative. A meditative mind can use logic with compassion. Compassion is the fruit of meditation. Logic has no compassion, but compassion can use logic. Logic has no wisdom. We need logic and we need intellect. We also need love and compassion. According to Āyurveda, we must use intellect and knowledge with love. Āyurveda is the science of love, intuition, and intellect. A mano sāra person maintains a balance of the physical and spiritual worlds.

Witnessing Awareness

The mind is the only sense organ that has the capacity to see itself. The ears cannot hear themselves. The eyes cannot see themselves, unless there is a mirror. The tongue cannot taste itself. Nevertheless, the mind can see itself. It has double-arrowed attention. The mind can look outside and, at the same time, it can look inside. In the kingdom of the senses, the mind is king. Mind has the capacity to choose and is a powerful instrument of experience.

Right from this moment, bring discipline and watch the mind. Watching the mind means looking at your thoughts as they are, looking at your feelings and emotions as they are, without identifying them as "this is my fear, this is my thought." Without identification, justification, evaluation and notification, you can see a clear-cut gap between two thoughts, a space between two memories, a distance between two emotions. In that space, there is a door. Enter into that door.

Thought is like a lingering cloud in the sky of consciousness. You are not the cloud; you are only watching the cloud. In between two clouds, there is a vast space. Remember that no cloud can stay in the sky. In the same way, no thought can stay in the consciousness. Just sit quietly or lie on the floor and watch the total movement of thinking. Let the mind think what it wants. It may think about good things or bad things. It does not matter; do not judge. Just observe the thinking. When you go on observing your thinking in this way, within one week you will see that thinking becomes slower. You can clearly see a space between two thoughts. If you enter that space, you will forget your body and your problems and you will be in a dynamic space.

Take care not to name it. The vast, incredible, immeasurable space is your true nature. Your true nature is endless and boundless existence. Live in the present, in the state beyond time and aging, which can be reached through sensitive awareness. You can remain in that vast space 24 hours a day. External sounds—the cry of a child, the barking of a dog, or a musical sound—all come into the ear and dissolve. You become the center of the whole universe, the whole existence, the whole presence.

To maintain such a state is pure love. When you are in the state of love, it is joy and bliss, which is your true nature. The molecules of bliss start flowing into your body. All disease is wiped out. You can achieve radical transformation of your brain cells simply by watching the movement of your mind at every moment.

Mano vaha srotas is profound, because it has its root in the universe and its fruit in the heart of every human being. Your heart, the fruit, and the universe, the root, merge together. Then you flower. The flowering of bliss and love takes place when the fruit and the root merge together.

Conclusion

We have studied the srotāmsi from the viewpoint of body, mind, and spirit. We studied 16 channels—three to receive, seven to maintain, three to eliminate urine, feces, and sweat, mano vaha srotas for the mind, plus stanya vaha srotas and rajah vaha srotas, which are present only in women. There is one last thing I would like to convey about srotāmsi. Diet and lifestyle that supports the dhātus and balances the doshas also allows a healthy flow in the srotas. For instance, a pitta person eating a pitta pacifying diet and maintaining good tissue nutrition will have healthy srotāmsi. The same is true for vāta and kapha types. Functional integrity of the doshas, dhātus, and srotāmsi, including mano vaha srotas, is the basis of good health.

Chapter Six

7

Ojas, Tejas, Prāna

आयुर्वेद

The three doshas are combinations of the five elements. Ojas, tejas, and prāna are the subtler, energetic forms of the doshas. As with the tridosha, ojas, tejas, and prāna are comprised of all five elements. However, each relates to the more subtle of the two predominant elements that make up the corresponding dosha.

⁕ Ojas is the pure essence of kapha dosha, and of the Water element in particular.

⁕ Tejas is the pure essence of pitta dosha, and of the Fire element in particular.

⁕ Prāna is the pure essence of vāta dosha, and of the Ether element in particular.

Ojas, tejas, and prāna should all be at an optimal level, which corresponds to the doshic prakruti. In the same way, ojas, tejas, and prāna can each be disturbed by quality (dushti), decreased in quantity (kshaya), or increased in quantity (vruddhi). In addition, they can be displaced, which is called *visramsa*. (see "Disorders of Ojas, Tejas, and Prāna" on page 287)

Ojas

Ojas is the essence related to vitality and immunity. It is like honey. As the honeybee collects the minute molecules of the essence of hundreds of flowers and accumulates them in the honeycomb, ojas, the pure essence of all bodily tissues, circulates via the heart and throughout the body to maintain the natural resistance of the bodily tissues. Ojas fights against aging, decay and disease. A person who has good ojas rarely becomes sick.

Ojas is a superfine biological substance, and the biological strength of the tissues depends upon it. Ojas is not a poetic or romantic concept, it is a protoplasmic, biological substance that includes albumin, globulin, and many hormones. It is formed during the biosynthesis of bodily tissue, that is, during the creation of the sthāyi dhātus. As ghee is the pure essence of milk, in the same way ojas is the pure essence of the dhātus (tissues). In the churning process to make butter, agni (heat and electricity) is created and it ionizes and separates the molecules of butter from the milk. By further heating the butter, the pure essence, which is ghee, separates. In the same way, the end product of digested food plus agni creates the nutritional precursor called āhāra rasa.

This āhāra rasa is then transformed into rasa dhātu, during which rasa by-products and ojas are also created. It is the tejas of rasa agni that separates out the pure essence of rasa (rasa sāra), the other by-products (lactation, menstruation, top layer of skin, poshaka kapha), and ojas. The same process occurs in all bodily tissues, because every dhātu has the capacity to create its own ojas. The ojas present in a single cell or dhātu is known as localized ojas. Collective ojas is the name given to the pure essence of all dhātus. If the ojas of a particular dhātu is depleted, its dhātu agni will be affected, because the ojas of a dhātu supports agni in the dhātu dhara kalā.

Modern medicine talks about the immune system, which includes the hematopoietic, endocrine, nervous, and digestive systems. The Āyurvedic concept of ojas corresponds to the modern medical concept of the immune system, including gamma globulin, which maintains the immunity of the liver.

Ojas also includes the endocrine, nervous, skeletal, muscular, hematopoietic, and digestive systems. When all these systems perform their physiological functions, ojas is maintained. Therefore, ojas is the potential source of strength, power, and natural resistance against illness, which is called natural immunity.

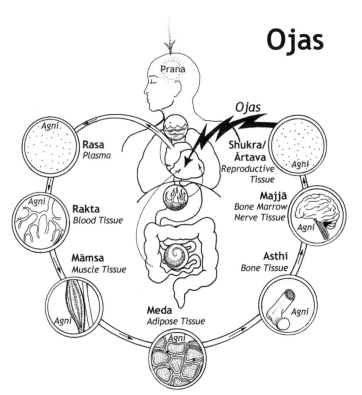

Ojas

Prana

Ojas

Rasa
Plasma

Shukra/
Ārtava
*Reproductive
Tissue*

Majjā
*Bone Marrow
Nerve Tissue*

Rakta
Blood Tissue

Asthi
Bone Tissue

Māmsa
Muscle Tissue

Meda
Adipose Tissue

Agni

"Ojas is the pure essence of all bodily tissues."

Immunity depends upon the quality of digestion, the quality of liver function, and the integrated function of all hormones in the endocrine system. There are two types of immunity—natural or inborn immunity and acquired immunity. When you receive a vaccination against smallpox or polio, that is acquired immunity, which is not ojas. Ojas is the natural resistance to fight infection.

Every disease has a capacity to cause disorder that depends upon how acute the infection is, the number of tissues involved, and the strength or weakness of the tissues. The disease process is classified as acute, sub-acute, or chronic. Disease can also be classified as due to internal causes (such as repressed emotions) or external causes (such as working all day under the hot sun). The strength of ojas is what determines whether these internal or external factors create a disease. For instance, if ojas is weak and a virus or bacteria are overwhelming, a person can develop a chronic illness. It is as if the body becomes a storehouse for invaders who think it is their body. They are the hosts instead of the guests, and when guests become hosts the power of ojas is diminished. Some pathologies are mild and others are serious, such as meningitis, encephalitis, or myocarditis. Every disease has a power and the power of ojas works against the power of disease. Ojas has the capacity to counteract the etiological factors or causes of disease.

Ojas is influenced by the power of agni, which determines digestion and the quality of assimilation and nutrition. The quality of ojas also depends upon lifestyle, stress, traumas, and the quality of relationships. If our relationships are not good, our ojas will not be good. A healthy relationship is a good tonic.

Inferior and Superior Ojas

Ojas is of two types: *apara*, which is inferior or unprocessed; and *para*, superior ojas. Tejas creates ojas and ojas protects prāna, the vital force of life that maintains the respiration of the cell. There is intelligence in the cell. That intelligence is tejas, but the flow of intelligence is prāna, and the medium through which the flow happens is ojas. Ojas is the seat of prāna and the superfine essence of all bodily tissues. This description applies to both apara and para ojas.

Apara ojas, which is raw ojas, is measured as half an añjali (equal to the size of an individual's cupped hand). Para ojas is measured as eight drops and is considered superfine ojas. It is colloidal (glue-like and submicroscopic) in nature, liquid, slimy, cooling, and sweet to the taste—like honey. It smells like *lāja*, roasted rice. It looks like ghee and is slightly yellowish-white in color. Ojas is rich in soma, which gives a blissful state of consciousness. There is cosmic soma and there is individual soma. Soma is released in samādhi and becomes bliss. It can be compared to serotonin. Certain neurotransmitters and hormones, such as serotonin and melatonin, are governed by the fire element in the majjā dhātu (nervous system). The pineal gland (*shiva granthi*) may be the seat of that agni and plays an important role in the production of soma.

Apara ojas moves throughout the body but para ojas stays in the heart. Para ojas stimulates the pacemaker sinoatrial (SA) node and maintains the life activity of the heart. Therefore, the function of apara ojas depends upon para ojas. If the heart stops, apara ojas stops flowing and this stagnation of ojas is death.

Apara ojas is mobile but para ojas is stable. Para ojas promotes stability of the tissues. The moment a red blood cell is born, it is moved through the body by prāna with apara ojas. Para ojas maintains the span of life of the red blood cell and every cell in the body. It gives strength and is capable of permeating the semi-permeable membrane of the cell wall, thus acting both inside and outside the cells.

One of the functions of ojas is to maintain the quality and quantity of all seven dhātus, three malas (wastes: urine, feces, and sweat), and three doshas. In addition, para ojas maintains consciousness. Our consciousness has a definite border, a definite frontier, and it has content. Container and content are the same. For example, a pot is the container and clay the content. In the same way, consciousness is the container, and thoughts, feelings, and emotions are the content. Because of its content, the container is limited.

Meditation empties the content, creating a space in the consciousness. When you empty the consciousness of its content, then the consciousness loses its border, its frontier, and it becomes all-inclusive awareness. In awareness, everything is welcome, because space is all-inclusive. Love is all-inclusive. Love says "yes" to every thought, feeling, and emotion. Fear and anger say "no." To say "no" means resistance and resistance breeds fear and anger, making the consciousness heavy and rigid. Then the consistency of consciousness becomes solid and such a solid and heavy consciousness creates depression.

To say "yes" means to allow a thought or circumstance to flower, to let go and expand. We say "yes" to some things and "no" to other things. Our "yes" and our "no" are opposite. But there is "yes" beyond "yes" and that "yes" is existence. The trees say "yes" to every season. When spring comes, they say "yes" and they flower. When summer comes, they say "yes" and become dry and thirsty. When fall comes, they say "yes," change color and are ready to drop their leaves. To say "yes" means to surrender—to every thought, feeling, and emotion. It means to let go, and letting go is a journey toward the heart. The word "yes" looks so simple. The dictionary gives a simple meaning. But to say "yes" to pain means to be with it and to be with something is to love it. To love some person means to be with that person. So to say "yes" means to be with it. Saying "yes" with awareness helps to stimulate ojas.

Para ojas brings stability but that stability has its own tremendous expansion and movement. It is like a jet plane moving through the air at 40,000 feet. You feel the plane is stable but the plane is not stable. It is moving with tremendous speed. Mobility and stability go together in para ojas. There is freedom and freedom is love, freedom is awareness. Therefore, awareness is love. Awareness is an all-inclusive state of consciousness. It is expansion. Therefore, love is expansion and selfishness is contraction. The moment one becomes selfish, one contracts the mind. This contraction dries ojas. Awareness enhances ojas, because para ojas becomes awareness.

Meditation needs very little effort. At 7:00 o'clock in the morning brush your teeth, drink a little water and herbal tea, and then sit quietly. This much effort is required. But the real meditation is effortless. We are tremendously full of effort. We try to get rid of anger, which is an effort; we try to get rid of fear, which is an effort. All efforts build stress and that stress diminishes ojas. During the day put out your effort but in the evening when you come home from work, practice a moment of effortless awareness. Sit quietly. Just float. That floating state of your mind is the effortless state of awareness through which you will glimpse God, you will glimpse Purusha, because Purusha is effortless awareness.

In that effortless state the mind becomes absolutely quiet and para ojas becomes active. In that effortless state of awareness, you realize your true nature, which is peace and love, and that state is supported in every cell by para ojas. In other words, para ojas opens the door to God consciousness, which is non-judgmental awareness. Then para ojas becomes soma, which releases molecules of bliss throughout the body.

Para ojas and soma are always present and accessible, but we are not always available for it to flow through us. We are stuck with fanaticism, emotions, anxieties, responsibilities, and effort. Our every effort denies peace, denies God, because God is not the product of effort or achievement. We do not know the art of looking at "what is." "What is" is the flow of enlightenment, which is quantum. "What should be, could be, would be" is the product of desire, mind, thought, and feeling. Therefore, "what should be, could be, would be" is an idea. An idea is not reality but is another name for illusion. Reality is "what is."

Your pain is "what is." Your pleasure at this moment is "what is." At this moment, the thought going on in your mind is "what is." Be with it. Listen. In that act, there is total surrender to "what is." "What is" is the flow of apara ojas. When you surrender to "what is" the apara ojas is transformed into para ojas. At every moment, "what is" comes to you to transform you but we become the barriers to our own enlightenment. Enlightenment is not tomorrow, not after 12 years, not after 12,000 years. The path of God is at every moment. Para ojas is at every moment. God is now, God is here, and God is also there. However, the division between here and there must cease. Then you will actually perceive para ojas. By remaining with this moment, these things will manifest at the cellular level.

Disorders of Ojas

The disorders of ojas are divided into four categories: *ojo visramsa* (displaced ojas), *ojo vyāpad* (disturbed ojas), *ojas kshaya* (depleted ojas), and *ojo vruddhi* (increased ojas).

Ojo Visramsa (Displaced Ojas). Ojo visramsa is the impairment of the distribution of ojas by the heart, due to leakage and escape through one or more of the *srotāmsi* (channels of the body). This kind of disorder of ojas is due to an improper function of vyāna vāyu, which circulates ojas to all the dhātus, and to vishama (imbalanced) dhātu agni in a particular dhātu. Ojo visramsa moves from dhātu to dhātu, manifesting where dhātu agni is weak. It is responsible for a wide variety of symptoms, including loose joints and inert extremities, and can lead to ojo vyāpad.

Both para and apara ojas keep vāta in the colon, pitta in the small intestine, and kapha in the chest. When the kapha from the chest goes into the sinuses, that is a displacement of ojas. When vāta from the colon goes into the sciatic nerve, that is a displacement of ojas in majjā dhātu. Ojas starts leaking from the srotas (channel) and this ojas becomes a foreign body. It is tejas that maintains the normal quality of ojas in the srotas, by regulating cellular permeability and metabolism. As long as ojas is in the srotas, it is healthy. When ojas leaks out of the srotas (channel), it becomes toxic. For instance, if blood oozes out of the blood vessel in rakta dhātu, it can create septicemia or a hematoma that leads to abscess and fever. That happens in ojo visramsa. Because of ojo visramsa there is impairment of tissue function. For example, ojo visramsa of the liver impairs the tissue and causes the person to develop episodes of hepatitis or mononucleosis.

Ojo Vyāpad (Disturbed Ojas). The second disorder of ojas is ojo vyāpad, which means ojas disturbed by one or more doshas. Also known as *ojodushti*, it is qualitative change in ojas. Either vāta, pitta, or kapha becomes aggravated and it disturbs the quality of ojas. In this condition, we find vāta ojo dushti, pitta ojo dushti, and kapha ojo dushti. Ojo vyāpad may be connected to one or several dhātus. If māmsa dhātu (muscle tissue) is leaking ojas, the person will develop symptoms connected only to that dhātu. But in ojo vyāpad more than one dhātu is usually involved.

In cases of a kapha ojas disorder, a person will be influenced by the entry of kapha into ojas. The circulation of ojas will be slowed and there will be a feeling of heaviness and dullness in the mind. This leads to a high level of unprocessed or raw ojas, which is described later as ojo vruddhi (increased level of unprocessed ojas).

Ojo vyāpad caused by vāta can create emaciation and the early signs of ojo kshaya. It becomes difficult to put on weight. Too much vāta in ojas can lead to extreme tiredness, tuberculosis, and the vāta type of chronic fatigue syndrome.

When pitta goes into ojas, tejas can burn ojas and the person is susceptible to autoimmune dysfunction. The immune system is effectively burned out. The person may develop rheumatic fever, mononucleosis (Epstein Barr virus), multiple sclerosis, HIV, or sickle cell anemia, a genetic immune dysfunction due to pitta. The liver is usually affected, because the liver is the seat of pitta. When pitta burns ojas, the person may also develop gout, lupus, psoriasis, eczema, or dermatitis.

Autoimmune diseases may be due to vāta, pitta, or kapha, but AIDS and most other autoimmune illnesses begin with high tejas and high pitta. The majority of AIDS cases begin with repeated flu, fever, lung infection, and/or pneumonia, but it develops into ojas kshaya. Please understand, ojo vyāpad is more serious than ojo visramsa, but ojas kshaya can be even more serious. Ojo visramsa is localized, but ojo vyāpad affects the entire immune system of the body.

Ojas Kshaya (Depleted Ojas).   Kshaya means depletion. The condition of ojas kshaya is the result of loss and wasting of ojas, which is a serious condition because ojas is lost both in quality and in quantity. Normally apara ojas is half an añjali and para ojas is eight bindu (drops). When that quantity is reduced, the result can be unconsciousness or various types of coma, such as uremic, diabetic, hepatic, encephalitic, or meningeal coma. These conditions mean that ojas is gone and, when ojas leaves the body, the person loses consciousness. This is why the teachings of Āyurveda say that prāna, semen, orgasmic fluid, and ojas should be protected.

Some signs of depleted ojas are chest pain, palpitations, breathlessness, fear, dehydration, muscle wasting, osteoporosis, and loss of muscle mass. Ojas kshaya can lead to pitta type of chronic fatigue syndrome (CFS), which means ojas in the liver is affected. In CFS the person feels extreme tiredness that is not cured by rest, and has various other symptoms, such as poor digestion, muscle pain, and mental sluggishness. Such a person may even have hepatitis B or C. An even more serious condition of ojas kshaya is full blown AIDS.

Note that ojas kshaya begins with ojo vyāpad. For instance, increased pitta can affect ojas and cause mononucleosis (Epstein Barr virus) or HIV infection. These are both pitta ojo vyāpad. However if these conditions are not treated, they can develop into ojas kshaya, which would be chronic fatigue syndrome or AIDS respectively.

Ojo Vruddhi (Increased Ojas). Vruddhi means increase. In ojo vruddhi, ojas is not fully processed and builds to an excessively high level. Increased kapha can increase ojas and this raw ojas can in turn increase kapha dosha. This happens in many kapha conditions, such as obesity and diabetes. The person may feel heaviness in the extremities, the joints become loose, swollen, and painful, there might be high triglycerides and high cholesterol, hypertension, and even a sudden heart attack. Glaucoma, generalized swelling, lymphomas, and lipomas are also conditions of ojo vruddhi. (Note that the suffix "oma" means tumor.)

Causes of Disorders of Ojas

What are the causes of ojas disorders? One cause is too much sexual activity. When there is excess indulgence of sex and a person has multiple orgasms in one night, ojas becomes depleted. Another cause is physical trauma, such as a severe car accident. Psychological trauma such as intense grief is also a contributing factor. Overexposure to bacteria, viruses, and parasites, as well as vigorous exercise beyond one's capacity, also affect ojas.

Chronic wasting diseases such as tuberculosis, chronic ascites, diabetes, chronic asthma, rheumatoid arthritis, cancer, typhoid fever, and ulcerative colitis are depleting of ojas. In some families, there is a genetic weakness of ojas that causes a deterioration of the tissues. During pregnancy a mother's wrong diet, lifestyle, and emotional stress can also affect the unborn child.

Tejas can disturb the intelligence of ojas, causing your own bodily cells to create antibodies that start destroying the healthy cells. When you go away and your dog is lonely, the dog becomes nervous, angry and depressed, and starts biting itself. Similarly, in our bodies, nervousness and anger destroy cellular intelligence, causing the creation of antibodies that start attacking our healthy cells. The molecules of ojas can become toxic and act as a foreign body or antibody.

Tejas

Tejas is the burning flame of pure intelligence. The principle of tejas embraces both light and heat. The illumination of the sun is tejas, which is also responsible for heating the Earth. In our food there is also solar energy (tejas) as well as life energy (prāna) and vital protective energy (ojas). Tejas is the primary energy involved in the digestion and transformation of everything that we take in and experience. This includes food, liquids, thoughts, actions, emotions and all else that comprises our human life.

Table 23: Functions of Tejas

Cellular biosynthesis of tejas gives:	
Deha Agni	Fire component of entire body
Bala	Strength
Ārogya	Positive health
Āyuh	Longevity
Prāna	Vital life force
Varna	Color complexion
Upachaya	Nutrition, tone of muscles
Prabhā	Glow, intelligence, luster
Ojas	Natural immunity

The term *deha agni* refers to the balanced fire component of the entire body. The essence of digestive fire is tejas, which manifests physically as enzymes, hormones, and amino acids, all of which govern cellular metabolism. Tejas is responsible for all the functions of life listed above, including the maintenance of optimal prāna and ojas. It is necessary to understand all of these components so that we can see the relationship between ojas, tejas, and prāna. If tejas is low, there is undue production of raw ojas. If tejas is high, it will dry and burn ojas. Therefore, the nature of ojas depends upon the quality of tejas.

Ojas, tejas, and prāna are not readily available to our system from raw wheat, corn, millet, or rice. We need the help of transformative processes to utilize the nutrients and ojas, tejas, and prāna from food. Cooking, chewing, fermentation, and sprouting are examples of these processes. With physical cooking, the tejas in the heat that cooks the food causes it to become soft, light, and smooth. This cooked food is easily broken down in the delicate lining of the intestinal folds and readily available for the gastric fire to transform the energy of the food into pure consciousness. The end products of digested food and the pure essences of all dhātus are ojas, tejas, and prāna, which are the basic, vital requirements for the life of every single cell.

Tejas is the energy of biological intelligence; ojas is the vital protective energy, a subtle substance; and prāna is the life force, the flow of intelligence. We will examine the qualities of tejas in human life. These qualities will help us to better understand the transformation of molecules of food, water, and air into pure consciousness.

Qualities of Tejas

Rūpa. Tejas has *rūpa*, which means color. The color of the skin, hair, and eyes, even the color of muscles and bones are all expressions of tejas. The seven rainbow colors are divine, cosmic tejas coming from the sun, which is the source of tejas. Because of the sun, the chlorophyll of plants gives color. The color of a flower changes because of tejas in the sunlight. A newly born leaf looks pink, transparent, delicate, and dances with the wind. As the leaf becomes mature, it becomes green. When the leaf ages, it becomes yellow, then brown and finally drops to the ground. This process is also tejas and what is true outside is also true inside. Tejas also gives color to the aura. The color spectrum of the auric field is the radiant energy of tejas.

A glowing color is called *prabhā*, which means luminous, shining, and lustrous. People with a prabhā personality have good tejas. Their eyes look bright and their skin is shiny. If tejas is depleted, the person has the opposite qualities of prabhā, which is *chāyā*, or shadow. That person looks dull, gloomy, and lusterless, as if in the shadow, even when wearing makeup. So one of the qualities of tejas in the body is to maintain prabhā; intelligence, glow, and a shiny and luminous personality. Please understand that these qualities are connected to digestion, metabolism, and nutrition.

Sparsha. The second quality of tejas is *sparsha*, which means touch. Why is touch related to tejas? The qualitative understanding of touch is governed by tejas, because tejas is cellular intelligence. Touch as a sensation is a movement of prāna, but the quality of the touch, whether it is cold or hot, is determined by the presence or absence of tejas. Tejas maintains optimum temperature, which is required to perceive touch. We perceive tejas with the eyes as color, but with the skin as touch.

Sānkhya. The third quality is *sānkhya*, which means number. Number implies division—one cell multiplying into

Tejas

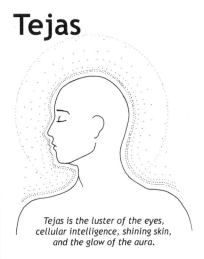

Tejas is the luster of the eyes, cellular intelligence, shining skin, and the glow of the aura.

two, two cells into four, four cells into 16. This multiplication of cells is most important in the formation of new tissues. Tejas is responsible for the appropriate number of X and Y chromosomes, which determine the sex of the fertilized ovum. According to Āyurveda, the human body contains a fixed number of dhātus (tissues), their upa-dhātu and mala (by-products), and their functional representatives, srotāmsi (channels). One of the functions of tejas is to maintain the appropriate number of doshas, dhātus, srotāmsi, and mala. So it is tejas which creates sānkhya, number.

Parināma. Sānkhya depends upon *parināma*, which means dimension. There is no dimension without expansion and contraction. Heat expands Ether and the absence of heat contracts Ether. The three-dimensional picture of a cell is created by tejas. The distance between two molecules—horizontal, vertical, and diagonal—is dimension. It is profound that tejas in the body governs the dimension of the size and shape of the body and this quality is called parināma.

Pruthaktva. *Pruthaktva* means separation; to create a passage by separating two molecules or cells. Tejas creates separation of a membrane from what it encases. Separation comes from the *tīkshna*, sharp or penetrating, quality of tejas. A peptic ulcer is a disorder created by this quality of separation in tejas and, if it is not treated, the ulcer becomes perforated.

Samyoga. *Samyoga* means conjugation or union. Molecules of similar quality have an affinity for one another, thus they unite to create a compact mass, which is governed by kapha. Kapha receives this intelligence of union from tejas. However, if tejas is too high, kapha cannot perform this function of union because it becomes too dry. In the case of ulcers, we need healthy, normal, physiological tejas to heal the ulcer. If tejas is too high, the person may develop ulcerative colitis. If tejas is optimal, it will kill the bacteria and viruses and create new cells and tissue to heal the ulcer. This quality is called samyoga: conjugation, conjunction, or union.

Vibhāga. Next is *vibhāga*, which means distinction. Vibhāga defines the size, shape, and margin in order to give a distinct form. Every organ and cell has a distinct form. Under a microscope, a red blood cell or a white blood cell has its own distinct form and imbalanced tejas can distort the form. This is a quality of tejas in the body.

Paratva. *Paratva* means priority, which is a subtle intelligence at the time of crisis. The body knows how to heal. When there are toxins moving in rasa dhātu, the priority of the body is to burn the toxins and the temperature becomes elevated. A person with fever has no appetite, because the priority of the body is to burn the toxins. When we interfere with the body by following our desires, we interfere with the dosha. When a child has a fever, never eat candy, cookies, or chocolate in the presence of that child. The child will be tempted and, if that desire is satisfied, more toxins will enter the system. The healing capacity of the body is the priority of supreme intelligence. Every cell has tejas and the body knows what is to be done at the moment of crisis. That is cellular intelligence.

Aparatva. The opposite of priority is *aparatva*, postponement. In the presence of fever, the priority of the body is to burn the toxins. When going through a bad time, have patience. When the crisis is over, normal functions can resume. Before taking off, a pilot knows the weather at his destination. If the weather is bad, he does not take off. He postpones the time of departure. The intelligence of aparatva comes from tejas. Always listen to the body.

Suppose a person awakens at 4:00 o'clock each morning and is diligent in the practice of yoga, meditation, and prānāyāma. Perhaps in the due course of life, this person does not follow a proper lifestyle and toxins build in the body. The body becomes toxic and says, "Today I can't do yoga." That is aparatva. The body wants to fight those toxins but our ahamkāra says, "No, I want to become an enlightened soul and a perfect yogi. I'm not going to listen to you." We torture the body and compel it to do certain things. In that way, we destroy the intelligence of the cells.

We have priorities, such as a job and making money, but we never listen to the priority of the body. When the body goes on strike and a person gets a fever or flu, then the body controls us. Priority is paratva and postponement is aparatva. Both of these qualities come from tejas, which is the supreme intelligence present in pitta and supreme order present in agni.

Dravatva. *Dravatva* means fluidity or liquefaction. Tejas has the capacity to liquefy mucus or any toxic substance. For example, if butter is placed near a fire, the tejas of the fire melts the butter and liquid butter flows easily. The same thing happens in the body. Liquid kapha is easily eliminated from the body. If wax is stuck at the bottom of a bottle, hold the bottle over the fire and the wax will liquefy. Then wash it with hot water. Hot water removes impurity faster than cold water, which is the whole purpose of oleation and sudation. Oleation is a treatment for stimulating the dravatva quality of tejas. This automatically pacifies vāta and stimulates the liquefication of toxins that then can drain out of the system.

Gati. As a quality of tejas, *gati* means velocity. Vāta has *vega*, which means random movement. Another meaning of vega is the creation of natural urges, such as urination, defecation, and sneezing, which is a function of vāta. But pitta has gati, which means movement with vector, in a particular direction. It is tejas that helps the doshas to move with focus. The elimination of sweat, urine, and mucus is stimulated by tejas.

Bhāsvara. Another property of tejas is bhāsvara. *Bha* means illumination. That is why the sun is called bhāsvara, that which illumines every object. *Svar* means self. Every cell is governed by the self-illumination of tejas.

Ūrdhva gamitva. Another quality of tejas is ūrdhva *gamitva*. Ūrdhva means up. Ūrdhva gamitva is upward movement. We rise up because of tejas, not only physically but also mentally. Going beyond the problem, not getting stuck with a conclusion, judgment or depression, transcending even fear, anxiety, and insecurity are also upward movements. Tejas helps us go into a transcendental state. Meditation, which helps to awaken the upward energy, uses tejas. If tejas is good, one transcends without effort. If tejas is dull, there is no awakening.

Nitya. Tejas is *nitya*, eternal, the flame of life. Life never dies. The body has birth, growth, and death. But tejas as a flame of life is eternal.

Manifestations of Tejas
Tejas takes the form of visible or perceptible heat but it is more than visible fire. Visible fire is a gross element but tejas is subtle energy. The intensity of illumination that is called luminosity is at its highest near the flame and diminishes as distance increases. In the process of digestion, every molecule of food comes in contact with tejas. Tejas governs optical and tactile perception and is responsible for understanding all objects of perception.

Bhaumī tejas is the subtle energy present in the agni of the Earth. In the same way, *apya tejas* is the subtle energy of the agni of water; *agni tejas*, the energy of the agni of fire; *vāyu tejas*, of the agni of air; and *divya tejas* of the agni of ether or space, which includes the sun, stars, moon, and lightning. All of these forms of tejas are present in the liver, which is the seat of bhūta agni. According to Sānkhya philosophy, the bhūta agni of the liver is the fire component of the five elements of Ether, Air, Fire, Water, and Earth. Bhūta means element and each of the elements has its own agni. Tejas is the subtle energy present in these bhūta agni. Āyurveda looks at every human being as a microcosm of the universe. We are the world and the world is us.

When walking in the sunlight, the tejas particles coming from the sun go directly into the liver and kindle the liver tejas. With certain types of anemia, when the liver does not process the gastric intrinsic factor, medicated bitter oil is applied all over the body and the person is asked to lie in the sun. This treatment improves liver function. In this condition, the divya tejas is weak in the liver. However, when a newborn baby develops jaundice within the first week of life, it is *āpya tejas* that is depleted. The baby is placed under a blue light, which clears the air, pacifies pitta, and helps to improve liver function. The liver is healed by this blue light.

Dravyamaya tejas means the tejas found in matter with form, shape, and color. Tejas is the potential energy of fire, light, which comes from sattva. Tejas is the subtle energy within agni. Agni is the kinetic energy of fire, the movement of light. This is a manifestation of rajas. The consolidation of tejas creates matter, which derives from tamas. From this one can see that matter is actually a form of crystallized light, slowed in vibrational frequency. It is nothing but trapped tejas. There is potential energy in both sattva and tamas. In sattva, the potential energy is light. In tamas, the potential energy is darkness. For example, wood (matter) is made up of many atoms and these atoms are moving (rajas). Wood has potential agni, which is light (sattva), and Vaisheshika philosophy calls this tejas. Tejas keeps these molecules together as wood.

The tejas of the stomach is called *udaraka tejas*. This is the energy present in jāthara agni, which is the gastric fire. Jāthara agni releases the tejas in food by breaking it down into smaller and smaller pieces, so that it is available to the cells, systems, and organs. This tejas principle within food is called *karaja tejas*. In Western terms, we are talking about the action of enzymes in the body. Then it is the tejas principle in bhūta agni that continues to transform the atoms of food into the biological atoms of the body.

Tejas and Karma

We postpone meditation and enlightenment but we never postpone our addictions. The moment there is a desire to smoke, people smoke. They never delay. But when there is a thought of meditation we say, "It is too late. I have to go to the office. I will do meditation tomorrow." We postpone good things. If we carry death in our breath every day, then every breath becomes an offering to God. God is awareness, God is eternity, God is life. And that life is tejas. That is why tejas is *nitya*, eternal. Nothing is eternal in this world. Famous people come and go. Only their memory remains in the collective consciousness.

Thought is a movement of prāna, but the form of thought is tejas, which is intelligence. *So'ham* is not a thought, it is not a word, and it is not a symbol. It is the inner, profound vibration of prāna, that pure consciousness which is *spanda*, or pulsating. A particle moves like a wave, but the perception of this movement is relative to the observer. When the observer looks at it as a wave, it is a wave. When the observer stops looking at it as a wave, it becomes a particle. It is a wave but it is also a stable particle. The vibration of consciousness is so'ham. It is in-breath, out-breath. So is higher consciousness, which goes in. Ham is the ego, which goes out. So'ham is the pure state of choiceless, passive awareness. There is a silent gap between so and ham, between ham and so. In that silent gap, one transcends so'ham into pure blissful awareness.

Everything happens spontaneously by Nature's law. The eyes see, the ears hear, the nose breathes, the heart beats, and the stomach digests. *Prārabdha karma* is accumulated past life karma that we have to burn through, whether we like it or not. *Pra* means previous and *arabdha* means accumulated—the accumulated seeds of past lives that we must experience in this lifetime. According to prārabdha karma, one person is attracted to another person's prārabdha karma and therefore chooses that person as his father or mother, or someone they have a close relationship with during the lifetime.

We are here for a set period of time. Life continues even though one becomes enlightened, just as a fan continues to move after it is switched off. The force that continues one's life is prārabdha karma. Even though a person becomes enlightened, his body goes on as long as prārabdha karma is there. Once prārabdha karma is exhausted, he simply dies and he is not afraid of dying. He dies with bliss. He knows that when his shirt is worn out, he has to drop that shirt (the body) and buy a new one.

The pure essence of prārabdha karma is tejas, which unfolds the intelligence to burn the past life karma. That is why conscious living and conscious dying is a blissful state. Unconscious living and unconscious dying is illusion. When a person's prārabdha karma is exhausted, he has no reason to live and life withdraws. Whatever he has done in this life is accumulated and added to the storehouse of karma, called *sañchita karma.* A part of the sanchita karma then becomes prārabdha karma for the next life. That is the theory of karma.

Tejas and Kundalinī

Kundalinī is the bio-spiritual combination of tejas, ojas, and prāna. When a person meditates, the energy rises up from the root chakra to the crown chakra along the ascending track of tejas. The kundalinī shakti has ascending and descending tracks along the spinal cord. It is a dormant neuro-electricity potentially present at the root of the spine. Shakti awakens and moves up by the grace of the guru, kundalinī yoga, prānāyāma, meditation, prayer or puja. There are certain signs of the awakening of kundalinī. A person develops goose bumps, spasms, or a surge of energy moves up.

The anterior passage of kundalini is the descending path from the crown down to the heart and stomach, via the vagus nerve. The vagus accelerates cardiac activity and stimulates hydrochloric acid secretion in the stomach. The posterior passage of kundalini is the ascending path governed by the sympathetic and parasympathetic nervous systems. Both the anterior and posterior pathways belong to kundalini.

Meditation opens the door to higher consciousness and life without meditation is a futile, meaningless game. Life with meditation is bliss. Meditation blesses us even during times of pain or intense moments of grief and sadness. We enjoy that grief and sadness, because bliss is not the opposite of grief. Grief merges into bliss and bliss and love are contagious. Anything that touches love becomes love. Love is infectious and transformative—love transforms fear, anger, grief, and sadness. Without transformation there is no creation. Love is creative.

We do not know unconditional love. Our love is a shoddy little affair. If we really love someone, we love his hate, his anger, and his jealousy. And if we love that anger, hate, and jealousy, they are transformed into love. That is why love has no opposite, bliss has no opposite. Remember that enlightenment is not the opposite of unenlightenment. But the opposite of unenlightenment is enlightenment. Light is not the opposite of darkness. The moment darkness meets the light, darkness disappears and becomes light.

Even an enlightened person suffers, but their suffering is different from ours. When we suffer, we suffer. When an enlightened person suffers, they don't take the suffering as a personal thing, but as the suffering of humanity. Can you do that from this moment? When you have anger or fear, do not say it is "my" anger or "my" fear. When you are suffering from cancer, do not say it is "my cancer." It is the cancer of the whole of humanity.

Out of suffering can come great compassion and love. The root meaning of the word suffering is love. But we don't want that kind of love, because our kind of love is a romantic thing. In our meaning of love, there is only joy, happiness, giving, and receiving. Our love is an idea, a concept. It is not real love. It is an emotional affair. True love goes with pure awareness which is light, tejas. Therefore, love is tejas, love is intelligence. Once intelligence dawns then pleasure and pain become the same. In the state of bliss, pleasure and pain are welcome. In the state of unconditional love, love and hate are welcome. You simply say "yes" to everything. Tejas becomes the auric field; it becomes light. In that expanded tejas of the aura, people are bathed with bliss and joy. Tejas is glow and has the quality of being eternal.

Tejas is the burning flame of pure intelligence. Keep that flame alive and bright. It is a flame that burns without wick or fuel. It has no smoke. That light is your true nature. That light is tejas.

Prāna

Prāna is the life energy that performs respiration, oxygenation, and circulation. It also governs all the motor and sensory functions. The vital pranic force enkindles the central bodily fire (agni) and the natural intelligence of the body is expressed spontaneously through this activation by prāna. One seat of prāna is in the cranial space. Prāna governs all higher cerebral activities, including the functions of the mind, memory, thoughts, and emotions. The physiological functioning of the heart (another seat) is also governed by prāna and from the heart prāna enters the blood (another seat), thus controlling oxygenation in all the dhātus and vital organs.

Prāna governs the biological functions of the two other subtle essences, ojas and tejas. During pregnancy, the navel of the fetus is the main door through which prāna enters the womb and the body of the fetus. This prāna also regulates the circulation of ojas in the fetus. Thus, in all human beings, even in the unborn, a disorder of prāna may create an imbalance of ojas and tejas, and vice versa.

One of the functions of prāna is respiration. We inhale cool air and exhale warm air. The warm air is solar, the sun, and the cool air is lunar, the moon. We inhale the cool moon and it goes behind the belly button. When the moon meets the sun

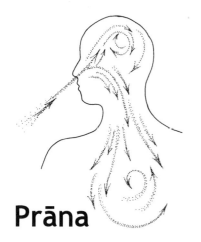

Prāna

behind the belly button, it becomes the new moon. The new moon is solar. On exhalation of the solar energy of that new moon, it merges into cosmic space about 12 finger widths from the tip of the nose, the spot where exhaled air stops. The moment exhaled air merges into outer space it becomes the full moon. This is a mystic, yogic, tantric concept. Understanding your new moon and your full moon will help you to understand the secret of life.

Every human body is bilaterally symmetrical. There is a right brain and a left brain, right arm and left arm, right ear and left ear. Everything is divided into two, including the genital organs—right testicle and left testicle; right ovary and left ovary. The right side of the body is governed by the left brain and the left side by the right brain. The right side is solar, male; the left side is lunar, female. All the prānic currents (movements of energy) coming from the left side go into the right hemisphere, so the right brain is associated with the feminine. Female energy is intuition, surrender, and compassion. When a poet writes a poem, he uses the right brain. The left brain is masculine and masculine energy is ambitious, aggressive, and competitive. The left brain is the mathematical, calculating, logical, scientific brain. A scientist investigates secrets under the microscope by using the logical, skeptical mind.

Prāna is a bridge between Purusha and Prakruti, male and female, solar and lunar energies. When we refer to Purusha and Prakruti as male and female, it is not a reference to gender but rather to energy—the polarity of positive and negative. Without the positive pole there is no negative, and without negative there is no positive. Even in a woman there is Purusha and in a man there is Prakruti. This concept is much more than gender. It is the male aspect of energy and the female aspect of energy.

Prāna is both masculine and feminine. Respiration is a bridge between male and female energies. When we breathe through the right nostril, we are charged with solar energy, which makes us more skeptical and logical, because the right nostril stimulates the left brain. Breathing through the left nostril stimulates the right brain, increasing compassion and intuition.The breath cycle changes approximately every 90 minutes. Inhaling through the left nostril is inhaling through the lunar (feminine); exhaling through the right nostril is mixing moon and sun. Likewise, when we inhale through the right nostril, we inhale the sun (masculine), and when we exhale through the left nostril, the sun is meeting the moon.

Meditation begins with awareness of the breath. When we inhale, the cool air touches the nostrils and fills the lungs, moving the diaphragm down, expanding the chest. The up and down movements of the diaphragm are governed by prāna. On inhalation, prāna goes behind the belly button. The belly button is important, because it connects the fetus to the mother. From this connection, the fetus receives prāna, ojas, and tejas from the mother.

Prāna is located in the hypothalamus of the brain. The hypothalamus sends a message to the sympathetic and parasympathetic nerves, to the intercostal muscles, and to the diaphragm. When the diaphragm descends, the external intercostal muscles contract, a vacuum is created, and air goes in. When the lungs are full of carbon dioxide, the hypothalamus is stimulated and sends a second message to contract the diaphragm, and it rises up. The internal layer of the intercostal muscles contract and the ribs move and work, as if pressure is created from outside, and the lungs exhale. This is the mechanism of respiration. It appears to be mechanical, but Āyurveda says that respiration is full of life, mind, feelings, enthusiasm, and inspiration. When a poet is inspired to write poetry, there is a connection to the cosmic prāna during inspiration, and during expiration the individual prāna goes out, takes the nectar of life and rushes back into the lungs, heart, and belly button.

Breath is a common factor between the animal kingdom and the plant kingdom. Oxygen, the food of prāna, is necessary for life. Cosmic prāna gives life energy to the whole universe and to all organisms present on the Earth. Prāna is made up of both Ether and Air elements, but primarily Ether. Vāyu (Air) is dry, light, cold, rough, subtle, mobile, and clear, which are all qualities of vāta. Ākāsha (Ether) is clear, subtle, light, expansive, omnipresent, and has the same qualities as Consciousness, which is the origin of the five elements. In Sanskrit, the soul is called Ātman, which is Awareness, Pure Consciousness, or Self. Ātman is the source of Awareness. Without Ātman, there is no Consciousness, no Awareness. When Ātman goes, Awareness is gone.

In a way, ākāsha (Ether, Space, or pure void) is our existence. We are all afraid of the void within. There is vast space outside and there is space within ourselves. Ether and Awareness seem identical, but they are not the same. Ether is material space and carries tamasic attributes, but Awareness is timeless and alive. Space is time. The space between each of us is time. To cover the space between two people requires time.

Time and space are one. Time is a product of our perception. But there is no concept of time in Pure Awareness. It is pure existence, which is beyond time and space. Pure Awareness has no attributes, but all attributes belong to it. That is why Awareness is everything; yet Awareness is nothing. To enter into nothing, one enters into everything. In Awareness, there is not one single attribute; all attributes are there.

Awareness in action with a different frequency of time yields a different quality. Therefore, the attributes of Ether, Air, Fire, Water, and Earth are different manifestations of Awareness. Awareness is manifested from tamas into Ether, Air, Fire, Water, and Earth. Through rajas, Awareness is manifested as thought, feelings, and emotions. Through sattva, Awareness is manifested as happiness, joy, bliss, and contentment.

Personality is the psychosomatic response of tridosha to internal and external stimuli—environmental, relational, and emotional. The subtle movement of the emotions is the movement of prāna. Emotions are held in the lungs. Just as we consume our food, so we inhale the emotions in the air and the emotions of the universe. When there is deep-seated grief and sadness (vāta), the upper lobes of the lungs do not function properly. When there is deep-seated anger and hate (pitta), the middle lobes of the lungs are affected. When there is deep-seated attachment and greed (kapha), the lower lobes are involved.

There is a corollary between the accumulation of prāna and emotional stagnation. The stagnation of deep-seated emotions, or suppressed emotions, results in division. These emotions become harmful when they are seen as separate from the self. Only when they are seen as one with the self do they become harmless, that is, the harmlessness which has no duality. When there is no division, there is transformation. Observe emotions from beginning to end, without judging, without comparing, and without needing to dispose of them. Simply observe what is occurring and do not label them as fear, grief, sadness, or anger. Watch the stream of emotions without "keeping a distance." The realization of the emotion is the ending of the emotion. To look without distance is to see the observer and the object as the same. To look at anything without separation is the cleansing, opening, and clearing of prāna vaha srotas (the channel of prāna), the healing of symptoms.

The Functional Integrity of Prāna, Tejas, and Ojas

We will now shift our attention to the functional integrity of prana, tejas, and ojas. From the time of physical birth until physical death, we are faced with the aging process. Because the continuous breakdown of the bodily tissues and organs causes deterioration and degeneration at the cellular level, it is at the cellular level that rejuvenation must take place.

The tridosha play an important role in the maintenance of cellular health and longevity. Each dosha plays a vital part in upholding the function of each of the billions of cells that constitute the human body. Kapha maintains longevity. Pitta governs digestion and nutrition. Vāta, which is closely related to the pranic life energy, governs all life functions.

On a deeper level, to combat aging it is necessary to balance the three subtle essences within the body: prāna, tejas, and ojas. The functions of prāna, tejas, and ojas correspond, at a subtler level of creation, to the functions of vāta, pitta, and kapha respectively. Proper diet, exercise, and lifestyle can create a balance among these three subtle essences, ensuring long life.

Ojas, tejas, and prāna must have functional integrity. A balance of ojas, tejas, and prāna constitutes one's aura, the defense shield against any intrusions from outside. Ojas is the substance of the aura, tejas is the color of the aura, and prāna is the movement in the aura. The stronger the aura, the more the things of this world can be thrown off and one can be happily and joyously "in the world but not of the world." Weak ojas hinders the proper transmission of tejas. This in turn weakens the digestion and aids in the production of āma. Too much āma seals out prāna, which weakens the entire system and opens the door for disease.

There is an apple hanging from the tree. We chew the apple, swallow it and within a few hours the apple becomes rasa dhātu, the plasma. The apple goes into the blood and into the muscle; it becomes a part of the bone tissue and even a part of consciousness. So the consciousness of the apple hanging in the tree becomes the consciousness of a human cell. When the body dies, all the elements are buried in the earth and another apple tree is born.

Soma, sūrya, and anila maintain global life. Soma is the moon, lunar energy, cosmic plasma; sūrya is the sun, solar energy, the source of heat and light; and anila is cosmic prāna. Vishnu means cosmic prāna, which is present in the atmosphere and protects global life. The movement of the Earth is governed by prāna and we can refer to cosmic prāna as ozone, a highly oxidizing agent. The molecule of ozone, O_3, yields into oxygen, O_2, and that oxygen is the food of prāna.

The human body has divine energy and intelligence. Cosmic intelligence and the intelligence of the body are one. The word intelligence means order and there is a mathematical order in the cosmos. The movement of the Earth around the sun and the rotation of the Earth about its axis are responsible for the rising and setting of the sun and for the seasons. This is cosmic order, mathematical order. Just as mathematics can be applied to simple sums, it can also be applied to the seasons and celestial events. Therefore, mathematics is the language of the entire universe.

Chaos is disorder and the cosmos is order. Āyurveda says that within disorder, there is order and that order is virtue. Dharma means order, virtue. The sun, moon, and prāna are all doing their dharma. Our human body is a beautiful chemical order, the order of universal chemistry confined in a small microcosm. The same order is present in a single cell and every cell is a center of awareness, a center of consciousness.

Soma

Soma and oxygen are the food of prāna. Many times people misinterpret oxygen as prāna, but if oxygen is pumped into a dead body life will not return, because that oxygen cannot be used by prāna. Prāna is life force, the flow of intelligence. Every cell has cytoplasm, the cellular material inside the plasma membrane and outside the nucleus, and that cytoplasm is the cellular rasa dhātu. This contains cellular soma. Within the cytoplasm, the molecules of food, water, and air undergo a transformation. Outside of the cell membrane, the molecules of food, water, and air are lifeless āhāra rasa. The moment they enter the cell, the molecules are transformed into an energized living cell. That transformation of lifeless molecules into living cells is governed by tejas. From the food precursor, āhāra rasa, the pīlu agni (and pīlu tejas) transforms soma into cellular food. Pīlu agni is the digestive fire present in the membrane of every cell, and pīlu tejas is the subtle energy of pīlu agni.

Charaka says that ojas is the pure essence of all bodily tissues and the superfine essence (para ojas) becomes soma. Soma is transformed by tejas into prāna, which is the flow of supreme intelligence. One could say, soma is the mother of prāna and tejas is the father of prāna. Global consciousness is maintained by the sun (sūrya), the moon (soma), and cosmic prāna (anila). In the same way, the life of a single cell is governed by a microform of these as tejas, ojas, and prāna. The tejas principle transforms soma into pure consciousness in the nucleus of the cell.

Modern quantum physics observes that matter and energy are one. Soma is the subtlest matter. It is the food of a cell, of RNA/DNA molecules, chromosomes, and genes. Soma is not a structure, it is a particle, and many particles get together to create a structure. Structure means the arrangement of the molecules and function is the energy flow through that arrangement. There is no structure without function and there is no function without structure. A change in structure due to change in function is called morphology.

A particle is material, a wave is not. When a particle becomes a wave, it becomes consciousness. Soma is a particle, and when it becomes a wave it becomes consciousness. This is key to understanding the relationship between soma, ojas, tejas, and prāna. If we remove a living cell from the body and put it under a microscope, that cell will die within two minutes because the plasma has been removed. If the cell is kept in the plasma, it will remain alive for a longer time. This cellular plasma is soma. Soma is the consciousness that nourishes the cell. Without cellular plasma, the cell has no consciousness and dies.

The body has a supreme intelligence comparable to that of the universe, the cosmos. Soma is transformed into sattva, rajas, and tamas, which are the qualities of consciousness. Through meditation, one can change the quality of soma and therefore change the qualities of one's consciousness. Kanāda gave us this information five thousand years ago.

We are applying modern physiology and psychology to explain these terms. It is difficult to translate these words. However, I will give the following definitions: Soma is cytoplasm, cellular food, a food of consciousness, a food of mind. Ojas is the cellular immune mechanism. Tejas is the body's enzymes, amino acids, and hormones. It is the pure energy of intelligence, which transforms soma into prāna. Prāna is the flow of intelligence or life force. If we remember these definitions, that is enough.

If tejas is not strong enough to transform soma into prāna, then intelligence will be uncooked. This raw intelligence may create incredible desires. The root cause of desire is unprocessed soma. When the desire is satisfied, agni will be kindled and one will receive satisfaction. Soma is the mother of intuition, and intuition and intelligence need to go together. The biological need is the intelligence of the cell and that intelligence is cellular intuition. Scientists use intuition but they intellectualize, measure, and make it into a logical sequence of knowledge; that knowledge becomes science, as it is known in the West. Vedic knowledge incorporates both intellect and intuition.

The Vedas speak a great deal about soma, which is a transcendental state of awareness, an expansion of consciousness or bliss. Soma is peace and love. So'ham is a mantra that is often used in meditation to quiet the mind. In a sense, so'ham is soma. So'ham means: I am that pure consciousness; I am that pure awareness; I am that pure, eternal, witnessing consciousness. A chattering mind becomes quiet by chanting the holy name of God. When a chant goes on and on, all your cells, all your molecules of ojas, pick up that vibration and start pulsating with the rhythm. Then there is a chant without a chanter that is an expansion of consciousness. In that state, the chant unfolds into soma. Chanting with love brings awareness and beauty. The holy name of God unfolds and showers soma upon you. You chant in dreams and in deep sleep. Then it is a chant without effort, which unfolds into effortless awareness.

Every sound has a different vibration, frequency, and action. Primordial sound flows through para ojas and leads to the soma state of consciousness. In the same way that every individual has a different prakruti (constitution), every individual also has his or her own prakruti sound. If you know your prakruti, if you know your sound, you will be liberated through para ojas. That is a profound and ancient Vedic secret. As an Āyurvedic physician knows your prakruti and vikruti, he also has the insight to tell you the sound of your prakruti, which is your basic vibration of ojas, tejas, and prāna. That sound leads to inner peace. That sound vibrates in your cells, in your RNA/DNA molecules, and in your consciousness.

Awareness

We all need healing. We as individuals must bring awareness to our feelings and emotions. Otherwise, we never take responsibility for our healing. We always hold the other person responsible for our suffering—either our mother, father, or someone else. We need to accept the responsibility that "I am the pain and the pain is me. My pain is my creation, my reflection; it is me." We must understand our relationship with our suffering and in that understanding, we maintain our ojas. In that ojas, there is the beautiful light of tejas, which is the perception. And in the flame of attention, grief and sadness burn and we become totally free.

We have to protect our ojas, tejas, and prāna through awareness, because tejas is the flame of attention that is the luminosity of awareness. Prāna directs attention to the spot, creating perception. Attention plus prāna is perception. There are many things waiting for our perception but we cannot perceive everything at one time. Perception is a product of time and our perception is a learned phenomenon, which is directed by knowledge and experience. In the perception of observer, object, and observation, this trinity becomes one when ojas, tejas, and prāna are balanced. This balanced state is perfect health.

When we are honest with our feelings and emotions, ojas is building, tejas is glowing, and prāna is flowing. That is a state of good health, which exists at every moment, in every event of life. Āyurveda says every breath, every moment, and every event should be with total awareness. When listening to someone, at the same time listen to the listener. When looking at an object, at the same moment look at the looker. When you look at me, my body is an object and you are the observer. When I am looking at you, your body is the object and I am the observer.

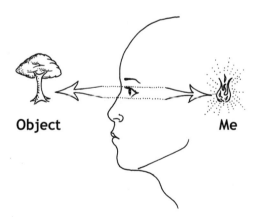

Object   **Me**

When you look outside, one arrow goes out. At the same time, a second arrow goes into the heart to look at the looker. This is called double-arrowed attention. In double arrowed attention, a third phenomenon happens, which is called witnessing. If you remain in witnessing, you will never get hurt. Forget about your past life. Forget about your future life. Your past is recorded in your astral body. When practicing thi awareness, that light, that flame of witnessing attention will burn and heal the memories of parents' illnesses and past life hurt, as well as hurt from this life. Just take responsibility, sit, and meditate. Unless you open your heart, unless you jump into the inner abyss, you are not going to become enlightened. Ultimately, you have to knock on your own door and come back to yourself. Love is within you. God is within you.

Chapter Seven

8

Digestion and Nutrition

आयुर्वेद

Rasa (Taste)

Ra means "to relish, praise, or taste;" *sa* means "juice, sap or secretion." *Rasa* is the taste associated with secretions in the mouth. The moment a substance (food, medicine, or herb) touches the tongue, the first experience is taste or rasa. Any substance, be it pepper or milk, creates salivation and thereby taste. The word rasa has many profound meanings. Rasa means taste, melody, experience, comprehension, interest, enthusiasm, appreciation, emotion, juice, plasma (rasa dhātu), mercury (a heavy, liquid metal), semen, and essence.

According to Āyurvedic philosophy, the moon is the mother of water and the sun is the father. Water in the atmosphere is cool, clear, and without any taste. The sun causes evaporation of water droplets from the ocean, causing clouds to form that are carried by the wind to the mountains, where they create precipitation. At the moment a water droplet is formed in a cloud, it has no taste. However, the electrochemical reactions that occur during the creation of thunder and lightening that accompany cloud formation and rain, mean that each molecule of water attracts molecules of the five elements in a unique combination. The six tastes are formed from the various permutations of the elements. Although each taste contains all five elements, the particular combination determines the nature of the taste. For instance, sweet taste has a predominance of Earth and Water. The water molecules containing the tastes eventually fall to the ground and enter plants. Hence, it is said that the nectar of the moon creates various tastes in each plant and water is the mother of all tastes. This is shown by the fact that taste is perceived through the tongue, the sense organ related to the Water element, and a dry tongue cannot taste accurately.

Table 24: Five Elements and Foods

Earth	Most kinds of seeds and nuts. Meat. Mushrooms. Root vegetables. Beans. Wheat, rice, and many other grains. Coconut meat. Hard dried fruits. Minerals.
Water	Milk and dairy products. Juicy fruits, such as plums, watermelon, grapes, cantaloupe, oranges, papaya, and peaches. Coconut water. Juicy vegetables, such as cucumbers, zucchini, and tomatoes. Salt.
Fire	Spices, such as hot peppers, black pepper, cinnamon, cloves, ginger, asafoetida (hing), garlic, and onions. Sour fruits, such as pineapple, lemons, grapefruit, tamarind, and sour berries like cranberries. Alcohol. Tobacco.
Air	Dried fruits. Raw vegetables. Rough vegetables such as broccoli, cabbages and sprouts. Nightshades like potatoes, tomatoes and eggplants. Many beans, such as black beans, pinto beans, and chickpeas.
Ether	Sprouts. Fresh vegetable juices. Algae and spirulina. Intoxicating and narcotic drugs, such as alcohol, marijuana, LSD, cocaine, and tobacco. Anesthetic drugs, such as ether.

How Taste Relates to the Elements

Every substance is made up of some combination of th five basic elements, so these elements are present in all s tastes. The relationships between the tastes and their tw predominant elements are given in the table below.

The Fire, Air, and Ether elements are light and tend move upward. Hence the tastes containing these elements al move the doshic energies to the upper parts of the bod producing lightness. Conversely, the Earth and Water elemer are heavy and move downward, so those tastes affect the lower part of the body more and can produce heaviness.

Table 25: Taste and the Five Elements

Taste	Predominant Elements
Sweet (madhura)	Earth + Water
Sour (amla)	Earth + Fire
Salty (lavana)	Water + Fire
Pungent (katu)	Air + Fire
Bitter (tikta)	Air + Ether
Astringent (kashāya)	Air + Earth

Relation of Rasa to Tongue and Organs

If you look at a tongue, you can apportion different areas to the different tastes and also to particular organs. Āyurveda says there are specialized taste buds on the tongue and the moment we put food into the mouth, bodhaka agni allows us to experience its taste. When you eat something sweet, the taste buds on the tip of the tongue become active and send a message to the related organs, which are the thyroid gland and apical area of the lungs. Sour taste is related to the middle and lower lobes of the lungs, and salty to the kidneys. Pungent relates to the stomach and heart, bitter taste to the pancreas, spleen, and liver, and astringent to the colon.

That is why there can be immediate reactions in the body after eating food. You can see this when you give a baby something with a strong flavor; their whole body responds to the taste. Even as an adult, the moment you eat something pungent, your heart starts beating faster and your stomach starts growling because these organs are stimulated through the taste buds. Similarly, the moment you taste sour, a message is sent by the chemo-receptors to the lungs and your body creates more bronchial secretions.

Hence a person who eats a lot of sweet foods tends to have a sluggish, underactive thyroid and can put on weight, leading to obesity. Over-intake of sour foods may lead to pulmonary congestion. Frequent use of salty taste can weaken the kidneys and cause water retention. People who are addicted to pungent foods and spices increase their circulation through the heart, become excessively hungry, and have burning

Tongue: Related Tastes & Organs

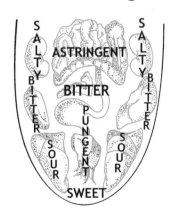

sensations in the stomach. They are also prone to gastritis. Abnormal consumption of bitter taste can weaken the pancreas, liver, and spleen, and excess astringent taste can cause constipation in the colon.

Table 26: Tastes and Their Related Organs

Taste	Associated Organs
Sweet	Thyroid and upper lungs
Sour	Lungs
Salty	Kidneys
Pungent	Stomach, heart
Bitter	Pancreas, liver, spleen
Astringent	Colon

Pharmacological and Psychological Actions of the Six Tastes

Some substances have only one taste while others contain many tastes. The three fruits that combine in the herbal compound called triphala have *pañcha rasa alavana*. This means five tastes (*pañcha rasa*) without salty (*alavana*). If you take triphala daily, half a teaspoon at bedtime, you will experience these different tastes at different times, depending on the state of your rasa dhātu. One day you may taste triphala as bitter, because your rasa dhātu is lacking bitter taste. Another time you might take triphala and it is sour, which means your rasa dhātu is missing sour taste. The same thing if you taste pungent, astringent, or sweet. There are very few conditions where triphala tastes sweet. When there is no āma (toxins) in the body and all seven dhātus are perfectly balanced, triphala tastes sweet, and that is the time to stop triphala.

Every substance's unique combination of attributes will influence its actions in the body. Taste can have a long-standing effect on the doshas, creating either therapeutic or unbalancing actions on body and mind. Each taste has a psychological component, creating positive or negative influence, which becomes apparent with frequent usage. We will now examine each of the *shad rasa* (six tastes) in detail.

Sweet

The word *madhura* means pleasant, charming, beautiful, agreeable, and melodious, as well as sweet. Earth and Water are the elements that make up the sweet taste. Its qualities are heavy, cooling, and oily. Sweet pacifies both vāta and pitta, but increases kapha. The sweet taste is strongly present in foods such as sugar, honey, dates, maple syrup and licorice, as well as more mildly in foods such as milk, rice, and wheat. The sweetness of rice is so mild that you may not taste the rice as sweet, but if you eat something bitter and then some rice, you will taste the relative sweetness.

Love is madhura, so you call a person you love "honey." You never say "Oh, my chili pepper." This is because love is associated with sweet taste, not pungent. Sweet is appealing to our taste buds. If you dip one finger into honey and a second finger into a bitter herb, then offer these two fingers to a baby, the baby will grab the finger with sweet honey and go on sucking it, but will hate the bitter finger.

Sweet taste enhances the vital essence of life (ojas). Samādhi may be called sweet because it unfolds the love divine. When used moderately, sweet is wholesome to the body and anabolic, promoting the growth of all seven dhātus—plasma, blood, muscles, fat, bones, marrow, and reproductive fluids. Proper use gives strength and longevity. It encourages the senses, improves complexion, promotes healthy skin and hair and a melodious voice. Sweet taste relieves thirst and burning sensations, enhances blood sugar, is nutritive to body tissues, helps to heal emaciation, and has a sustained cooling effect. If your tongue is burnt by chili pepper, eat a little sugar and it will cool down that burning sensation. Sweet can bring stability and gives energy, vigor, and vitality.

In spite of all these good qualities, excessive usage can produce many disorders involving any of the doshas. Sweet foods especially aggravate kapha and cause cold, cough, congestion, heaviness, loss of appetite, laziness, and obesity. They may also cause abnormal muscle growth, lymphatic congestion, tumors, edema and diabetes. Sugar or any extreme sweet taste creates thirst because it enhances kapha, which clogs the water channels of the body (ambu vaha srotas). Over-intake of sweet increases the need for sleep and can make the person sluggish. The person's healing capacity diminishes because sweet is the best media for bacteria, fungi, and parasites to grow. It also can adversely affect the heart, brain, kidneys, and pancreas leading to diabetes, nephrotic syndrome, or high triglycerides. If sugar accumulates in the brain, the person can get stroke paralysis. Too much sweet makes the blood viscous, which can lead to high cholesterol, high triglycerides and arteriosclerotic changes. Sweet in moderation is nectar, but sweet in excess is poison.

Psychologically, sweet in moderation enhances love and compassion. Sweet taste has a natural affinity towards joy, happiness, and bliss. That is why sweet is the taste of holy prasāda. No one gives you chili pepper or pickles as prasāda. Prasāda means compassion, love, richness, holiness, and wholesomeness. However, excess sweet will create attachment, greed, and possessiveness. It is tempting to eat a lot of sweet and it is addictive.

Sour

Sour is called *amla*, and is comprised predominantly of Earth and Fire elements. Amla means sour, acidic, and that which easily ferments. Sour taste decreases vāta but increases pitta and kapha. Although sour taste initially burns kapha, when used over a long term or in excess it will increase kapha. Sour substances are liquid, light, heating, and oily in nature and stimulate metabolism. Sour taste is found in foods like sour cream, yogurt, vinegar, cheese, citrus fruits such as lemon and grapefruit, unripe mango, green grapes, and fermented foods.

The moment you put a sour substance on the tongue your senses become sharp and you close your eyes. It immediately makes the eyes, ears, and teeth sensitive. Sour taste increases salivary secretions, stimulates appetite, and to some extent it enhances secretion of digestive enzymes. A moderate amount of sour taste is anti-flatulent and antispasmodic. It is refreshing; it energizes the body, nourishes the heart, and enlivens the mind.

In a small quantity, sour increases secretions and eliminates excess kapha. This is the reason why a regular small dose of apple cider vinegar works well for some people, balancing cholesterol and eliminating congestion. However, in a large quantity sour dries the membranes and creates congestion. Suppose you have a cold. Vitamin C is ascorbic acid, which is sour, so a small amount can be used to burn kapha. Maybe 500 mg. of vitamin C twice a day will help to reduce congestion, but a large dose such as 10 grams will worsen congestion. Such a large dose may be toxic to the liver and cause inflammatory conditions, such as cystitis, urethritis, and so forth. In a pitta person, that amount of vitamin C can create acid indigestion or skin rashes.

Sour will tend to increase pitta in a person of pitta prakruti and kapha in a kapha prakruti person. If one uses sour taste in excess, it can cause sensitive teeth, excessive thirst, hyperacidity, heartburn, acid indigestion, gastritis, ulcerative colitis, and ulcers. As sour taste has a fermentation action, it is toxic to the blood and can cause skin conditions like dermatitis, acne, rashes, eczema, boils, and psoriasis. It may lead to acidic pH in the body and cause burning in the stomach, throat, chest, heart, bladder, and urethra. Excess sour can also lead to diarrhea, dysentery, edema, damp lungs, and it can worsen congestive disorders.

Psychologically sour taste brings comprehension, appreciation, recognition, and discrimination. Sour is sharp, so it makes the mind alert, sharp, and enhances the span of attention. However, excess sour can induce judgment, criticism, jealousy, and hate. It will make the mind agitated, hyperactive, and so discriminative that slowly the person becomes very critical. When a relationship ends, there is often a sour taste in the mouth, which is a sign of judgment and rejection.

Salty

Salty is called *lavana*. Water and Fire are the predominant elements. Salty taste is heating, heavy, oily, and hydrophilic in nature. When used moderately, it relieves vāta but increases kapha and pitta. Classical examples of the salty taste are table salt, sea salt, rock salt, sesame salt, seaweed, and tamari. Sodium chloride is the most common salt that provides salty taste. Āyurveda recommends mineral rock salt in preference to sea salt or table salt. It contains many minerals in addition to sodium and thereby balances the doshas if used in moderation.

Due to the Water element, salty taste is laxative and, owing to the Fire element, it is anti-spasmodic. Like sweet taste, salty is anabolic in nature. Just a little bit of salt enhances the flavor of food, but it is so strong that any more than a little nullifies the effect of the other tastes. It stimulates salivation, aids digestion, absorption, and assimilation, and helps the elimination of wastes. Salty taste has anti-flatulent action, removing gases from the colon. When taken in moderation, it promotes growth, gives energy, and maintains the water electrolyte balance. If a person is dehydrated or becomes tired, blood pressure often drops. A pinch of salt in food will equalize the blood pressure and enhance energy. People who work hard under the hot sun lose salt through their sweat. That is why in tropical countries like India, people need more salt in their diet. Salt is also necessary for muscle strength. If you lose salt because of sweating, your muscles feel fatigued. This is all the positive side of salt.

Too much salt in the diet may cause sodium retention, leading to aggravation of pitta and kapha. It makes the blood thick and viscous and causes thickening and narrowing of the blood vessels, producing hypertension (high blood pressure). That is why a hypertensive patient should not consume too much salt. Due to its hydrophilic nature, salt may induce water retention, resulting in edema and swelling, which is also related to high blood pressure. Heat sensations, fainting, wrinkles, ulcers, bleeding disorders, and hyperacidity may all be caused by overuse of the salty taste, and it often worsens skin conditions. Frequent salt consumption can also cause hair loss by increasing pitta. In high quantities, salt can induce vomiting, which can help to excrete excess kapha and pitta. In general, use of mineral rock salt does not cause these effects.

Psychologically, salt enhances spirit, confidence, courage, enthusiasm, and interest. If you eat a salt-free diet for one month, you will experience dullness and depression and lose your creativity. An inquiring, probing mind comes from salty taste. If you remove salt from your diet you will feel tired, fatigued, lack interest, and your whole life will become bland. Salty taste improves the flavor in a relationship. However, excess consumption of salt can, like sweet, create temptation, addiction, attachment, greed, possessiveness, and other kapha disorders, as well as pitta problems such as irritability. If you open a bag of salty chips, your hand automatically goes back to the bag and, unless somebody stops you, it is hard to stop eating them. This is the addictive power of salty taste.

Pungent

Pungent is called *katu* and it contains Fire and Air elements. It is light, drying and heating in nature. It pacifies kapha but excites pitta and vāta. If you eat a little bit of something pungent, its first action will be to pacify vāta because of the heat. However, long-term or excessive consumption of pungent taste creates dryness and increases vāta as well as pitta. The pungent taste is present in many common spices, such as cayenne pepper, chili pepper, black pepper, mustard, ginger and asafetida, as well as foods like onion, radish, and garlic.

When used in the diet in moderation, it kindles agni, improves digestion and absorption, and cleans the mouth. Pungent taste clears the sinuses by stimulating nasal secretions and dissolving kapha dosha. It aids circulation, breaks up clots, removes fat from the body, and helps with the elimination of waste products. Most pungent substances are blood thinners, antispasmodic, anti-parasitic, and anthelmintic (dewormers).

Pungent taste may cause negative reactions when it is overused in the daily diet. It can kill sperm and ova, causing sexual debility in both sexes. It may induce burning, choking, fainting, hiccoughs, and fatigue with thirst. If it leads to pitta aggravation, it can cause diarrhea, heartburn, and nausea. With vāta provocation from overuse of pungent taste, giddiness, tremors, insomnia, and muscle pain may occur. Peptic ulcers, colitis, and skin conditions may also result from excessive use. The sharp, penetrating action of pungent taste will create inflammation, irritation, and ulceration and can be carcinogenic. Anything that is a strong irritant is potentially carcinogenic. For instance, a chronic ulcer that is irritated by pungent chilies can result in cancer. For that reason a patient of cancer should stay away from extremely hot, pungent food.

Psychologically, pungent taste brings enthusiasm, vitality, and vigor. It removes obstructions and brings clarity of perception. Pungent taste is hot, sharp, and penetrating, so it will help the mind to probe, investigate, inquire, explore, and concentrate. The mind becomes sharp, focused, attentive, and determined. However too much pungent will make the mind angry, violent, irritable, envious, jealous, aggressive, and competitive. These are rajasic qualities of pitta in the mind. If a person is often angry, they should stay away from pungent and eat sweet, which is cooling and soothing.

Bitter

Bitter is called *tikta*. It has the Air and Ether elements and is cool, light, and dry in nature. Bitter taste increases vāta but decreases pitta and kapha. Examples of bitter taste are found in bitter melon, turmeric root, dandelion root, aloe vera, yellow dock, fenugreek, sandalwood, neem, and coffee. We must have all six tastes in our diet, but bitter is the taste most lacking in North American food. Bitter taste improves all other tastes, because if you have a little bitter then any food will taste good. That may be the reason that coffee, which is bitter, became so popular in the West. In the East, there are many bitter vegetables—bitter gourd, bitter melon, bitter cucumber—and many bitter herbs.

Though bitter flavor is not delicious in itself, it promotes the flavor of the other tastes. It is anti-toxic and kills germs. It helps to relieve burning sensations, itching, fainting, and obstinate skin disorders. Bitter is anti-inflammatory, antipyretic (reduces fever), laxative, and cleansing to the liver. It stimulates firmness of the skin and muscles. In a small dose, bitter taste can relieve intestinal gas and it works as a digestive tonic. It is drying to the system and causes a reduction in fat, bone marrow, urine and feces. Bitter is good for supporting therapy to the pancreas, which is why bitter herbs such as neem and turmeric are given to a person with high blood sugar. Bitter is cleansing, because it does *lekhana*, which means scraping of fat and toxins. It actually kindles agni due to its dry and light qualities and pacifies pitta by its cold quality. Therefore, it is good for high pitta conditions with low agni due to increased liquid quality.

By itself, bitter is nauseating. Over-consumption of the bitter taste may deplete any of the dhātus and can induce dizziness and unconsciousness. Extreme dryness and roughness, emaciation, and weariness are often the result of excessive eating of the bitter taste. Bitter taste is antibacterial and antiviral. That is why most antibiotics are bitter. Over-consumption of bitter taste can reduce bone marrow and lead to osteoporosis. Certain antibiotics, such as chloramphenicol and tetracycline, are bitter and they can create blood disorders and bone marrow depression. Bitter taste inhibits sexual energy. Bitter kills worms; sperm is a micro-worm, so an excessive amount of bitter taste inhibits the production of sperm. In moderation, bitter taste can promote celibacy and aversion to worldly attachments. That may be the reason that many yogis in India take bitter neem juice for austerity and celibacy.

Psychologically, bitter taste makes your mind celibate. You withdraw your mind from temptation and your mind becomes more introverted. It creates aversion to desires and you become more self-conscious and self-aware. Bitter taste can help to unfold the withdrawing of the mind and senses from the outer world into the inner world, which is introspection. However, too much bitter taste will make a person cynical and boring and can lead to rejection. It can create aversion, separation, isolation, and loneliness.

Astringent

Astringent taste, which is *kashāya*, is derived from the Air and Earth elements and is cooling, drying, and heavy in nature. It reduces both pitta and kapha, but increases vāta. Unripe banana, pomegranate, chickpeas, green beans, yellow split peas, okra, goldenseal, turmeric, lotus seed, alfalfa sprouts, mango seed, arjuna, alum, and most raw vegetables are all examples of astringent taste. If you eat something astringent it creates a dry, choking sensation in the throat.

Astringent taste improves absorption and creates binding of the stool. So, whenever a person has diarrhea or dysentery, use an astringent herb like kutaja or arrowroot, or an astringent fruit such as cooked apple pulp or cooked, unripe banana. If you eat these, it will bind the stool and correct the diarrhea. Astringent taste is also anti-inflammatory and decongestant. It aids in healing ulcers and it does lekhana, the scraping of fat. Astringent taste also stops bleeding by promoting clotting and constricting the blood vessels.

In excess, astringent taste can create spasms, griping sensations in the intestines, and constipation. Extreme astringency creates coagulation and clotting, so if a person has blood clots astringent herbs are not good. The astringent taste absorbs water and causes dryness of mouth and difficulty of speech. Frequent use of astringent foods may cause choking, absolute constipation, distention, cardiac spasm, and stagnation of circulation. It may affect the sex drive and lead to depletion of sperm. It can give rise to emaciation, convulsions, Bell's palsy, stroke paralysis, and other neuromuscular vāta disorders.

Psychologically, astringent taste is supportive and grounding, because of the Earth element. It brings things together and makes the mind collected and organized, putting everything in its right place. These are the good qualities of astringent when eaten in appropriate amounts for your own constitution. However too much astringent taste makes the mind scattered and the person becomes disorganized. It can create insomnia, fear, anxiety, and nervousness, as well as fixation, rigidity, harshness, and emotional stagnation. Depression is also related to excessive use of astringent taste, because the person holds on to emotions and becomes depressed.

Table 27: Effects of Tastes on the Doshas

Taste	Effects[a]		
Sweet	V ↓	P ↓	K ↑
Sour	V ↓	P ↑	K ↑
Salty	V ↓	P ↑	K ↑
Pungent	V ↑	P ↑	K ↓
Bitter	V ↑	P ↓	K ↓
Astringent	V ↑	P ↓	K ↓

a. ↑ = increases and may lead to aggravation, ↓ = decreases and calms

According to Āyurveda, each taste used collectively or individually in the appropriate dose brings about balance of all the bodily systems and yields happiness and good health to all living beings. But if used improperly, much harm can result. So one should learn the normal and abnormal effects of these six tastes and make use of them properly in daily cooking.

Cravings

Craving for certain tastes is related to increased or decreased doshas. Healthy cravings are related to the response of cellular intelligence to an increased dosha without formation of āma (toxins). Other cravings can be due to increased doshas slowing agni, resulting in the production of āma. These toxins clog the cell membranes and disturb cellular intelligence, generating perverted cravings. Generally, an increased dosha without āma produces healthy cravings and disturbed doshas with āma create perverted, unhealthy cravings.

For example, if pitta is increased the person can become hypoglycemic and crave sweet taste. This is a healthy craving that should be satisfied. Sweet taste pacifies the high pitta and normalizes the blood sugar. Similarly, low kapha can result in the body needing more sweet taste. However high kapha can also lead to sweet craving, due to kapha and āma creating confused cellular intelligence. That is an unhealthy sweet craving that should not be satisfied, because the sweet taste will only further increase kapha dosha.

Students of Āyurveda should pay attention to whether a craving is healthy or unhealthy. Cravings can be due to biological need or from psychological desire. The type of craving can be determined by clinical assessment, such as examination of the tongue or pulse. Healthy cravings are created by cellular intelligence and are biological needs that should be satisfied. Perverted cravings are desire and should not be satisfied.

Vīrya (Potent Energy)

When any medicinal herb or food substance is put on the tongue, the first experience is its taste. Rasa has action through bodhaka kapha, prāna vāyu, and sādhaka pitta. Soon afterwards, you often feel a heating or cooling energy in the stomach or small intestine. This is due to the potent energy of the substance, called *vīrya*. Vīrya means "energy, strength, power, potency, and active principle." Vīrya operates through jāthara agni and its field of action extends to all the dhātu agnis.

In the same way that each rasa can be described by its gunas (qualities), vīrya can also be expressed in terms of the effects of the twenty qualities. In particular, there is a system used in Āyurveda that is called *ashthavidhā vīrya*, the eight types of vīrya. These are eight qualities from the list of twenty gunas that tend to have the most prominent effects on the body. They are the pairs of hot-cold, heavy-light, oily-dry, and the soft and sharp gunas. However out of these eight, it was found that hot and cold are the two qualities that have a direct effect on agni (digestive fire) and therefore immediately influence metabolism. The remaining six qualities mentioned above have effects that are experienced later or in a more subtle way.

Table 28: Functions and Effects of Vīrya

Normal Functions of Ushna (Heating) *Vīrya*	Normal Functions of *Shīta* (Cooling) *Vīrya*
Pacifies vāta and kapha, stimulates pitta	Pacifies pitta, builds kapha and vāta
Promotes metabolic activity (digestion)	Promotes anabolic activity (growth)
Kindles agni (dīpana)	Slows agni
Promotes digestion (pāchana)	Relieves burning, irritation, and inflammation
Increases body temperature	Decreases body temperature
Enhances blood circulation	Enhances lymphatic circulation
Abnormal Functions Due to Excessive Use	**Abnormal Functions Due to Excessive Use**
Burns ojas, reduces kapha, builds vāta	Inhibits pitta
High or tīkshna (sharp) agni	Low or manda (dull) agni
Promotes catabolic activity (destruction)	Abnormal growth
Hypoglycemia	Slow metabolism, obesity
Inflammation, ulceration, perforation	Poor digestion and malabsorption
Bleeding	Āma formation

By self-experience, one can form general rules about what a particular taste "feels like" in the body, which is its vīrya. For example, the sweet taste generally has a cooling energy, which provokes kapha but is pacifying to pitta. There are exceptions to the rule. Honey and molasses are sweet, which is normally cooling, but both have heating energy. Similarly, sour taste is usually heating, but limes are sour and they are cooling.

However, most substances usually follow the guidelines shown in the following table.

Rasa	Vīrya	Action[a]	Other gunas increased
Sweet	Cooling	3	Heavy, oily/unctuous, soft
Sour	Heating	1	Light, oily/unctuous, sharp
Salty	Heating	2	Heavy, oily/unctuous, sharp
Pungent	Heating	3	Light, dry, sharp
Bitter	Cooling	2	Light, dry, sharp
Astringent	Cooling	1	Heavy, dry, soft

a. Heating or Cooling action: 3 = Strongest; 2 = medium; 1 = weakest

Vipāka (Post-Digestive Effect)

The final post-digestive effect of taste (*vipāka*) occurs in the colon and has an action on the excreta: urine, feces, and sweat. However, its field of action extends to the dhātus and the cellular level. Vipāka can be observed by its action on both the excreta and on the dhātus. To make it simple, Āyurveda uses three post-digestive tastes (sweet, sour, and pungent) to summarize the qualities of vipāka. Generally, sweet and salty rasas have a sweet vipāka, sour rasa has a sour vipāka, and the vipāka of pungent, bitter, and astringent is pungent. Once again, there are exceptions.

Vipāka takes the molecules of food, water, and air to the cell membrane, in conjunction with the bhūta agnis. When a cell is isolated from the body and investigated under a microscope, it dies within a few minutes because the cell is separated from the nutrients that are the end products of vipāka. Vipāka transports these superfine products of digestion in āhāra rasa (digested food precursor of bodily tissues) for further transformation into living cellular components. Pīlu agni, the agni in each cell membrane, chooses appropriate molecules for that cell and they then become part of the cell. The same process occurs for each dhātu, whereby the dhātu agni selects appropriate nutrients from those yielded by vipāka. So vipāka precedes *dhātu pāka* (nutrition) at the dhātu level and pīlu pāka at the cellular level.

Each of the three vipākas has slightly different effects from those of the rasas of the same name. Sweet vipāka promotes tissue growth and anabolic functions of the body, so it increases kapha. It also helps to eliminate feces, urination, and sweat. Sour vipāka promotes metabolic functions and increases pitta. It makes the stools loose (possibly causing diarrhea) and creates acidic pH of urine, feces, sweat, and other bodily secretions. Pungent vipāka enhances catabolic activity and increases vāta dosha. It can cause constipation and block the flow of the bodily excretions.

Table 29: Effects of Rasa and Vipāka on the Doshas

Rasa	Vipāka	Actions	Effects on Doshas
Sweet, Salty	Sweet	Anabolic	Increases kapha
Sour	Sour	Metabolic	Increases pitta
Pungent, Bitter, Astringent	Pungent	Catabolic	Increases vāta

Sugar and salt are the same in that they promote anabolism, water retention, and can lead to obesity, hypertension, and diabetes if used in excess. In the digestive process in the small intestine, the Fire component of salt nourishes agni, leaving the Water component predominant by the time it reaches the colon. This Water element results in salt having a sweet vipāka. Hence sweet vipāka resulting from sweet and salty tastes has the same action. However, the pungent vipāka has slightly differing actions, depending upon whether the rasa of the substance is pungent, bitter, or astringent. All types of pungent vipāka are catabolic and dry bodily secretions, but each has its own additional effects.

The pungent vipāka derived from pungent substances tends to cause hemorrhoids, irritation of the colon, and dry, irritating skin conditions. Additionally, there is often diarrhea preceding the constipation that commonly occurs from pungent vipāka. Pungent vipāka from bitter rasa is more antipyretic (cooling) and has a particularly strong effect on the reproductive system, diminishing sperm formation and causing low libido. Finally pungent vipāka from astringent rasa is more likely to produce fissures and fistulae, osteoporosis, and pain in the joints.

Prabhāva (Unique, Specific Action)

When two substances of similar rasa, vīrya, and vipāka show different actions, this is called *prabhāva*. Prabhāva means a dynamic action that cannot be explained by the logic of rasa, vīrya, and vipāka. For instance, ghee (clarified butter) with milk in doses of two teaspoons per cup is laxative, but in a smaller dose, like half a teaspoon, it is constipating. Why? The answer is prabhāva. All gemstones, crystals, and mantras aid healing due to their prabhāva. Prabhāva is the specific, dynamic, hidden action of awareness present in a substance. It has a direct action on pithara agni inside cells.

Prabhāva is *achintya vīrya*, which means an unpredictable action of a substance. Every substance has a unique permutation and combination of five elements yielding a rasa, vīrya, and vipāka. If two substances have similar rasa, vīrya, and vipāka but different atomic structural arrangements, they are called *vichitra pratyaya ārabdha*. This means we obtain different experiences from each substance, even though rasa, vīrya, and vipāka are similar. This difference in their pharmacological action is due to prabhāva.

Examples of prabhāva include:
1. Chitrak and Danti. These two Āyurvedic herbs both have pungent rasa, heating vīrya, and pungent vipāka. However danti is a laxative and chitrak is not. Why? Because of prabhāva.
2. Rock salt and sea salt both possess salty rasa, heating vīrya, and sweet vipāka. Yet sea salt is more kapha-increasing and therefore not good for hypertension, whereas rock salt is okay in that condition. Prabhāva is the only explanation.
3. Fresh cayenne pepper and fresh pippali (pepper longum) are both pungent, heating, and with a pungent vipāka. (Note that pippali's vipāka changes to sweet when it ages.) However, cayenne aggravates hemorrhoids whereas pippali does not. Again, this is due to prabhāva, because the rasa, vīrya, and vipāka are all identical.

Actions of Rasa, Vīrya, Vipāka, and Prabhāva
The fields of action of rasa, vīrya, vipāka and prabhāva can be studied on a clinical basis. The first subjective experience of a substance on the tongue is rasa (taste); a short time later, one feels vīrya (heating or cooling energy); finally, the substance has an action on urine, feces and sweat, which is vipāka (the post-digestive effect of the substance). If an individual eats hot chili pepper, he or she will immediately experience its pungent taste, then its heating energy. The next day the person can observe a burning sensation in the feces and urine.

Rasa directly relates to the tongue and bodhaka kapha, and its field of action is the digestive process up to rasa dhātu. The āhāra rasa (digested food precursor of bodily tissues) is unprocessed rasa dhātu and it contains all five elements, *shad rasa* (the six tastes), *ashtavidhā vīrya* (the eight qualities of potent energetic effect), as well as nutrients for all seven dhātus. Rasa dhātu contains all twenty gunas (the ten pairs of opposite qualities), but those that have the most powerful effects are the eight that comprise vīrya, particularly hot and cold.

Bodhaka agni brings forth the rasa (taste) of a substance and jāthara agni its vīrya (potent energy). Bhūta agni creates vipāka, the post-digestive effect, in conjunction with the agni in the colon. Then pīlu agni and dhātu agni take the partially digested substance and transform it into cellular material, and prabhāva (unique, specific action) can occur through pithara agni. The vīrya of a substance has a more slow, sustained action than its rasa. It works via the media of agni and acts with vipāka through to the cellular level. Vīrya is responsible for digestion, absorption, and assimilation of food and yields into vipāka. Each phase of digestion is dependent on the previous phase, so without vīrya, vipāka is not possible. If one knows the rasa, vīrya, and vipāka of a food or medicinal herb, it is simple to understand its action on bodily systems. This knowledge is essential for both healing and cooking.

Table 30: Digestion: Fields of Experience and Action

	Field of Experience	Field of Action
Rasa	Tongue	Rasa dhātu
Vīrya	Stomach & small intestine	Dhātu agni
Vipāka	Colon	Excreta and pīlu pāka (cell membrane)
Prabhāva	Specific areas of the body	Pithara pāka (inside cells)

Digestion

The food we ingest undergoes the process of digestion and absorption through the action of agni. Every substance has rasa (taste) and every stage of digestion also has a distinct taste associated with it. As we will see, there are sweet, sour, salty, pungent, bitter, and astringent stages of digestion. The six stages of digestion act on the food as it progresses through the gastrointestinal tract. The end product of digested food is called āhāra rasa, the juice of the food, which becomes the food precursors for the dhātus. These food precursors are acted on by bhūta agni from the liver, because at this point the five elements from the food need to be turned into a form that can nourish the tissues. Then the various dhātu agnis further transform the food and split it into *prasāda* and *kitta*. Prasad is poshaka (essential) and creates sthāyi (mature) dhātu, while kitta is poshya (non-essential) and creates asthāyi (immature) dhātu.

Digestion is called *pāchana*. *Pāchana* is a process of biochemical transformation of complex, larger food particles into a simpler form suitable for absorption and assimilation. The primary digestion occurs in the gastrointestinal tract by the action of the agni subtypes of the three doshas along with the various agnis, such as jāthara agni, bhūta agni, and dhātu agni. Eventually food is transformed into energy in the tissues, which then yields into consciousness.

The digestive process is governed by agni and certain subtypes of each of the three doshas. It begins with bodhaka kapha, in the mouth, then jāthara agni in the stomach, which is the functional integration of kledaka kapha, pāchaka pitta, and prāna vāyu. Digestion in the duodenum is governed by rañjaka pitta, pāchaka pitta, samāna vāyu, and kloma agni (pancreatic juices). Samāna vāyu continues to predominate to the ileocecal valve. When the foodstuff comes through the ileocecal valve into the cecum, apāna vāyu predominates. As discussed in the section on agni, these doshic subtypes each have their own agni. It is the same agni, but expressed through the various functions of the doshas.

The Stages of Digestion

Usually six or more hours are required for the digestion of a meal. The six tastes each relate to one stage of the digestive process lasting approximately one hour. Every taste nourishes rasa dhātu during its respective stage of digestion, resulting in rasa dhātu containing all six tastes. The tastes also travel in āhāra rasa to nourish the asthāyi dhātu that is related to that taste, as we will discuss shortly.

The process of digestion begins when you put food into the mouth and you chew. There are four types of food, called *ashita*, *khadita*, *peyam*, and *lehya*. Ashita means a soup or jelly-like thing that you do not have to masticate, just swallow. Khadita means mastication and food you have to chew to make soft. Peyam means drink, like water or fruit juice, or very thin gruel. Lehya means that which you lick, such as ice cream or pickles. (If you bite a pickle, your teeth will become sour.) The moment that any kind of food or substance comes in contact with the saliva (bodhaka kapha), the first experience is taste

Āyurveda says that taste has direct action on the doshas, so the moment you start eating food the process of digestion begins. Prāna vāyu helps the process of mastication by sending an order to the muscles of the tongue and chewing occurs. The food bolus becomes soft, warm, oily and easy to swallow.

The digestion of carbohydrates begins in the mouth, with the help of ptyalin (an enzyme) in the saliva and chewing. Saliva is bodhaka kapha, which makes food easy to swallow and helps perception of taste, along with prāna vāyu and sādhaka pitta. Saliva helps the digestion of carbohydrates and maintains water electrolyte balance and oral temperature. If the tongue is totally dry, it becomes cold. The fire component that maintains oral temperature is called bodhaka agni. Bodhaka kapha secretion increases with happiness and joy, which is why children always drool. However, if an adult drools in deep sleep it can be an early sign of diabetes. Excess salivation is a kapha disorder that is a sign of either too much kledaka kapha in the stomach or pancreatic dysfunction, which is a pre-diabetic condition. Excess salivation also happens in Parkinson's disease and Bell's Palsy, which are vāta disorders affecting the facial muscles. If you have fear, anxiety, and stress, there is insufficient secretion of saliva and the tongue becomes dry, leading to poor taste perception. Saliva kills bacteria. That is why first thing in the morning we should brush our teeth and scrape the tongue to remove any dead bacteria.

The taste of food stimulates jāthara agni and aids digestion by stimulating prāna vāyu in the hunger center of the brain. Pleasing food smells also stimulate this center. Prāna also governs the movement of food down the esophagus into the stomach and, along with samāna vāyu, initiates churning in the stomach. Kledaka kapha in the stomach liquefies the food, allowing the molecules to come into contact with jāthara agni. Kledaka kapha and pāchaka pitta combine in jāthara agni through their oily and liquid qualities, along with prāna vāyu and samāna vāyu.

The first hour of digestion is the stage called *madhura avasthā pāka*, the sweet stage. All six tastes are present during this first hour, but the sweet taste is predominant. Earth and Water are the elements of the sweet taste, so it provokes more kapha secretions. The moment food enters the stomach, kledaka kapha from the greater curvature (or fundus) of the stomach is released, making the food sweet. The fundus of the stomach secretes gastric mucosal secretions. The food is broken down into smaller and smaller pieces, so agni can contact every food particle. Simple sugars are digested at this stage and released by the stomach to general circulation, so blood sugar rises.

The first two or three hours increase kapha, but the first hour (the sweet stage) is the most kaphagenic. For that reason, one may feel heavy and dull after eating. Although not yet digested, the ingested food brings contentment and groundedness due to kledaka kapha nourishing all kapha in the body. Additionally, the Water and Earth elements give a sense of fullness and satisfaction by stretching the stomach wall. If food quantity is increased over time, the stomach stretches and we need even more food to stimulate the stretch reflex. How does undigested food give you energy? The sweet taste of kledaka kapha goes through āhāra rasa into rasa dhātu, whose function is prīnana, which means nourishment and a sense of contentment. So, in this stage the sweet taste nourishes asthāyi rasa dhātu.

The second stage of digestion is called *amla avasthā pāka*, the sour stage. The Earth and Fire elements are predominant and the food continues to break into smaller and smaller pieces. In the first hour, the stomach is heavy due to Earth and Water elements, but in the sour stage the stomach becomes a little lighter due to the Fire element. Food in the stomach becomes sour because of the secretion of hydrochloric acid from the lesser curvature of the stomach, as well as other enzymes. Kledaka kapha provides the lining that protects the stomach from these acids, so if kledaka is decreased, heartburn, gastritis, and gastric ulcer can result. Agni secretes sour taste into rasa dhātu, so this sour stage in the rasa often aggravates any hives, rashes, urticaria, itching, or eczema, because the body builds up pitta dosha.

In the sour stage of digestion, the hormone gastrin stimulates the release of pepsin, which is an enzyme that begins the digestion of proteins. Rennin is a specialized enzyme also released at this time to coagulate milk protein. It is produced in high amounts in babies, but much less is present in adults. Prāna vāyu operates in both the sweet and sour stages. In this second stage, the sour taste is yielded into rasa dhātu and nourishes asthāyi rakta dhātu.

The third stage of digestion is the salty stage in the duodenum (the first part of the small intestine). It is called *lavana avasthā pāka*. The Water and Fire elements of the salty taste create emulsification. Samāna vāyu, pāchaka pitta, and rañjaka pitta from the liver are responsible for this stage of digestion. The salty stage in the earlier part of the duodenum relates to māmsa dhātu and salty stage in the latter part of duodenum to meda dhātu. Once the pyloric valve opens and food enters the duodenum, bile from the gallbladder (rañjaka pitta) and pancreatic enzymes (kloma agni) mix with the food. Bile and pancreatic juices are alkaline and the food coming from the previous stage in the stomach is sour, which is acidic. Acid plus alkali is equal to salt and water. This simple chemical equation shows that food here becomes salty. The salty taste has a buffering action, which assists further digestion of fats and protein. Enzymes such as amylase, trypsin, and lipase are released in the pancreatic juice. If there is low kidney energy, swelling and edema can occur in this stage. This salty stage of digestion yields salty taste into the rasa dhātu and nourishes both asthāyi māmsa dhātu and asthāyi meda dhātu.

The fourth stage relates to the pungent taste, and takes place in the jejunum, the second portion of the small intestine. It is called *katu avasthā pāka*. Air and Fire are predominant in this stage. The Fire component makes the food more yellowish-brown and is used for the digestion of food. The enzymes in the upper part of jejunum are more pungent and have a lot of Fire element with its hot, sharp, and subtle qualities. The Fire component of pungent also causes increased heat and circulation, and if there is high pitta it can irritate hemorrhoids, skin rashes, and bleeding disorders. Air makes the bones porous and is necessary for absorption of nutrients. Most absorption happens in the ileum and colon, but initial absorption of chyle begins in the jejunum. Air also results in production of gases and intestinal peristalsis, via samāna vāyu. In this stage, the pungent taste is yielded into rasa dhātu and nourishes asthāyi asthi dhātu.

The fifth stage of digestion is the bitter stage, called *tikta avasthā pāka*. It takes place in the ileum, the last (and longest) portion of the small intestine. Further digestion occurs in the ileum and there is still some presence of bile, which is bitter. Ether and Air are the components of bitter taste and they create most of the absorption of food through the villi of the ileum wall. The Air element continues to stimulate samāna vāyu, maintaining peristalsis. Due to the light quality of Ether and Air, the stomach and intestines become light, which can create false hunger. However, it is not a good time to eat. One should not eat again until the completion of the astringent stage an hour or so later. Tikta avasthā pāka also cools the body and can calm high pitta symptoms. In this stage, the bitter taste is yielded into rasa dhātu and nourishes asthāyi majjā dhātu.

When foodstuff comes to the ileocecal valve, apāna vāyu opens the valve with the help of samāna vāyu, which pushes the

Six Phases of Digestion

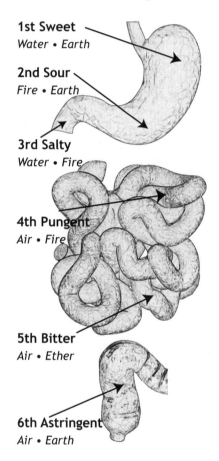

1st Sweet
Water • Earth

2nd Sour
Fire • Earth

3rd Salty
Water • Fire

4th Pungent
Air • Fire

5th Bitter
Air • Ether

6th Astringent
Air • Earth

food through into the cecum. The cecum, a pouch that forms the first portion of the large intestine, is sometimes called the second stomach because the food stays there for a while. In the cecum, the food becomes astringent, called *kashāya avasthā pāka*. This is the sixth stage of digestion. The elements of astringent are Earth and Air. The Air element helps further absorption, while Earth is heavy and rough and gives bulk to the stools. The liquid foodstuff becomes thicker and thicker as it passes through this stage. The astringent taste is necessary for the absorption of certain vitamins, minerals, and water, which takes place in the ascending colon and the first half of the transverse colon. Kleda (liquid) is absorbed through the colon and eliminated via the kidneys and bladder as urine. In the second half of the transverse colon, the food becomes solid and heavy, developing into well-bound fecal matter in the descending and sigmoid colon. The astringent stage of digestion stimulates mass peristalsis. The Air element nourishes *poshaka vāta* in the colon, and apāna vāyu stimulates the urge to defecate, ideally once or twice a day, depending upon the quality and quantity of foodstuff. Down to the pyloric valve, movement is governed by prāna vāyu. From the pylorus to the ileocecal valve, samāna vāyu governs movements. However, from the ileocecal valve throughout the large intestine, apāna vāyu governs all movement. True appetite returns during this stage, due to the Air component of astringent taste stimulating prāna in the hunger center of the brain. Astringent taste is yielded into rasa dhātu and nourishes asthāyi shukra or ārtava dhātu.

The timing of the various tastes is not fixed. It varies from person to person, from constitution to constitution. To simplify, the first hour of digestion is sweet, the second is sour, then salty, pungent, bitter, and astringent. So, within six hours all six tastes enter āhāra rasa. In this way, the six stages nourish the asthāyi dhātus within 6 to 12 hours after eating. However, the nutrition inside the cells in the sthāyi dhātus takes much longer—5 days per dhātu. Thus, sthāyi rasa dhātu is nourished 5 days after eating a food and 35 days must pass before sthāyi shukra/ārtava receives full nourishment.

Phases of Digestion and the Doshas

❊ Kapha: predominant for the first 1-2 hours, nourishes all bodily kapha

❊ Pitta: predominant for the next 2-3 hours, nourishes all bodily pitta

❊ Vāta: predominant for the final 2-3 hours, nourishes all bodily vāta

Stages of Digestion *(about 1 hour per stage)*

Madhura avasthā Pāka (Sweet stage). Digestion is stimulated by prāna vāyu and begins in mouth with bodhaka kapha (saliva), which regulates oral temperature, maintains lubrication, and begins digestion of starches. Chewing and lubrication break down food particles in the mouth. Bodhaka, prāna vāyu, and sādhaka pitta are responsible for taste perception. Prāna governs the movement of food down the esophagus into the stomach and, with samāna vāyu, initiates churning. Kledaka kapha in the stomach liquefies food, and combines with pāchaka pitta, prāna vāyu, and samāna vāyu within jāthara agni. Water and Earth elements stretch the stomach to give a sense of fullness and satisfaction. Absorption of simple sugars occurs, promoting energy and contentment. Sweet taste is yielded into rasa dhātu (plasma).

Amla avasthā Pāka (Sour stage). Hydrochloric acid (pāchaka pitta) is secreted in the stomach and makes the food acidic. Kledaka kapha protects the stomach from the acidic secretions. Stomach is still heavy, due to Earth element, but increasingly lighter from Fire element, which promotes digestive enzymes. Digestion of protein and fat begins. The sour stage can exacerbate pitta conditions, such as itching and skin rashes. Sour taste is yielded into rasa dhātu.

Lavana avasthā Pāka (Salty stage). Pyloric valve opens and food enters duodenum. Acid foodstuff from the stomach mixes with alkali pancreatic secretions and bile, yielding salts. Intestinal digestive enzymes are released. Digestion of carbohydrates, proteins, and fats occurs. This stage maintains water-electrolyte balance. Salty taste is yielded into rasa dhātu.

Katu avasthā Pāka (Pungent stage). Occurs in the jejunum. Most intestinal enzymes are pungent. Protein, fat, and carbohydrates continue to be digested. Fire component of pungent causes increased heat and circulation. Air component results in gases and intestinal peristalsis. Pungent taste is yielded into rasa dhātu.

Tikta avasthā Pāka (Bitter stage). Food enters the ileum. The Air element continues to create peristaltic movement along with samāna vāyu, and there is rapid absorption. Stomach and intestines become light, which can create a sense of hunger. However, it is not good to eat now. This stage cools the body and calms pitta symptoms. Bitter taste is yielded into rasa dhātu.

Kashāya avasthā Pāka (Astringent stage). Apāna and samāna vāyu open the ileocecal valve and food enters the cecum. Absorption of remaining minerals and liquids occurs. Feces are formed by the Earth component of astringent taste, stimulating peristalsis and resulting in elimination through the downward energy of apāna. Hunger returns as the Air component stimulates prāna and jāthara agni. Astringent taste is yielded into rasa dhātu.

How to Eat a Balanced Diet

Āyurveda regards food and its role in daily life in a unique and integrated way. Understanding some basic principles will help one to recognize foods that help keep the doshas in balance. Each dosha has certain attributes or qualities, such as dry, hot, or heavy. In the same way as the doshas, each kind of food is made up of certain qualities. For example, popcorn is light and dry, whereas cheese is heavy and oily. The qualities in a particular person combine with the qualities inherent in the food to determine how the body accepts and digests that food. Even one's emotional outlook can be directly affected by the food one eats, such as the mind feeling sharp and irritable after eating hot chili peppers.

Table 31: Examples of Attributes of Certain Foods[a]

Attribute	Food	Attribute	Food
Heavy	meat, cheese, peanuts	**Light**	rice, popcorn, sprouts, ginger
Cold	wheat, milk, mint	**Hot**	chili pepper, alcohol, eggs
Oily	cheese, avocado, coconut	**Dry**	millet, rye, dry cereal
Slow	meat, yogurt, tofu	**Sharp**	chili pepper, ginger, mustard
Stable	ghee, dry grains, dry beans	**Mobile**	alcohol, sprouts, popcorn
Slimy	yogurt, avocado, ghee	**Rough**	salad, popcorn, raw vegetables
Dense	cheese, meat, coconut	**Liquid**	milk, fruit juice, vegetable juice
Soft	ghee, avocado, oils	**Hard**	coconut, almonds, sesame seeds
Gross	meat, cheese, mushrooms	**Subtle**	ghee, honey, alcohol
Cloudy	yogurt, cheese, urad dal	**Clear**	fresh water, algae, vegetable juice

a. See "Food Guidelines for Basic Constitutional Types" on page 291 for a list of foods classified according to the doshas.

Āyurveda offers a logical approach for determining a correct diet based upon an individual's constitution. This approach is quite different from the current Western definition of a balanced diet, based on eating proportionately from various food groups. Āyurveda believes that understanding the individual is the key to finding a truly balanced diet. It teaches that agni in the digestive tract is the main gate through which nutrients enter the tissues and then pass along to individual cells, maintaining the life functions.

In general, when the qualities of a food are similar to the qualities of a dosha, this will tend to aggravate that dosha, such as when a vāta (dry) person eats popcorn (dry). Opposite qualities tend to be balancing, such as when a pitta (hot) person drinks mint tea (cooling). This fundamental principle can help you select foods that are balancing to your own unique constitution. The qualities can be determined to a large extent by consideration of the rasa, vīrya, and vipāka of a substance. For instance, a food that has sweet rasa, cooling vīrya, and sweet vipāka will strongly aggravate kapha, which is inherently sweet and cool, but pacify pitta dosha. Sometimes a food can be a mixture of doshic qualities. For instance, fresh ginger has pungent taste, heating vīrya, and sweet vipāka. This results in an action of pacifying all three doshas in moderation, but increasing pitta in excess.

Nutritional Disorders

In Āyurveda there are five basic types of nutritional disorders:

1. **Quantitative Dietary Deficiency:** malnutrition due to insufficient food or even starvation.
2. **Qualitative Dietary Deficiency:** results in malnutrition, toxic conditions, and lack of essential nutrients. Includes poor food combinations, which disturb the normal functioning of agni and interfere with the state of our doshas.
3. **Quantitative and Qualitative Over-nutrition:** includes emotional overeating. Can result in obesity, high cholesterol, high triglycerides, and hypertension, and even lead to heart attack or paralysis.
4. **Toxins in food:** certain foods or harmful residues in foods, such as pesticides and synthetic hormones, can directly cause toxemia and lead to digestive disorders.
5. **Foods unsuitable for one's constitution:** imbalance the doshas and ultimately leads to disease.

An individual's agni largely determines how well or poorly food is digested. Quantitative malnutrition is rare in the West and is addressed by giving the person more food. However, overeating, emotional eating, eating unsuitable foods, and even toxic food are common throughout the world. They create āma (toxins), which is the root cause of many diseases. Each of these conditions can be dealt with to a large degree by a robust and balanced agni.

While it is true that all five types of nutritional disorders should be considered, food combining and inappropriate diet for the constitution are of special importance. It is no surprise to see on the market today so many digestive aids, along with pills for gas and indigestion. Most of these conditions begin with poor food combining. Diet is much discussed and there are many theories on the topic.

Food Combining

Every food has its own taste (rasa), a heating or cooling energy (vīrya), and a post-digestive effect (vipāka). Some also possess prabhāva, an unexplained effect. When two or more foods having different taste, energy, or post-digestive effects are combined, agni can become overloaded, inhibiting the enzyme system and resulting in the production of toxins. Yet these same foods, if eaten separately, might well stimulate agni, be quickly digested, and even help to burn āma.

Poor food combining can produce indigestion, fermentation, putrefaction and gas formation, and, if prolonged, can lead to toxemia and disease. For example, eating bananas with milk can diminish agni, change the intestinal flora, produce toxins, and cause sinus congestion, cold, cough, and allergies. Although both of these foods have a sweet taste, milk has cooling energy and bananas are heating. Additionally, their vipāka is different—bananas are sour while milk is sweet. This causes confusion to our digestive system and results in those imbalances. Similarly, milk and melons should not be eaten together. Both are cooling, but milk is laxative and melon diuretic. Milk requires more time for digestion. Moreover, the stomach acid required to digest the melon causes the milk to curdle, so Āyurveda advises against taking milk with sour foods.

These incompatible food combinations not only disturb the digestion but also cause confusion in the intelligence of our cells, which can lead to many different diseases. Before you say "This is much too complicated, how will I ever figure it out?" there are some useful guidelines to help you understand these concepts. And remember that Āyurveda is a strong proponent of the "go slowly" school of thought. You might want to introduce yourself to food combining by initially eating fruit by itself, as many fruits create a sour and indigestible "wine" in the stomach when mixed with other food. Once you have adopted this change into your eating habits, try other suggestions from the list below. Above all, a strong digestive fire (if we are so blessed) can be the most powerful tool of all to deal with "bad" food combinations, so always respect your agni.

❋ As a general principal, avoid eating lots of raw and cooked foods together.

❋ Don't eat fresh foods with leftovers and minimize your use of leftover foods from the previous day.

❋ If foods with different and possibly aggravating qualities are cooked together in the same pot, they are predigested together, so agni can better handle them without problems.

❋ Spices and herbs are often added in Āyurvedic cooking to help make foods more compatible or to ease undesirable effects. For instance, adding cooling cilantro to hot, spicy food can help it to be digested.

❋ Different quantities of each food involved in a combination can sometimes be significant. For instance, equal quantities *by weight* of ghee and honey are a bad combination; this is approximately 3 parts of ghee to 1 part honey by volume. Any other ratio of the two is not toxic.

❋ If we have become accustomed to a certain food combination through years of use, then it is likely that our body has made some adaptation to this. This is not to say that we should continue the practice, which still produces toxic effects, but to explain why the newcomer to a bad combination (such as apples and cheese) may experience a strong case of indigestion whilst the "old-timer" digests it adequately.

❋ Antidotes, such as cardamom in coffee, or ghee and black pepper with potatoes, often help to alleviate some of the negative effects inherent in those foods. (Coffee is stimulating and ultimately depressing to the system, but cardamom helps to neutralize these effects. Potatoes generally cause gas, but the ghee and black pepper pacify vāta and stimulate agni, helping to counteract that effect).

❋ Eating a "bad" combination *occasionally* usually does not upset the digestion too much.

The Three Laws of Nutrition

Nutrition of the tissues in Āyurveda is called *dhātu poshanam*. There are three laws that govern nutrition. One is called *kedāra kulya nyāya* (irrigation), the second is called *khale kapota nyāya* (selectivity), and the third one is *kshira dadhi nyāya* (transformation).

Kedāra kulya nyāya is irrigation. The end product of digested food, called āhāra rasa, is carried throughout the body via the circulatory system, in the same way that a field is supplied with water by an irrigation system. This law describes the initial digestive process through to the point that the bhūta agnis break down the food into biological elements that are circulated in the āhāra rasa.

Then by khale kapota nyāya, which is selectivity, every dhātu selects the elemental components that nourish that particular tissue. *Kapota* means pigeon. You could visualize this process as a field and seven trees, and in each tree there is a pigeon. Each pigeon flies to the field, takes its grain, goes back and feeds its young one. The field is the body, which has been irrigated by the gross digestion of food. The pigeons are the asthāyi dhātus and their young are the sthāyi dhātus. The intelligence of the pigeon enables it to choose suitable food for its baby. Likewise, every dhātu agni has intelligence, which is necessary for selectivity.

For example, rasa agni selects plasma cells, while rakta agni chooses iron molecules that build hemoglobin in the red blood cells. Protein molecules are chosen by māmsa agni, while meda agni selects fat molecules, asthi agni selects minerals, and so forth. We can look at this through the eyes of Āyurveda and say that rasa chooses predominantly Water element; rakta chooses mainly Fire and Water; māmsa selects Earth, Water, and Fire; meda chooses Water and Fire; asthi selects predominantly Air and Earth; majjā takes Ether, Air, and Water; while shukra and ārtava select all elements.

The third law is kshira dadhi nyāya, which governs the transformation of the tissue precursors into the tissues themselves. This is the conversion of asthāyi (immature, unprocessed) dhātu into sthāyi (mature, processed) dhātu and it is governed by the respective dhātu agni. Rasa agni acts on āhāra rasa, which is asthāyi (immature) rasa dhātu, and transforms it into sthāyi (mature) rasa. Similarly rakta agni transforms asthāyi rakta into sthāyi rakta dhātu. This process occurs in every dhātu and the end product of tissue nutrition is ojas. Ojas is the pure essence of all dhātus. It goes to the heart and eight drops of para (supreme) ojas stays there, while the apara ojas is circulated throughout the body and mind.

Three Laws of Nutrition

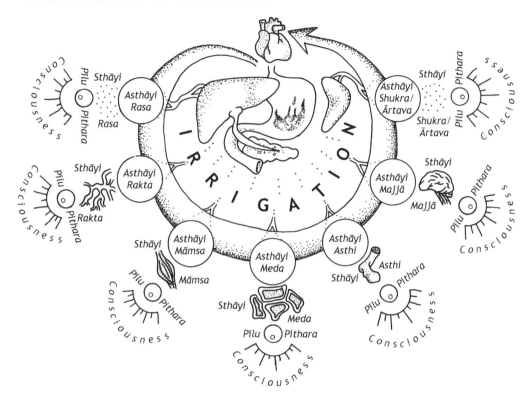

Nutrition Begins at Conception

The development of each dhātu is governed by ojas, tejas, and prāna and begins at the moment of conception. Shukra (the male seed) and ārtava (the female egg) carry ojas, tejas, and prāna from each parent's body. Prāna splits the fertilized cell—one into two, two into four, four into sixteen, and so forth. An ancient Vedic saying states "eko'ham bahusyam," meaning "I am one, I want to be many." Each of us was once a sperm, which looks like the tail of the Sanskrit letter Aum (or Om). Aum is the first primordial sound of creation. When you feel Aum, udāna moves up, kundalinī moves up. Any mantra without Aum has no potential to produce any fruit. That is why Aum is called the primordial seed of creation. First there was one seed, then out of that seed billions were born.

The fertilized ovum is called *kalala*. The Sanskrit meaning of kalala is "the first expression of creation." *Kali* means bud; kālā means time, movement, and order. In pregnancy, the kālā is approximately nine months and nine days. Kalala is the primordial expression of prakruti, the union of male and female.

The Three Laws of Nutrition: Irrigation, Selectivity, and Transformation

Law of Irrigation (kedāra kulya nyāya): circulation of nutrients to dhātus; governed by prāna and jāthara agni.

Law of Selectivity (khale kapota nyāya): each dhātu selects appropriate nutrients; governed by tejas and bhūta agni.

Law of Transformation (kshira dadhi nyāya): transformation of asthāyi into sthāyi dhātus; governed by ojas and dhātu agni.

It is potential creativity. Within that fertilized ovum there are maternal and paternal ojas, tejas, and prāna. Prāna divides kalala, tejas maintains its integrity, and ojas maintains its immunity. All of this happens at the subtle level of a *bija*, the seed. As the entire tree is present in its seed, so the whole person is present in the human seed.

From that kalala, the child's seven dhātus are manifested. The fetal rasa, rakta, māmsa, meda, asthi, majjā, and shukra/ārtava are formed in sequence, reflecting order within the development of the fetus. Within the first month, rasa reaches maturity; in the second month, rakta; and the third, māmsa. In a like manner, every tissue is developed, so that within seven months all tissues reach maturity. Ojas, tejas, and prāna maintain the nutritional transformation of immature dhātu into mature dhātu and are vitally important in the development of the seven dhātus within the body of the fetus.

Depleted ojas may manifest as chromosomal defects in the fertilized ovum and can cause congenital anomalies. If the ojas of the baby is depleted, the child may be born with a defect in the heart, a cleft palate, atrial septal defect, or ventricle septal defect. During pregnancy, ojas is unstable as it moves between the mother and fetus. For this reason, it is good for the mother to take ghee during pregnancy, because ghee can help to stabilize the ojas in the fetus and thus avoid some chromosomal defects.

Modern science understands that the gender of a child is determined by chromosomal combination at conception and is unalterable. While the following techniques may seem unbelievable to modern ways of thinking, one could think of them as enhancing the gender characteristics of the unborn child. According to ancient Āyurvedic texts, shukra and ārtava are initially dormant in the fetus and gender is not expressed until the third month of pregnancy. It can be changed during the first two months of pregnancy by using the fresh juice of the bud of the root of the banyan tree. Grind the bud into pulp and squeeze it through cheesecloth. Put five drops of that fresh juice into the right nostril of a pregnant woman. Then the fertilized ovum will become a male child. Put it into the left nostril and the fertilized ovum will become a female child. This is profound Āyurvedic genetics. Although these concepts are not accepted in current western genetic theory, research using these techniques might reveal very interesting results.

We do not have fresh banyan roots in the West, but we can use ashvagandha or shatāvarī ghee. Putting five drops of ashvagandha ghee into the right nostril of a pregnant woman in the early morning may produce a male child. If you want to have a female child, put five drops of shatāvarī ghee into the left nostril. The five drops relates to one drop for each element: Ether, Air, Fire, Water, and Earth. These drops should be used in early morning before sunrise and in the evening for the first two months of pregnancy.

Cellular Metabolism (Pīlu Pāka)

The Sanskrit word *paka* means the biochemical process of digestion. Pīlu pāka is cellular digestion and metabolism at the molecular level. Each cell is breathing and that breathing is of two types: aerobic and anaerobic. Anaerobic breathing takes place in the skeleto-muscular system using carbon dioxide rather than oxygen. Lactic acid is produced by anaerobic metabolic activity during glycogenesis, which is the absorption of glucose. Oxygen is necessary for aerobic breathing, which maintains metabolism, combustion, oxidation, and burns free radicals. Anaerobic breathing relates to apāna vāyu and enhances the span of life of a cell, while aerobic breathing relates to prāna vāyu and speeds oxidation and aging. Prāna moves in and apāna moves out. Inside the cell, vyāna vāyu circulates the nutrients and samāna stays within the cell membrane and maintains osmotic pressure. Udāna is in the cell nucleus. Even though it is a gaseous waste, carbon dioxide can be utilized through anaerobic breathing to enhance the life span of all cells. This is how yogis live hundreds of years. The body can actually thrive on limited oxygen. A person stops aging through anaerobic breathing, which is why prānāyāma is most important. In a transcendental state of meditation, breathing automatically becomes very quiet. In this state of blissful awareness, bodily cells are performing anaerobic breathing.

The rate of respiration is the rate of movement of prāna and apāna at the cellular level. The faster the breathing, the quicker the metabolism, and thus the quicker the rate of oxidation and combustion. Slowing down breathing slows down oxidation, slows metabolism, and enhances the span of life by slowing down the rate of death and destruction of cellular material. Although oxygen (prāna) is necessary for combustion, carbon dioxide (apāna) actually slows metabolism, to the point it can be as slow as a turtle. A turtle has extremely slow breathing, hence it can live for a larger number of years than most people. However, a dog breathes quickly, so its span of life is relatively short. In meditation, the rate of respiration diminishes to that of a turtle. In a normal, healthy condition, the respiration rate is about 15 per minute. In smokers, it elevates to 25 per minute. Joggers breathe fast while jogging but, if they are fit, their heart rate and breathing become slow when they are resting. When yogis do prāṇāyāma, they can easily hold prāna in the belly for one minute. When the breath stops, it is being held in the abdomen and the chest. The oxygen inhaled is more fully utilized, which stimulates anaerobic breathing in the cells of the deep tissues and can enhance the span of cellular life.

In Empty Bowl Meditation, one can just sit quietly and let the lungs do their job. The moment you interfere, the breathing pattern will change. Simply sit and observe the breath. The lungs inhale and air goes in. The lungs exhale and air goes out. In that movement, the breathing becomes quiet and the gap of silence between inhalation and exhalation increases. When one has the sudden sense of "Aha!" at the beauty of a sunset or a sunrise, breathing stops. In a moment of total awareness, there is a suspension of breath. Breathing becomes silent and the mind merges into the pure space of awareness.

Pīlu Pāka and Pithara Pāka

The elemental components of food are split up by jāthara agni and bhūta agni into finer and finer parts of Ether, Air, Fire, Water, and Earth, and then circulated in āhāra rasa, which is the law of irrigation. Pīlu agni, the agni in the cell membrane, selects certain elemental molecules, which is the law of selectivity applied at the cellular level. These digested molecules of food, water, and air enter into the cell with the help of prāna and cellular waste is thrown out with the help of apāna. Pīlu agni, like dhātu agni at the tissue level, then transforms these elements from the asthāyi (immature) form into the sthāyi (mature) cellular components. Within a cell there is soma, the pure essence of ojas and a substratum of consciousness. The role of pithara agni within the cell nucleus is to transform this soma into consciousness. Pīlu pāka takes place through the cell membrane into the cytoplasm, but outside the cell nucleus. Pithara pāka occurs inside the nucleus.

Kanāda, a great *rishi*, talked about pīlu pāka in detail. He discovered the atom and called it *anu*. Pīlu is another word for atom. Thousands of years ago there were no microscopes, but the rishis' description of *anu vaha srotas* is exactly the description of a cell. Anu means atomic; srotas means channel or pathway. So anu srotas is the pathway of atoms, which is the cell. Every cell has its own pathway and these pathways have their own agni, ojas, tejas, and prāna. Pīlu pāka is the subtle transformation at the atomic level caused by heat (agni). (see also "The Amino Acids and 20 Gunas" on page 98)

Kanāda was an enlightened soul and founded Vaisheshika philosophy. At the time of his death, he asked

"What is death? It is the disintegration of atoms of the body into the universe." Earth molecules go to earth, Water molecules to water, Fire to fire, Air to air, and Ether to ether. The dying person gasps, as if prāna is leaving the body, the senses do not function, the pupils are dilated, the heart beats feebly, and the pulse becomes impalpable. The body temperature rises, as if fire is leaving the body. Before death, the person sweats, as if water is leaving the body. Kanāda was a great enlightened soul. He never cried for the mortal frame.

In pīlu pāka every cell is nourished, as the agni of the cell nourishes the cellular cytoplasm. In pithara pāka the tejas of the cell nucleus (including nucleic acid) nourishes chromosomes and RNA/DNA molecules and transforms soma into consciousness. This concept is most important. Pithara agni is a manifestation of tejas in the body in its pure energetic form. In pithara pāka, every RNA/DNA molecule is nourished. Vaisheshika philosophy says that our food nourishes the mind and consciousness. This is the process of molecular digestion, through which the molecules of food, air, and water become part of our cells and our consciousness. At this level of nutrition, matter becomes energy. If we eat sattvic food, through pithara pāka we will have sattvic qualities in the mind and consciousness, which are love and peace. If our food is rajasic, it will create more rajasic qualities in the mind, producing agitation, temptation, and restlessness. If we eat mushrooms, meat, or other tamasic food, the mind will be dull, heavy, and depressed. It is difficult to produce superfine, spiritual thinking while eating tamasic food. At pithara pāka, the sattvic, rajasic, and tamasic qualities of food are transformed into the finer part of the mind and consciousness, so the quality of mind depends on the quality of food. (see "Relationship of Sattva, Rajas, and Tamas to Foods and Behavior" on page 290)

Consciousness is a subtle space within and between cells, which corresponds to the Ether element. The energy that maintains intercellular or synaptic space is Ether. The subtle vibration in this space is the mind, which relates to Air. Cellular intelligence is buddhi (intellect), which is Fire. When cellular mind becomes the emotional mind (manas), it expresses through the Water element. The rigid, hard ahamkāra (ego or self-identity) at the cellular level is from the Earth element, which gives form to the cell. Earth is solid, like the ego, and the consolidation and crystallization of consciousness is from Earth molecules. We all have the feeling of "I am" and that "I" of every cell consists of Earth molecules. At a grosser level, Earth includes proteins and minerals; Water relates to all liquids; Fire

Meditation is harmony between pilu agni and pithara agni.

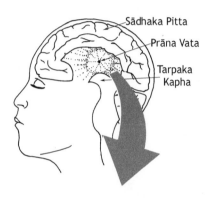

Sādhaka Pitta
Prāna Vata
Tarpaka Kapha

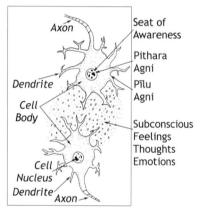

Axon
Seat of Awareness
Pithara Agni
Pīlu Agni
Dendrite
Cell Body
Subconscious Feelings Thoughts Emotions
Cell Nucleus
Dendrite
Axon

includes enzymes and amino acids; Air includes oxygen and all movement; and Ether is space. What is true on the gross, physical level is also true on the subtler, cellular level, because each cell is the basic unit of life. Every cell has consciousness, every cell is a center of awareness, and the Ether molecules of food nourish consciousness of the cell.

We carry subconscious thoughts, feelings and emotions from time immemorial. Within each cell, we carry the memory of our parents' and ancestors' illnesses. If your grandfather had diabetes, there is the cellular memory of diabetes within you and you may have been born with a weak pancreas. This phenomenon is called *khavaigunya*. *Kha* means space; *vaigunya* means defective or weakened. If there is a family history of hepatitis, the grandchild may be born with a weakness in the liver and the liver becomes a defective space within the body. Similarly, if there is a history of rheumatism in the family, the cells of the joints and bones carry a memory of rheumatism.

Day-to-day memory is recorded in majjā dhātu (bone marrow, nerve tissue, and related connective tissue) and genetic memories are recorded inside the cells within the genes. Subconscious memories are recorded within the etheric space between cells of the connective tissue throughout the body. Tarpaka kapha includes the connective tissue between the brain cells, which is a specialized part of majjā dhātu. Past life memories are a complex network of trans-neural energy pathways within tarpaka kapha. At the time of death, these memories—subconscious, genetic and past life—gather within the astral body, which is carried from one life to the next.

The role of pithara pāka is to digest *every* thought, feeling, and emotion and thereby nourish cellular consciousness. Thoughts, feelings, and emotions move through the connective tissue to the cell membrane. If pithara agni is low, these thoughts, feelings, and emotions touching the cell membrane are not assimilated or processed. Unprocessed thoughts, feelings, and emotions are then stored within the intercellular space of the connective tissue, and that becomes the subconscious mind. This unprocessed material that stays within the connective tissue can also be described as mental āma (toxins).

Desire
Spirituality, life, religion, and consciousness are all connected to the quality of agni and tejas in pīlu pāka and pithara pāka, and to the food we eat. Some families, including many in India, have not tasted meat for generations. However, in the West, the majority of people are meat eaters. At present in

America and other Western countries, many people are becoming vegetarian. Sometimes when the chain of eating meat is suddenly broken, cellular metabolism is affected and the body faces shocks to its system, including the cell membranes and RNA/DNA molecules. For that reason, there is sometimes intense craving for meat. According to Āyurveda, we need to satisfy that desire in some way. Desire can reflect a biological need and needs must be satisfied. Once biological needs are satisfied, one can better enter a state of freedom from all desire. If the body is depleted of protein, which creates symptoms such as spaciness, a person can sometimes benefit from eating meat, such as chicken, turkey, or fish, just to take care of the needs of the body. There are also many vegetarian substances that provide rich sources of protein, such as tofu and other soy products, soaked almonds, goat's milk, cow's milk, and cheese. Some people do not consider milk a suitable food for a vegetarian. They say it is a product of the cow, the upadhātu of the rasa dhātu of the cow. Āyurveda considers fresh milk from a healthy cow to be a sattvic and healing food.

The teachings of Āyurveda say to allow a break in your thoughts and concepts and be a normal human being. Āyurveda is a science of the golden mean. Try to find the golden mean of everything and do not be a fanatic. Fanaticism creates suppressed desires and fanatical people never reach enlightenment. They become stuck with desires and their own ideologies. Suppressed desires keep the soul in the wheel of time, the wheel of birth and death.

Many religious philosophies say that, when a person dies, whatever that soul loves should be offered. The Bhagavad Gītā says that if there is no desire at the time of death, the soul is liberated. The Koran and Egyptian teachings also state this belief. Desire is a powerful drive. If there is unsatisfied desire or some unfinished business, the person will take birth again to complete that circle of desire. In the RNA/DNA molecules within the cell nucleus there is a specific genetic code, which records genetic cellular memory through a set pattern of amino acid molecule chains. These molecular chains are unprocessed soma, which produces desire and may be the source of cellular khavaigunya (weakened or defective space).

So, unprocessed soma is the source of all desires, but processed soma brings satisfaction. An ordinary person's soma has intense desires. For instance, when there is a deficiency of calcium or iron, children eat clay. If there is a deficiency of protein, the person can have a strong desire for meat or other high protein food. A deficiency of oily substances creates a craving for fats or cheese, and if there is a deficiency of sweet taste, the person craves sugar. Soma tries to satisfy the natural needs of every cell, whether it is a plasma cell, a red blood cell, a muscle cell, or any other type of cell. In that way, soma communicates with the body.

The most important thing is to understand desire. Desire is timeless and ancient, but the understanding of desire is the ending of it. Desire leaves a residue of neurological memory, which creates sensation. That is okay. Remain with these sensations as you go about your life. This is true awareness. Do not let thoughts come and take charge of the sensations. To stop thoughts taking control is not suppression; it is the key. Then soma is transformed into love, which is pure awareness.

Thoughts, Feelings, and Emotions

To summarize, the intercellular space in the connective tissue may be the seat of the subconscious mind, while within the space of the cell is the seat of genetic memory. The connective tissue is made up of specialized cells. In between these cells are intercellular spaces that accumulate the crystals of subconscious—unresolved thoughts, feelings, and emotions. These crystals are the substratum of the subconscious mind. The moment subconscious emotions touch the cell membrane, we become conscious of them. We become conscious of our fear, anger, grief, or hurt. However, if pithara agni is low, it is incapable of dealing with this material; or if pīlu agni and pithara agni are not synchronized, they cannot process the emotions.

In both these cases, pithara agni sends a message to pīlu agni to reject these emotions and once again the conscious becomes subconscious. Hence, the cell membrane is a bridge between conscious and subconscious. When one becomes aware of subconscious fear, those crystals of fear are actually touching the cell membrane. If pithara agni is too low, it sends the message "Hey, I can't deal with it. Throw it out!" and pīlu agni becomes rigid. Then that subconscious fear is thrown back into the connective tissue. This repressed emotion accumulated in the connective tissue is called stress, and it burns ojas and affects immunity.

Pithara means parents, so pithara pāka is genetic digestion. However, pithara also means continuous, constant meditation. Meditation is the awakening of your pithara agni. By opening communication between pithara agni and pīlu agni, any thoughts, feelings, and emotions that touch a bodily cell will be digested and transformed into cellular intelligence. When pithara agni transforms every thought, feeling and emotion into awareness, your cells remain healthy. Digestion of unresolved emotion is the function of pithara agni and when it is functioning perfectly, there is no precipitation. The moment there is precipitation in your awareness, that precipitation settles to the bottom and creates intercellular or mental āma of unresolved grief, sadness, or other emotion.

Thought is the response of memory. It is a biochemical vehicle through which we can communicate with our cells. Therefore, positive thinking and affirmation are the art of kindling pithara agni, so that it becomes strong and vibrant and starts burning unwanted, unresolved emotions. The subconscious mind is our own creation, a black hole created by us. The material we do not want to deal with is contained in the subconscious mind. We dump this unwanted "stuff" down into the basement, into the intercellular space of the connective tissue, which is the seat of the subconscious mind.

Everything is universal and personal. There is universal consciousness and there is personal consciousness; universal mind and personal mind; universal Self and individual self. These are the two energy fields—local and non-local, individual and universal. Enlightenment means to remove the fence and go beyond the frontier of your consciousness. Your consciousness is a tiny enclosure and you live in your own small world. The drop sees itself only as a drop, but the drop eventually becomes the ocean. In fact, the drop is the ocean. Bhakti yoga means letting the ocean come to the drop. When the ocean floods the drop, it is bhakti, love. When the drop becomes the ocean, it is jñana, pure knowledge. Through pure knowledge this drop, which is your individual consciousness, merges into universal consciousness. Meditation is a way of emptying the consciousness of its content. You can do this by using pithara agni to bring a transcendental state of awareness. Meditation means bringing harmony between pīlu agni and pithara agni. It breaks down the crystals of unresolved emotions. In pañchakarma cleansing we stimulate pīlu and pithara agni and try to remove excess doshas and āma (toxins). When āma goes into a cellular energy field, it becomes cellular āma or mental āma. Through the actions of *snehana* (oil massage), *svedana* (sudation or sweating), and pañchakarma cleansing therapies such as basti, we kindle pīlu agni and pithara agni and help to burn the āma stuck in the intercellular energy fields.

Modern physics speaks of the unified field and the Vedas speak about unity in observation. When you observe fear through the eyes of a cell, your first attitude is to judge that fear. The pithara agni of your millions of cells judges and says "This is fear; fear is bad and unwanted." Therefore, you become the observer or subject, and fear becomes the observed or object. This division between observer and observed creates a miscommunication between pīlu and pithara agni, resulting in pīlu pāka getting clogged and building more āma. The moment you label fear as fear is the beginning of suppression. It creates an image of fear that is recorded within the intercellular space of the connective tissue. To kindle your pithara agni is to look at every feeling and emotion without labeling it or naming it. Then what happens? The observer and observed become one. Then, when a molecule of fear enters the cell, pithara agni transforms that fear into mind, memory, intellect, and into pure consciousness. Then even fear nourishes consciousness and it is no longer fear but pure awareness. There is a real ending of fear when you give complete freedom to the fear and allow it to flower. The flowering of fear is the ending of fear. This is the real meditation, the only meditation—to observe your every thought, feeling, and emotion with total awareness, without division between object and subject.

There are many ways to communicate with a single cell. Polarity, craniosacral work, marma point therapy, *abhyanga* massage, and many herbs may create and access different pathways to communicate with pithara agni. Psychology can bring comfort by giving labels, which is a way of bringing about familiarity. Recognition gives comfort, but recognition is a limitation of experience. Naming and labeling is a process of isolation. The moment you name or label something, you become separate from that thing. In that process, your pithara agni becomes weaker and gives the wrong message to pīlu agni to reject that thing. The standard Western psychological approach makes a person feel comfortable, because fear of the unknown becomes fear of the known. The view seems to be, if you have pain, take painkillers; if you have insomnia, take tranquilizers. Similarly, if you have fear, label it, pack it and store it. Each of these actions is a way of suppressing the experience so the person can avoid pain, but this does not allow the person to process it completely. It then remains in the tissues and cells as unprocessed experience or āma.

But we are not here to suppress. That is all symptomatic treatment, where you label the symptoms to learn how to live with the emotion. It does not eradicate the emotion. The Āyurvedic approach goes one step beyond labeling symptoms. We must find our true relationship with the emotion. For instance, fear is my projection, my resistance, and my own reaction; so it is me. The moment we realize that I am the fear and the fear is me, that realization kindles pithara agni and starts burning the toxic molecules of fear. Then our cellular chemistry changes and fear matures into pure awareness and love.

We have to add a step to the approach of western psychology, and that is how we can use emotions as a springboard to jump into the transcendental state of meditation. In that transcendental state, when pīlu agni and pithara agni are balanced, every cell becomes a bliss cell and our bodies become bliss bodies. Bliss is not pleasure. Bliss is the transcendental state of pure awareness, where free radicals are completely neutralized and there is no āma in the cell. In such a cell, the *chitta* (mind stuff), buddhi, and manas of the cell merge into pure awareness. Bliss is contagious. If one cell becomes a bliss cell, it also makes neighboring cells full of bliss molecules. Daily practice of meditation enhances your bliss molecules and then meditation becomes automatic, subconscious. How long should one meditate? The answer is until meditation becomes subconscious and natural. Then life becomes a movement of meditation—in the way you walk, talk, eat, and listen. Every action is directly connected to your innermost pithara agni.

Conclusion

Digestion is a subtle process that transforms food into consciousness. Initial digestion takes place in the gastrointestinal tract, governed by jāthara agni. Rasa (taste) occurs on the tongue, due to bodhaka agni, and nourishes rasa dhātu. Vīrya (potent energetic effect) is experienced in the stomach and small intestine, due to jāthara agni, and acts on the dhātu agnis. Simultaneously, the six stages of digestion each directly nourishes one particular asthāyi dhātu, via the taste of that particular stage. The sweet stage nourishes rasa, sour nourishes rakta, and so forth. In the last of these six stages, astringent avasthā pāka, vipāka (post-digestive effect) begins in the colon, due to bhūta agni and colon agni, and acts on the excreta and cellular (pīlu) agni. The bhūta agnis take the gunas (qualities) yielded by rasa, vīrya, and vipāka and nourish the tanmātrās (sound, touch, form, taste, odor) at the cellular level, in conjunction with pīlu and pithara pāka.

The bhūta agnis from the liver govern the transformation of food, water, and air into the five elements. These elemental components of food are circulated in āhāra rasa, due to the law of irrigation. Pīlu agni at the cellular level or dhātu agni at the tissue level, then selects certain elemental components to nourish that particular cell or tissue. This is the law of selectivity. Pīlu agni or dhātu agni then transforms these elements from asthāyi (immature) form into sthāyi (mature) cellular or dhātu components. Finally, pithara agni within the cell nucleus nourishes consciousness via sattva, rajas, and tamas. This is the level where prabhāva (specific, unexplained action) can occur.

Vāta, pitta, and kapha are the physiological functional units of the body and prāna, tejas, and ojas are their representatives at the molecular level, governing cellular activity. Ojas maintains cellular immunity, tejas governs the digestion, absorption, and transformation of food, and prāna maintains cellular respiration. When ojas, tejas, and prāna are harmonized, they produce soma. Soma is the pure essence of ojas and is a celestial, tranquilizing drink. In other words, *every cell receives nutrition and tranquility*. In the highest profound transcendental state of meditation, *every cell becomes a bliss cell*. That is the spiritual function of ojas. Soma is Shiva, the higher transcendental state of awareness. Soma is the moon, *amrita*. Amrita means eternity, immortality, ambrosia, or nectar. If you look at a picture of Lord Dhanvantari, the deity of Āyurveda, he carries a jar that contains soma. Your agni has the capacity to transform your food not only into gunas; not only into ojas, tejas, and prāna; but into soma. The ultimate fate of your food is to become bliss.

9

Conclusion

आयुर्वेद

सम दोषाः समाग्निश्च सम धातुमलक्रियाः ।
प्रसन्नात्मेन्द्रियमनाः स्वस्थ इत्यभिधीयते ॥

सु १५ ३८

sama doṣāḥ samāgniś ca sama dhātu mala kriyāḥ
prasannātmendriya manāḥ svastha ityabhidhīyate
(Sushruta Samhita, 15.38)

One who is established in Self, who has balanced
doshas, balanced agni, properly formed dhātus, proper
elimination of malas, well functioning bodily processes, and
whose mind, soul, and senses are full of bliss, is called a
healthy person.

The Āyurvedic Definition of Health

Āyurveda considers health to be a state of perfect balance
between vāta, pitta, and kapha, corresponding to one's
individual prakruti, and a balance of the seven dhātus (tissues)
and three malas (waste products). Health does not mean

absence of defined disease. When doshas, dhātus, and malas are in proper functional relationship, there is a perfect balance of the body, senses, mind, and consciousness. There is clarity, happiness, joy, peace, and love. Good, robust agni allows this state of health to manifest and balanced agni is also the outcome of balanced doshas, dhātus, and malas. At a cellular level, this translates as a perfect balance of ojas, tejas, and prāna, and a predominance of sattva in the mind. One's sense of well-being reflects this inner state of health. Practically speaking, the most important aspect is harmony between the doshas, which results from dealing with the physical and emotional factors in one's life.

The Doshas

Pitta dosha governs metabolism, that is, the physical and biochemical transformations that take place within the body. Through this process, food and thoughts are transformed into energy, heat, and vitality. Pitta performs these functions throughout one's life, but is especially prominent during the adult years. All these activities of pitta depend upon agni. Poor agni means poor health. Wrong diet, wrong lifestyle, and repressed emotions can all alter the normal function of agni and pitta dosha.

Anabolism is the process of building up the body. It is the creation, growth, and repair of cells. This is managed by kapha and is most active from birth to the early teenage years. Kapha dosha can also be disturbed by poor diet and lifestyle, and unprocessed emotions. Catabolism is the destructive, but necessary, stage of transformation where larger molecules are broken down into smaller ones. For example, we constantly produce new red blood cells, which is anabolism. The maintenance of their activity is metabolism, governed by pitta through its fire component, agni. Eventually every blood cell dies, which is catabolism. This molecular death is governed by vāta dosha and is most active in old age. Vāta-provoking food and lifestyle, as well as emotional disturbances, can create imbalanced vāta and disturb health.

When anabolism is greater than catabolism there is growth. If catabolic activity is greater, there is emaciation or deterioration. Metabolism tries to achieve a balance between the anabolic and catabolic functions. Robust agni maintains this balance and gives a long, healthy life.

Vāta, pitta and kapha are present everywhere in the body, and these three doshas are the body's protective mechanism. They are constantly bombarded by time, in the form of age, time of day, and seasons. They are also impacted by the food we eat, our emotions, our relationships, the changes of the sun, moon, planets, and astral bodies, and even the place we live. All these factors affect the doshas and our sense of well-being, which is our inner state of balance. The state of agni and one's inner response to the outer world also challenge the integrity of vāta, pitta and kapha.

At the time of fertilization, the predominant dosha in both the male seed and the female egg is responsible for the creation of an individual's unique constitution, called prakruti. Prakruti reflects one's psycho-physiological temperament and disease proneness. The doshas have an affinity for one another and thereby support our prakruti. Where there is pitta, there is kapha and vāta. Where there is kapha, there is vāta and pitta. Without all three doshas, no one can exist on this planet.

The Interactions of the Doshas

If 100 buffalo and cows are put together, the cows will group with the other cows and the buffalo with the other buffalo. Like attracts like. Similarly, pitta and kapha are both liquid, so the liquid quality of pitta maintains the liquid quality of kapha, and the liquid quality of kapha nourishes the liquid quality of pitta. Likewise, the unctuous and oily qualities of pitta and kapha promote each other. However other qualities of pitta—hot, sharp, and light—counteract the other qualities of kapha—cold, slow, and heavy. With the hot, sharp, and light qualities, pitta penetrates into kapha and breaks kapha molecules into smaller and smaller particles, making them lighter. The light, spreading, and sharp qualities of pitta also attract vāta, because vāta is light, mobile, and subtle, which is similar to sharp.

Vāta and kapha both have cold quality, so if a person is exposed to the cold, kapha and vāta will both be increased. Vāta individuals with arthritic pain and kapha individuals with sinus congestion can both have worsened symptoms in cold weather. When a person is exposed to cold air, the first dosha increased is vāta, causing goose bumps and shivering. Damp cold creates increased kapha, causing congestion.

The predominant quality in a particular person inhibits the minor quality. If the hot quality of pitta is predominant, it will not only neutralize the cool quality of kapha, it will also warm vāta. The Air element is cold, even though physical air becomes hot in summer and cold in winter. Hence bodily air (vāta) is cold and dry. Cold has penetrating action, and along with sharp quality can cause frostbite. Mucus (kapha) can be cool or even warm, because water retains some heat. Therefore when comparing the two, vāta is cold and kapha is cool, in the same way that ice is cold and water is cool. In this way the cold quality of vāta and the cool quality of kapha have a relationship.

When vāta, pitta, and kapha are balanced according to the person's prakruti, their opposite qualities control each other and give health and happiness. If the doshas become imbalanced, their opposite qualities aggravate and provoke each other, creating disease and toxicity. This qualitative control by the doshas constantly maintains the individual's genetic code, when under the influence of normal, healthy agni.

The qualities of vāta when balanced create happiness, joy, creativity, and flexibility. Imbalanced vāta creates indecision and confusion, as well as restlessness, anxiety, fear, nervousness, insecurity, hyperactivity, and ungroundedness. The higher functions of pitta are knowledge, comprehension, appreciation, right judgment, recognition, and total understanding. Disturbed qualities of pitta give wrong judgment, prejudice, manipulation, anger, hate, and envy, leading to chemical depression and suicidal thoughts. The balanced qualities of kapha produce love, compassion, forgiveness, centeredness, groundedness, stability, and all-inclusiveness. When the qualities of kapha are disturbed, it can create ignorance, lethargy, delusion, laziness, attachment, greed, possessiveness, excess sleep, and depression.

Factors That Affect Our Health

Āyurveda is a way of healing and a way of life that always takes into consideration the whole person. According to the teachings of Āyurveda, every aspect of your life contributes to your overall health. Poor health seldom has a simple or single cause. Some factors will respond to changes, like diet, and some are beyond individual control, like the weather. With the latter, there are actions that can be taken to reduce or eliminate the impact. Of course, it is not possible or wise to try to change everything at once. Āyurveda says that slow and steady is the best route to successful change.

Most people find that diet is the best place to begin an Āyurvedic lifestyle. To this end, there are ten important dietary habits to avoid:

1. Overeating
2. Eating without real hunger
3. Emotional eating
4. Drinking fruit juice or excess water or no water during a meal

5. Drinking chilled water at any time
6. Eating when constipated or emotionally disturbed
7. Eating before 7 AM or after early evening
8. Eating too much heavy food or too little light food
9. Snacking on anything except fruit between meals
10. Eating incompatible food combinations, such as fruit with a meal

Choosing a Balanced Lifestyle

Lifestyle has its own rhythm in each person's life. Waking too early or late, irregular food habits, staying up late, job stress, untimely bowel movements, and suppression of natural urges are a few habits that can unsettle a person. Regularity in sleeping, waking, eating, and elimination brings discipline and helps to maintain the integrity of the doshas and overall good health.

The body's biological clock is regulated by the doshas. The time of maximum activity of kapha is during early morning and early evening, the pitta period is during midday and midnight, while vāta hours are dawn and dusk. This reflects the individual life cycle, where kapha rules the early childhood years, pitta governs from puberty to middle age, and vāta is predominant in later years. Similarly, there are three broad phases of digestion, each governed by a particular dosha. The first phase is kapha, the second is pitta, and the third is a vāta phase. Finally each season is ruled by one of the doshas. Health results from acting with awareness to do the right thing at the right time. That way our doshas will be in harmony.

Exercise, too, should be appropriate for one's own constitution. Kapha individuals can perform the most strenuous exercise, pitta a medium amount and vāta a small amount of gentle exercise. Walking, swimming, and yoga are probably the best types of exercise of all for any constitution. Adequate exercise stimulates the gastric fire, improves digestion, relieves constipation, and induces relaxation and sound sleep.

Āyurveda has definite suggestions about the role of sex in one's life. The role of sex is to bring creative energy into our relationships. With the right person at the proper time, sex can unfold higher love. Sexual activity should be avoided after heavy meals, when hungry, or if angry, for this could be detrimental to health.

Relationships, Emotions, and Meditation

Daily life is relationships, both the relationships we have with one another and the one we have with ourselves. Ideally, clarity, compassion, and love should characterize these relationships. It is often easier to love and respect others more than one's self. Relationships are mirrors to use for self-learning, enquiry, and investigation. Through that learning, inner transformation can take place. If our relationships are unclear, confusion and conflict will affect our well-being.

Emotions, like anger, fear, or anxiety, arise from reactions to our daily relationships. These reactions are due to inattention in the moment. Each person needs to pay total attention to his or her thoughts, feelings, and emotions. If they do not, these will be undigested and just as capable of poisoning the body as bad food combinations. Each emotion is a biochemical response to a challenge and may provoke the doshas. Fear and anxiety will provoke vāta, anger and hate upset pitta, and attachment and greed will aggravate kapha.

Meditation plays a most important part in daily life and is a powerful tool to help maintain health. While the dictionary says that the term meditation means "to think, to ponder, to go through and examine," this definition does not impart the profound meaning of the word at all. Meditation is an action of clear perception, an observation with total awareness and without any conclusion, judgment, or criticism. Meditation demands that you be utterly one with the moment. In this oneness, there is radical change in one's psyche. In this moment-to-moment awareness, there is a cleansing of the body, mind and consciousness. This will bring you to that state of peace that is joy, bliss, and enlightenment. At this point, life becomes a movement of spontaneous meditation.

Behavioral Medicine
Everything we do can bring us closer to our true nature, and Āyurveda is a means of bringing total awareness to every thought and action. This is behavioral medicine in its purest form. We will conclude with a sutra that shows us the path to good health, which means a state of balance between body, mind, and consciousness.

May your journey through life bring you truth and bliss. Namaste.

नित्यं हिताहारविहारसेवी समीक्ष्यकारी विषयेष्वसक्तः ।
दाता समः सत्यपरः क्षमावानाप्तोपसेवी च भवत्यरोगः ॥

वा. सू. अ. ६

nityam hitāhāra vihārasevī samīkṣyakārī viṣayeṣvasaktaḥ
dātā samaḥ satyparaḥ kṣamāvān āptopa sevī ca bhavat
yarogaḥ

(Vāgbhata Sūtrasthāna)

That person who always eats wholesome food, enjoys a regular lifestyle, remains unattached to the objects of the senses, gives and forgives, loves truth, and serves others, is without disease.

Appendix

The Twenty Attributes (Gunas) and Their Effects on the Doshas

Quality	Vāta	Pitta	Kapha	Agni	Actions
Heavy	↓	↓	↑	↓	Increases bulk nutrition and heaviness, creates dullness and lethargy.
Light	↑	↑	↓	↑	Helps digestion, reduces bulk, cleanses, creates freshness and alertness.
Slow	↓	↓	↑	↓	Creates sluggishness, slow action, relaxation and dullness.
Sharp	↑	↑	↓	↑	Immediate effect, promotes sharpness, quick understanding, creates ulcers.
Cold	↑	↓	↑	↓	Creates cold, numbness, contraction, unconsciousness, fear and insensitivity.
Hot	↓	↑	↓	↑	Promotes heat, digestion, cleansing, expansion, inflammation, anger and hate.
Oily	↓	↑	↑	↓	Creates smoothness, moisture, lubrication, vigor, compassion and love.
Dry	↑	↓	↓	↑	Increases dryness, absorption, constipation and nervousness.
Slimy	↓	↑	↑	↓	Decreases roughness, increases smoothness, love and care.
Rough	↑	↓	↓	↑	Causes cracking of skin and bones, creates carelessness and rigidity.
Dense	↓	↓	↑	↓	Promotes solidity, density and strength.
Liquid	↓	↑	↑	↓	Dissolves and liquefies, promotes salivation, compassion and cohesiveness.
Soft	↓	↑	↑	↓	Creates softness, delicacy, relaxation, tenderness love and care.
Hard	↑	↓	↑	↓	Increases hardness, strength, rigidity, selfishness, callousness and insensitivity.
Static	↓	↓	↑	↓	Promotes stability, obstruction, support, constipation and faith.
Mobile	↑	↑	↓	↑	Promotes motion, shakiness, restlessness, and lack of faith.
Subtle	↑	↑	↓	↑	Pierces, penetrates subtle capillaries, increases emotions and feelings.
Gross	↓	↓	↑	↓	Causes obstruction and obesity.
Cloudy, Sticky	↓	↓	↑	↓	Heals fractures, causes unclearness, and lack of perception.
Clear	↑	↑	↓	↑	Pacifies, creates isolation and diversion.

The Seven Bodily Tissues (Sapta Dhātu)

Dhātu (Tissue)	Function	Size	Upa-dhātu (Superior by-product)	Dhātu Mala (Inferior by-product)
Rasa (Plasma and lymph)	Nutrition, Affection (prīnana), Immunity	9 añjali	Top layer of skin Lactation (stanya) Menstruation (rajah)	Poshaka kapha
Rakta (Red blood cells)	Life function (jīvana), Oxygenation, Enthusiasm	8 añjali	Blood vessels and granulation tissue (sirā) Small tendons and sinews (kandara)	Poshaka pitta
Māmsa (Muscle tissue)	Plastering (lepana), Form, Movement, Support, Strength, Protection	varies	Six layers of skin (tvacha) Subcutaneous fat (vasā)	Ear wax, nasal crust, sebaceous secretions, tooth tartar, smegma (khamala)
Meda (Adipose tissue)	Lubrication, Personal love (snehana), Bulk to body, Insulation, Beauty	2 añjali	Tendons, sinews, ligaments, flat muscles (snāyu)	Sveda (sweat)
Asthi (Bone tissue)	Support (dhārana), Structure, Protection of vital organs	Approximately 365 bones	Teeth (danta) Cartilage (taruna asthi)	Hair (kesha) Nails (nakha)
Majjā (Bone marrow Nervous tissue Connective tissue)	Fills bone spaces (pūrana), Sensation, Communication, Learning, Memory	2 añjali	Lacrimal secretions (ashru)	Oily secretions in eyes (akshi sneha) Epithelial and mucous secretions that help discharge the bowel (vit sneha)
Shukra and Ārtava (Reproductive tissue)	Reproduction (prajanana), Produce ojas, Emotional release	½ añjali	Ojas	Apparently none but functionally is the pubic and axillary hair, secondary sexual characteristics

The 40 Main Types of Agni

Type(s) of Agni	Synonyms & Names	Sites	Functions
Jāthara Agni	Maha Agni Koshta Agni Kāya Agni Antara Agni	Āmāshaya (stomach)[a] Grahani (small intestine)[b]	Governs gross digestion in the gastrointestinal tract, the end product of which is āhāra rasa (chyle). The central fire, which regulates all other agnis in the body. All bodily agnis are flames of jāthara agni.
Kloma Agni		Kloma (pancreas and choroid plexuses)	Governs thirst, water metabolism, pancreatic enzyme secretions, and digestion of sweet taste.
Five Bhūta Agnis	Nabhasa Agni (Ether); Vāyavya Agni (Air); Tejo Agni (Fire); Āpo Agni (Water); Pārthiva Agni (Earth). Also called Pañcha (five) Bhūta Agnis.	Liver	Conversion of the five elements of ingested food into biologically available forms of the elements that can be utilized by the body. Represented by the various liver enzymes.
Jatru Agni		Ūrdhva jatru (thyroid) Adha Jatru (thymus)	Bridge between bhūta agni and dhātu agni. Regulates bodily metabolism; maintains immunity.
Seven Dhātu Agnis	Also called Sapta (seven) Dhātu Agnis.	Dhātu dhara kalā, the membrane which functionally separates each dhātu.	Nourishment of tissues; maintenance of tissue metabolism; transformation of immature into mature dhātu.
Pīlu Agni		Within the cell membrane	Maintains semi-permeability of cell membranes; converts extra-cellular molecules of food, water, and air into living cells; nourishes cells.
Pithara Agni		The membrane of the cell nucleus	Transforms cellular nutrients into consciousness.
Five Indriya Agnis	There is one agni for each of the five senses: Shabda (hearing) Sparsha (touch) Rūpa (vision) Rasa (taste) Gandha (smell)	Sense organs	Conversion of sensory input into a fully experienced, processed understanding.

The 40 Main Types of Agni

Type(s) of Agni	Synonyms & Names	Sites	Functions
15 Dosha Agnis	There is one dosha agni for each of the fifteen dosha subtypes.	The sites of each of the doshic subtypes. Includes rañjaka agni in liver, stomach, bone marrow, blood.	Functions of Rañjaka Agni, processing hemoglobin from old red blood cells; bile formation. To maintain the normal psychophysiology of each dosha subtype and their nutrition.
Three Mala Agnis	Mūtra (urine) Purisha / Kitta (feces) Sveda (sweat)	Primarily the bladder, colon, and sweat glands.	Processing of excreta (urine, feces, sweat).

a. **Major digestive functions of the stomach.** Churning of food bolus. Secretion of hydrochloric acid (HCl) and enzymes. Begins digestion of protein and fat. Absorption of water and glucose. Excretion of toxins and alkaloids.

b. **Major digestive functions of the small intestine.** Secretion of intestinal juices. Bile from gall bladder and pancreatic enzymes are secreted through their respective ducts into the duodenum, for further fat, protein, and carbohydrate digestion. Later digestion and absorption occurs in the jejunum and ileum.

Disorders of Ojas, Tejas, and Prāna

Ojas Disorders	
Ojo visramsa[a]	Cause is vishama dhātu agni (vāta or pitta). May be vāta pushing pitta or pitta blocking vāta.
Ojas kshaya[b]	Cause is tīkshna dhātu agni (pitta or vāta). Leads to vāta problems.
Ojo vruddhi[c]	Cause is manda dhātu agni (kapha). Raw ojas. Results in kapha problems.
Ojo vyāpad[d]	Ojo dushti. Any doshic disorder causing qualitative change in ojas.
Tejas Disorders	
Tejo visramsa	Cause is vishama dhātu agni (vāta) leading to vāta problems, *or* manda dhātu agni (kapha) leading to kapha problems.
Tejas kshaya	Cause is manda dhātu agni (kapha). Results in kapha problems.
Tejo vruddhi	Cause is tīkshna dhātu agni (pitta or vāta). Raw tejas. Leads to pitta problems.
Tejo vyāpad	Tejo dushti. Any doshic disorder causing qualitative change in tejas.
Prāna Disorders	
Prāna visramsa	Cause is vishama dhātu agni (vāta). Maybe from suppression of urges, shock. Leads to scattered energy.
Prāna kshaya	Cause is tīkshna dhātu agni (pitta or vāta). Leads to vāta problems. Similar symptoms to ojas kshaya. If low prāna, there is low tejas and low ojas. A common scenario is that weak ojas hinders proper transmission of tejas, leading to toxins, which block prāna flow and causes prāna kshaya.
Prāna vruddhi	Cause is manda dhātu agni (Kapha). Raw prāna. Leads to vāta problems. these include hyperactivity, breathlessness, A.D.D. May be from pitta or kapha blocking prāna.
Prāna vyāpad	Prāna dushti. Any doshic disorder causing qualitative change in prāna.

a.   Visramsa is a displacement of ojas, tejas, or prāna.
b.   Kshaya is a decrease or depletion in quantity of ojas, tejas, or prāna.
c.   Vruddhi is an increase in quantity of ojas, tejas, or prāna.
d.   Vyāpad means disturbed in quality.

Srotāmsi, the Systems and Channels of the Body

Srotāmsi	Functions	Mūla (Root)	Mārga (Passage)	Mukha (Mouth or Opening)
Prāna Vaha Srotas	Respiration, Emotions, Thinking, Communication (with higher self)	Left chamber of heart, GI tract (maha srotas)	Respiratory tract, bronchial tree including alveoli	Nose (nasa)
Ambu Vaha Srotas	Body temperature, Lubrication, Energy, Electrolyte balance, Selection of wastes	Pancreas (kloma), Soft palate (tālu), Choroid plexus	GI mucous membrane	Kidneys (vrukka), Tongue, Sweat glands (roma kupa)
Anna Vaha Srotas	Digestion, Assimilation, Absorption	Esophagus, Stomach - fundus (greater curvature)	GI tract (maha srotas) - lips through to ileocecal	Ileocecal valve
Rasa Vaha Srotas	Nutrition, Affection (prīnana), Immunity, Faith, Regulation of blood pressure and volume	Right chamber of heart (where all venous blood comes), 10 great vessels	Venous system, Lymphatic system	Venous/arterial junction
Rakta Vaha Srotas	Life function (jīvana), Oxygenation, Enthusiasm	Liver (yakrut), Spleen (pliha)	Arterial circulatory system	Arterial/venous junction
Māmsa Vaha Srotas	Plastering (lepana), Form, Movement, Support, Protection, Strength	Fascia and small tendons (snāyu), Mesoderm, 6 layers of skin (tvacha)	Entire muscle system including smooth, heart, involuntary muscles	Pores of skin
Meda Vaha Srotas	Lubrication (snehan), Personal love, Beauty, Insulation, Bulk to body	Omentum, Adrenal glands (vrukka)	Subcutaneous fat	Sweat glands (roma kupa)
Asthi Vaha Srotas	Support (dhārana), Structure, Protection of vital organs	Pelvic girdle, Sacrum	Skeletal system	Nails, Hair
Majjā Vaha Srotas	Fills bone spaces (pūrana), Sensation, Communication, Learning, Memory, Coordination	Brain, Spinal cord, Joints and junctions between dhātus (sandhi)	Central, Sympathetic, and Parasympathetic Nervous Systems	Synaptic space, Neuro-muscular cleft

Srotāmsi, the Systems and Channels of the Body

Srotāmsi	Functions	Mūla (Root)	Mārga (Passage)	Mukha (Mouth or Opening)
Shukra Vaha Srotas	Reproduction (prajanana), Produces ojas, Emotional release	Testicles, Nipples	Vas deferens, Epididymis, Prostate, Urethra, Urinogenital tract	Urethral opening
Ārtava Vaha Srotas	Reproduction (prajanana), Produces ojas, Emotional release	Ovaries, Areola of nipples	Fallopian tubes, Uterus, Cervical canal, Vaginal passage (yoni)	Labia minor/major (yoni oshtha)
Rajah Vaha Srotas	Menses	Fundus of the uterus	Endometrium Uterus	Cervix and vaginal passage
Stanya Vaha Srotas	Lactation	Lactiferous glands	Lactiferous ducts	Duct openings in nipples
Purisha Vaha Srotas	Absorption of minerals, Strength, Support, Formation and elimination of feces	Cecum, Rectum, Sigmoid colon	Large intestine	Anal orifice
Mūtra Vaha Srotas	Electrolyte balance, Elimination of urine, Maintenance of blood pressure	Kidneys	Ureter (kidney to bladder), Bladder, Urethra	Urethral opening
Sveda Vaha Srotas	Elimination of liquid wastes, Perspiration, Electrolyte balance, Body temperature, Lubrication	Sweat glands	Sweat ducts	Sweat duct, Openings in pores of skin
Mano Vaha Srotas	Thinking, Feeling, Inquiring, Deciding, Discrimination, Desire, Memory, Communication	Heart (cardiac plexus), 5 bilateral pairs nādi (pathways) - 1 pair (10) for each of the 5 senses	Entire body	Sense organs (ears, skin, eyes, tongue, nose), Marmāni (marma points)

Relationship of Sattva, Rajas, and Tamas to Foods and Behavior

Foods	Sattvic	Rajasic	Tamasic
Fruits	Mango, pomegranate, coconut, figs, dates, peaches, pears	Sour fruits: oranges, apples, banana, guava, tamarind	Avocado, watermelon, plums, apricots. *Note:* fruit overall is sattvic
Vegetables	Sweet potato, sprouts, leafy greens, zucchini, yellow squash, asparagus	Potatoes, nightshades, cauliflower, broccoli, spinach, winter squash, pickles	Mushrooms, garlic, onion, pumpkin
Grains	Basmati rice, quinoa, blue corn, tapioca, barley	Millet, corn, buckwheat	Wheat, brown rice
Beans	Mung beans and dal, red and yellow lentils	Brown lentils, lima beans, kidney beans, adzuki beans, tur dal, and small amounts of black, pinto, pink beans	Urad dal, and large amounts of black, pinto, and pink beans
Dairy	Fresh, unprocessed: cow's milk, ghee, soft cheese, homemade yogurt, goat's milk	Sour cream, salted or sour butter, cream, cottage cheese, ice cream	Cheese (hard, aged), processed milk, eggs
Nuts and Seeds	Almonds, white sesame seeds, fresh cashews	Most nuts, brown sesame seeds	Peanuts, rancid nuts, black sesame seeds
Spices	Saffron, turmeric, cardamom, coriander, fennel, cumin	Curry, chili, cayenne, and black pepper	Jalapeno pepper, nutmeg
Sweets	Fresh sugarcane juice, jaggary, raw sugar, raw honey (If bees are not harmed)	Processed sugar, artificial sweeteners, cooked honey	Molasses, soft drinks, stevia, extremely sweet tasting foods
Drinks, etc.	Certain herbal teas such as "Awareness tea," licorice tea	Coffee, black and green tea	Alcohol, marijuana, most drugs
Meats	None	Fish, shrimp, chicken	Beef, pork, lamb
Mental state and Behavior	Austerity, meditation, spiritual chanting, samādhi	Concentration, thinking, contemplation, excessive travel and movement	Unconsciousness, excessive sleep, coma
Emotions	Love, compassion, forgiveness	Fear, anxiety, envy, jealousy, anger	Attachment, loneliness, drowsiness, depression, destructive anger

Food Guidelines for Basic Constitutional Types

* OK in moderation ** OK occasionally	VATA		PITTA		KAPHA	
	AVOID	**FAVOR**	**AVOID**	**FAVOR**	**AVOID**	**FAVOR**
FRUITS[a]	Dried fruit Apples (raw) Pears Prunes (dry) Raisins (dry)*	Sweet fruit Bananas Berries, Cherries Grapefruit Grapes Lemons Limes Melons (sweet) Oranges Peaches Pineapple Plums Prunes (soaked)* Raisins (soaked)*	Sour fruit Apples (sour) Bananas Berries (sour) Cherries (sour) Grapefruit Grapes (green) Lemons Oranges (sour) Peaches Pineapple (sour) Plums (sour)	Sweet fruit Apples (sweet) Berries (sweet) Cherries (sweet) Dates Figs Grapes (purple)* Limes Melons Oranges (sweet) Pears Pineapple (sweet) Plums (sweet) Prunes Raisins	Sweet & sour fruit Bananas Dates Grapefruit Melons Oranges Pineapple Plums	Apples Cherries Figs (dry)* Grapes* Lemons* Limes* Peaches Pears Prunes Raisins Strawberries*
VEGETABLES	In general, dried, frozen or raw vegetables Broccoli Cabbage Cauliflower Celery Fresh corn** Eggplant Kale Mushrooms Onions (raw) Peas (raw) Peppers Potato (white) Squashes (winter) Tomatoes (raw); (cooked)**	In general, most cooked vegetables Asparagus Beets Carrots Cilantro Cucumber Green beans Leafy greens* Lettuce* Onions (cooked) Parsnip Peas (cooked) Potato (sweet) Pumpkin Spinach* Sprouts* Squashes (summer) Zucchini	In general, most pungent vegetables Beets (raw) Fresh corn** Eggplant** Mustard greens Onions (raw) Peppers (hot) Spinach (raw) (cooked)** Tomatoes	In general, most sweet & bitter vegetables Asparagus Beets (cooked)* Broccoli Cabbage Carrots (cooked)* Cauliflower Celery Cucumber Green beans Leafy greens Mushrooms Onions (cooked)* Peas Peppers, green Potato (sweet) Potato (white) Sprouts (most) Squashes Zucchini	In general, most sweet & juicy vegetables Cucumber Olives (black or green) Parsnips** Potato (sweet) Pumpkin Squashes (summer) Tomatoes (raw) Zucchini	In general, most pungent & bitter vegetables Asparagus Beets & greens Broccoli, Cabbage Carrots Cauliflower Celery Corn Eggplant Green beans Leafy greens Mushrooms Onions Peas Peppers Potato (white) Spinach* Sprouts Squashes (winter) Tomato (cooked)*
GRAINS	Barley Bran Bread (yeast) Buckwheat** Corn Granola Millet Oats (dry) Rice cakes** Rye	Amaranth* Oats (cooked) Quinoa Rice,(basmati, brown, white, wild) Wheat	Bread (yeast) Buckwheat Corn Millet Oats (dry) Rice (brown)** Rye	Amaranth Barley Bran Granola Quinoa Oats (cooked) Rice (basmati, white, wild) Rice cakes Wheat	Bread (yeast) Oats (cooked) Pasta** Rice (brown, white) Rice cakes** Wheat	Amaranth* Barley Bran Buckwheat Quinoa Corn Granola Millet Oats (dry) Rice (basmati)* Rye

Food Guidelines for Basic Constitutional Types

* OK in moderation ** OK occasionally	VATA		PITTA		KAPHA	
	AVOID	**FAVOR**	**AVOID**	**FAVOR**	**AVOID**	**FAVOR**
LEGUMES	Black beans Chick peas Kidney beans Lentils (brown) Miso** Navy beans Peas (dried) Pinto beans Soy beans Tempeh	Lentils (red)* Mung beans Soy cheese* Soy milk* Soy sauce* Tofu*	Miso Soy sauce	Black beans Chick peas Kidney beans Lentils (all) Mung beans Navy beans Pinto beans Soybeans Soy milk Soy cheese Tempeh* Tofu	Kidney beans Miso Soy beans Soy cheese Soy sauce Tofu (cold)	Black beans Chick peas Lentils (all) Mung beans* Navy beans Peas (dried) Pinto beans Soy milk Tempeh Tofu (hot)*

DAIRY	Cow's milk
	  (powdered)
	Goat's milk
	  (powdered)
	Ice cream**
	Yogurt (plain, w/
	  fruit or frozen)
		Most dairy is OK
		Buttermilk
		Butter, Ghee
		Cheese (hard)*
		Cheese (soft)
		Cow's milk
		Goat's milk
		Sour cream*
		Yogurt (spiced)*
			Butter (salted)
			Buttermilk
			Cheese (hard)
			Sour cream
			Yogurt (plain, w/
			  fruit or frozen)
				Butter (unsalted)
				Cheese (soft, not
				  aged, unsalted)
				Cow's milk
				Ghee
				Goat's milk
				Ice cream*
				Yogurt (freshly
				  made & diluted)*
					Butter (salted)
					Butter
					  (unsalted)**
					Cheese (most)
					Cow's milk
					Ice cream
					Sour cream
					Yogurt (plain, w/
					  fruit or frozen)
						Buttermilk*
						Cottage Cheese*
						Ghee*
						Goat's cheese
						  (unsalted & not
						  aged)*
						Goat's milk
						  (skim only)
						Yogurt (diluted)

ANIMAL FOODS	Chicken (white) Lamb, Mutton Pork Rabbit Venison Turkey (white)	Beef Chicken (dark) Eggs Fish (all) Shrimp Turkey (dark)	Beef Chicken (dark) Eggs (yolk) Fish (sea) Lamb Mutton Pork Turkey (dark)	Chicken (white) Eggs (white) Fish (freshwater) Rabbit Shrimp* Turkey (white) Venison	Beef Chicken (dark) Fish (sea) Lamb Mutton Pork Turkey (dark)	Chicken (white) Eggs (not fried) Fish (freshwater) Rabbit Shrimp Turkey (white) Venison
CONDIMENTS	Chocolate Horseradish	Chili peppers* Lemon Lime Mayonnaise Mustard Pickles Salt Seaweed Vinegar	Chili peppers Chocolate Mustard Mayonnaise Pickles Sea Salt Vinegar	Black pepper* Chutney, sweet mango Lime* Rock Salt* Seaweed*	Chocolate Lime Mayonnaise Pickles Salt Vinegar	Black pepper Chili peppers Horseradish Mustard Scallions Seaweed*
NUTS	None	In moderation: All nuts are good	No nuts except for those in "yes" column	Almonds (soaked and peeled) Coconut	Almonds** Coconut** All other nuts	Charole
SEEDS	Psyllium	Flax Pumpkin Sesame Sunflower	Sesame Tahini	Flax Psyllium Pumpkin* Sunflower	Psyllium** Sesame	Flax* Pumpkin* Sunflower*

Food Guidelines for Basic Constitutional Types

* OK in moderation ** OK occasionally	VATA		PITTA		KAPHA	
	AVOID	FAVOR	AVOID	FAVOR	AVOID	FAVOR
OILS	Flax seed	*Internal &* *external use:* Ghee Sesame Olive Most other oils *External:* Coconut	Almond Apricot Corn Safflower Sesame	*Internal &* *external use:* Ghee Sunflower Canola Olive *External:* Coconut	No oils, except for those in "yes" column	*For internal &* *external use in* *small amounts:* Corn Canola Sunflower *External:* Sesame
BEVERAGES	Alcohol (hard; red wine) Apple juice Caffeinated beverages Chocolate milk Cranberry juice Icy cold drinks Iced tea Prune juice** Soy milk (cold) Tomato juice** *Herb Teas:* Dandelion Ginseng Nettle** Red clover** Yerba Mate**	Alcohol (beer; white wine)* Almond milk Apple cider Carob* Grain 'coffee' Grape Juice Lemonade Orange juice Pineapple juice Soy milk (well- spiced & hot)* *Herb Teas:* Bancha Cinnamon** Fennel Licorice Peppermint Rosehips	Alcohol (hard; red wine) Caffeinated beverages Chocolate milk Cranberry juice Grapefruit juice Icy cold drinks Iced tea Lemonade Pineapple juice Tomato juice *Herb Teas:* Cinnamon** Ginseng Rosehips** Yerba Mate	Alcohol (beer; dry white wine)* Almond milk Apple juice Carob Grain 'coffee' Grape juice Orange juice* Pomegranate Prune juice Rice milk Soy milk *Herb Teas:* Chamomile Dandelion Fennel Licorice Mint Red clover	Alcohol (beer; hard; sweet wine) Almond milk Caffeinated beverages** Chocolate milk Grapefruit juice Icy cold drinks Iced tea Orange Juice Rice milk Tomato juice *Herb Teas:* Licorice* Marshmallow Rosehips**	Alcohol (dry wine)* Apple juice/cider* Carob Cranberry juice Grain 'coffee' Grape juice Pineapple juice* Pomegranate Prune juice Soy milk (hot & well-spiced) *Herb Teas:* Black tea, spiced Chamomile Cinnamon Fennel* Peppermint Yerba Mate
SPICES		Most spices are good!	Asafoetida (hing) Bay leaf Cayenne Cloves Garlic Ginger (dry) Mustard seed Nutmeg Oregano	Black pepper* Cinnamon Coriander Cumin Fennel Ginger (fresh) Saffron Turmeric Vanilla*	Salt	ALL spices are good.
SWEETENERS	Maple syrup** White sugar	Barley malt Honey (raw) Molasses Natural sugar Rice Syrup	Molasses White sugar**	Barley malt Honey* Maple syrup Rice syrup Natural sugar	Barley Malt Maple syrup Molasses Natural Sugar White sugar	Fruit juice concentrates Honey (raw & unprocessed)

NOTE: *Guidelines provided in this table are general. Specific adjustments for individual requirements may need to be made,*
e.g., food allergies, strength of agni*, season of the year, and degree of* dosha *predominance or aggravation.*
© 1994, 1997, 2001 Dr. Vasant Lad and The Ayurvedic Institute

The Ten Great Vessels

The ten great vessels are considered to have both a physical and an esoteric meaning. There are references throughout the ancient texts to them with varying interpretations of their meaning and significance. Here we offer a parallel of the two meanings.

The 10 Great Vessels

Physical	Esoteric[a]
Aorta	Cognitive Faculties
Inferior Vena Cava	Shabda (Hearing)
Superior Vena Cava	Sparsha (Touch)
	Rūpa (Seeing)
Right Pulmonary Artery	Rasa (Taste)
Left Pulmonary Artery	Gandha (Smell)
Right Pulmonary Veins	Organs of Perception
Left Pulmonary Veins	Ears
	Skin
Right Coronary Artery	Eyes
Left Coronary Artery	Tongue
	Nose
Coronary Vein	

a. The cognitive faculties and organs of perception carry the objects of perception to the heart.

Relevant Sutra

In the heart attached are ten vessels rooted there and of great significance. The words 'mahat,' 'artha' and 'hridaya' are synonymous. The body with six divisions, intellect, sense organs, five sense objects, self together with qualities, mind along with its objects are located in heart. (3-4)

Life known by the sense perception (reflexes) is located here. It is also the seat of the excellent ojas and reservoir of consciousness. That is why the heart has been said as 'mahat' (great) and 'artha' (serving all purposes) by the physicians.

From the heart as root, ten great vessels carrying ojas pulsate all over the body.

Charaka Samhita, Sutrasthana, Ch 30, verse 1-15

Glossary

A

āhāra rasa - Nutritive juice that is the end product of digested food, formed about 12 hours after eating; the nutritional precursor of all bodily tissues; asthāyi (unstable, unprocessed) form of rasa dhātu.

ajñā - The center point between the eyebrows related to the pituitary gland; the point where right hemisphere meets with left, alpha meets with omega, intuition meets with logic; the highest end point of human polarity; the center of cognition which is activated by light.

ākāsha - Ether or space element, the first of the five basic elements; the first expression of Consciousness; the subtle, light, expansive element which serves as the common factor or "home" for all objects in the universe and manifests as nuclear energy.

ālochaka - One of the subtypes of pitta dosha, situated in the sense organ of seeing; it is responsible for vision and color perception.

āmāshaya - The stomach; literally, the receptacle for undigested food.

ānanda - Bliss.

ānandamaya kosha - The sheath made of bliss.

āpas - Water; the Water element.

āpo agni - The fire component inherent in the water element.

āpta - Authoritative, truthful, trustworthy; authoritative testimony, one of the means of obtaining valid knowledge according to the Nyāya school.

āpya tejas - The fire component of water.

ārogya - Health.

ārtava - Female reproductive tissue, including ovaries, uterus, cervix, vagina, and the ova; closely associated with rasa dhātu due to its functional integrity with menstruation and lactation.

ārtava vaha srotas - The channels carrying nutrients for ārtava dhātu, or female reproductive tissue. The roots or governors of this channel are the ovaries and areola of the nipples. The pathway includes the fallopian tubes, uterus, cervical canal, and vaginal canal, and the opening is the labia of the vagina.

āsana - Yoga posture; one of the eight limbs of Yoga Philosophy; that which brings stability, strength, and ease to the body and mind.

ātman - The soul or Self.

āvila - Cloudy; characterized by cloudiness; confusion, loss of sensory perception; it increases kapha, decreases pitta and vāta.

āyuh - Life; longevity.

abhrak bhasma - Mica ash.

abhyanga - Full-body oil massage commonly given before pañchakarma to move doshas and toxins into the gastrointestinal tract where they can be removed by cleansing procedures; abhyanga is also done as part of a daily routine.

achintya vīrya - Unpredictable effect or action of a substance; a synonym for the word prabhāva.

adarshanam - Impaired visual perception, one of the signs of disturbed agni.

adhīrata - Impatience; living in the future; instability; all signs of impaired agni.

adho jatru granthi - The thymus gland.

agni - Fire element, the second of the five basic elements in the body; it regulates temperature, performs digestion, absorption, and assimilation of ingested food, and transforms food into energy or consciousness.

agni nārāyana - The fire that enters into the body of every human being and governs life.

agni tejas - The energy of the fire element.

Agnideva - The ancient Vedic deity of fire, both creative and destructive in nature; the energy of physical fire.

ahamkāra - A continuous feeling of "I am;" a center in the daily operating consciousness from where each individual thinks, feels, and acts as an independent being from his or her individual accumulated experience.

aharsha - Unhappiness, depression, signs of impaired agni.

akshi sneha - Oily secretions from the eyes; one of the inferior by-products of majjā dhātu.

alaukika - Supernatural; uncommon or unusual.

amātroshna - Loss of ability to regulate the body temperature, one of the signs of disturbed agni.

ambu vaha srotas - The bodily channels carrying water. The roots or governors of this channel are the pancreas, soft palate, and choroid plexus in the brain. Its pathway is the mucus membrane of the gastrointestinal tract, and the openings are the kidneys, tongue, and sweat glands.

amla - Sour taste; made of earth and fire, it increases pitta and kapha dosha, and decreases vāta dosha.

amla avasthā pāka - The sour stage of digestion that occurs in the second hour after eating.

amrita - Nectar; immortal nectar; anything strengthening, sweet, or beautiful.

anala - Fire; one of the synonyms for agni.

anāhata - The heart chakra; related to the thymus gland; the center of unconditional love; related to immunity; also denotes the cardiac plexus which governs heart activity.

anila - Cosmic prāna which maintains global life along with soma and sūrya; another name for vāta dosha; atmosphere.

añjali - A measurement formed when two hands meet together to make an empty bowl.

anna vaha srotas - The bodily channels that take in and carry food. This channel begins at the lips of the mouth, is governed by the esophagus and greater curvature of the stomach, continues through the entire gastrointestinal tract, and opens at the ileocecal valve.

annamaya kosha - Literally, the sheath made of food; the physical body.

antara agni - Internal fire; one of the synonyms for jāthara agni.

anu - Atom; also individual (as opposed to universal).

anu vaha srotas - The atomic channel or pathway; the pathway of atoms, which is the cell.

anumāna - Inference as one of the means of attaining valid knowledge according to the Nyāya system of philosophy.

apāna - The energy that governs outward movement; one of the subtypes of vāta dosha functioning mainly in the colon, it governs the elimination of feces, flatus, urine, menstrual blood, and other gross wastes, as well as subtle or cellular wastes.

apāna vāyu dushti - Disorder or disturbance of apāna vāyu; known by such symptoms as abdominal distention, diarrhea or constipation, gas, bloating, pain, and accumulation of wastes.

apakti - Indigestion; impaired digestion.

aparatva - Not beyond; postponement, a characteristic of tejas that gives the ability to know what is a priority and what may be done later, especially in a state of physical crisis.

ashauryam - Fear, anxiety, lack of courage, all signs of impaired agni.

ashita - One of the types of food; a soup or jelly-like thing that does not have to be masticated, just swallowed.

ashru - Lacrimation, tears; the superior by-product of majjā dhātu.

asthāyi - Unstable; immature; unformed; relates to stage in the process of tissue formation when food precursors have been selected by the tissue but have not yet been assimilated into the fully formed tissue.

asthāyi dhātu dushti - Entry of a dosha into the immature or unstable tissue causing qualitative disturbance; generally causes acute disorders, compared to those resulting from entry of a dosha into the stable, fully formed tissue.

asthavidhā vīrya - Eight qualities from the list of twenty gunas that tend to have the most prominent secondary effects on the body. They are the pairs of hot-cold, heavy-light, oily-dry, and the soft and sharp gunas. Hot and cold have the strongest effect on agni (digestive fire) and the remaining six qualities are experienced later or in a more subtle way.

asthi dhātu - One of the seven bodily tissues, asthi relates to bone tissue. Its major functions are supporting the body frame, giving protection, shape, and longevity, and making movement possible.

asthi vaha srotas - The channel carrying nutrients for asthi dhātu or bone tissue; its roots or governors are the pelvic girdle and sacrum. Its passageway is the entire skeletal system, and the openings or mouths of the channel are the nails and hair.

Atharvaveda - The fourth of the four Vedas, ancient scripture of India.

atipravrutti - Overflow; one of the three general categories of sroto dushti.

avalambaka - One of the five kapha subtypes present in the heart and lungs that supports all bodily kapha through circulation.

avyakta - Unmanifested; the pre-"big bang" state.

B

Bādarāyana - Name of the sage said to be the founder of Vedanta philosophy.

bala - Strength - physical, mental, and spiritual; a function of ojas and of healthy agni.

basti - Medicated enema, one of the five important cleansing measures of pañchakarma; it eliminates excess vāta via the colon, using herbal tea or oil enemas.

bhāsvara - Illumination; a characteristic of tejas.

Bhagavad Gītā - Name of a sacred celestial text that consists in a dialogue between Arjuna and Lord Krishna.

bhakti yoga - One of the main paths to liberation, the path of devotion leading to realization of the Divine in oneself.

bhasma - A specialized Āyurvedic preparation alchemically produced by fastidious purification and burning into ash; bhasmas are very potentized, easily absorbable, and release prāna into the system.

bhaumī tejas - Earthly tejas; The fire component present in the earth.

bhrājaka - One of the five types of pitta, located in the skin of the entire body. Its function is to give tactile sensation, color complexion, and luster to the skin, as well as digestion of any medications that are applied to the skin, such as oils, salves, or plasters.

bhrājaka agni - The fire component of bhrājaka pitta, which governs and organizes its functions.

bhrama - Faulty cognition, one of the three sources of invalid knowledge according to Nyāya philosophy.

bhūta - Element; the five basic elements of Ether, Air, Fire, Water, and Earth; that which manifests as matter

bhūta agni - The fire component of the five elements based in the liver, which manifests as the liver enzymes. It converts the five elements present in ingested food into biologically available forms of the elements that can be utilized by the body. There are five bhūta agnis, one for each of the five elements.

bindu - A drop; a point having no parts or magnitude; pulsating consciousness present at the time of fertilization of an ovum; the central point of a yantra.

bodhaka - The functions of kapha that are specifically related to the mouth and salivary glands, bodhaka protects and moisturizes the entire oral cavity and is related to taste recognition and secretion of saliva.

bodhana - Making known; understanding, knowledge.

brahmī - An herb similar to gotu kola.

brahma randhra - A small opening in the cranium located at the anterior fontanel of the brain and connected to the cosmic consciousness.

brahmanda - The expanding universal egg; the universe.

Brahman - The expansive, all-pervasive, universal consciousness; universal timeless existence; creative potential; the first in the Hindu trinity of gods: the creator of the universe (Brāhma).

Brahman agni - The fire of attention, awareness, and consciousness which is the ultimate higher function of agni; also known as dhyāna agni.

buddhi - The individual intellect.

buddhihāra - Lack of discrimination and reasoning power; indecisiveness; one of the signs of impaired agni.

buddhikāra - The creation of reasoning capacity, one of the functions of agni.

C

chāyā - Shadow; dullness; loss of luster; all signs of disturbed tejas or impaired agni.

chakra - The energy centers in the body, related to nerve plexus centers that govern the bodily functions. Each chakra is a separate reservoir of consciousness connecting the physical body to the astral body.

chala - Mobile; an attribute characterized by mobility and changeability; increases vāta and pitta, and decreases kapha.

chidākāsh - A space within the brain that is functionally connected to the synaptic spaces in between the neurons; the inner space of pure awareness present in the ventricles of the brain.

chikitsā - Treatment.

chitta - The mind; psychic energy; the psyche as a whole.

D

danta - Teeth; the superior by-product of asthi dhātu.

darshanam - Visual perception, one of the functions of healthy agni.

deha agni - Bodily fire; the general, non-specialized agni present throughout the body.

deha prakruti - The bodily constitution, incorporating the congenital state of the doshas. It results from changes in the doshas of the fetus during gestation, due to the mother's diet, lifestyle, emotions, and environment. Deha prakruti expresses congenital disorders and also any altered state of doshas that is so long-standing that it appears to be prakruti.

dhārana - The sixth limb in the Yoga system of Patañjali; the act of focusing attention on one object and mentally holding the object; one-pointed awareness.

dhātu - The elemental structural tissues that constitute the human body. There are seven basic tissues defined in Āyurveda: plasma, blood, muscle, fat, bone, nerve and bone marrow, and reproductive tissue.

dhātu agni - The agni component of each dhātu, located in the membrane that separates one dhātu from another. It nourishes the tissue, maintains tissue metabolism, and transforms immature tissue into mature tissue.

dhātu dhara kalā - The membranous structure between two dhātus that separates one dhātu from another.

dhātu dushti - Qualitative disorder of a stable, fully formed tissue.

dhātu kārshyana - Tissue emaciation; malnourishment; one of the signs of impaired agni

dhātu kshaya - Unduly decreased or diminished tissue.

dhātu poshana - Nutrition of the bodily tissues; one of the functions of healthy agni. Governed by the three laws of nutrition: irrigation, selectivity, and transformation.

dhātu vruddhi - Unduly increased or unprocessed tissue.

dhairyam - Patience; stability; confidence; all signs of healthy agni.

dhamanī - Artery.

dhī - Cognition; one of the faculties of buddhi, or intellect

dhruti - Retention; one of the faculties of buddhi, or intellect.

dhyāna - The seventh limb in the Yoga system of Patañjali; meditation; a continuous flow of attention without words or thoughts; a state of moment-to-moment, choiceless, passive awareness, or witnessing, without judgment, liking, or disliking.

dhyāna agni - The fire of attention, awareness, and consciousness which is the ultimate function of agni; also known as Brahman agni.

dig - Direction; one of the 9 causative factors according to Vaisheshika; vector, which is one of the factors influencing the creation and maintenance of the manifested universe.

dīpana - The action of kindling agni.

dīrgham - Appropriate span of life, maintained by healthy agni.

divya tejas - The fire component of ether or space.

dosha - Referring to vāta, pitta and kapha; the three psycho-physiological functional principles of the body, the ratio of which determines an individual's constitution at the time of conception. When functioning normally and present in normal quantities, the doshas maintain all healthy bodily processes. When out of balance, they create disease.

dosha dushti - Qualitative disturbance of any dosha, as opposed to quantitative disturbance.

dosha gati - The vector or direction in which a dosha moves.

dosha kshaya - Quantitative disturbance of any dosha wherein the dosha becomes depleted.

dosha prakruti - The ratio of doshas present at the time of birth, when the baby takes its first breath. The season, time, place, date, and planetary disposition at birth can all affect dosha prakruti.

dosha vruddhi - Quantitative disturbance of any dosha, wherein the dosha becomes increased.

dravatva - Fluidity or liquefaction, a function of tejas due to heat.

dravyamaya tejas - The tejas inherent in matter that has form, color, and shape; crystallized light.

dravya - Matter; substance; defined as that which has attribute and action, or guna and karma dwelling inseparably.

dravyashakti - The energy of matter; the energy of tamo guna (tamas).

duhkha - Literally, 'bad space'; a state of misery, pain, disease, unhappiness, or suffering of any kind.

dushti - Qualitative disturbance.

G

gandha - Odor; the tanmātrā relating to earth element; the subtle quality of the earth element that exists in objects, allowing them to be sensed by smell.

gati - Movement; gait.

Gautama - The founder of the Nyāya school of philosophy.

ghrita - A preparation of ghee (clarified butter) in which herbs are infused or boiled into the ghee.

grahani - The small intestine.

gulwel sattva - A preparation of the herb guduchi.

guna - Attribute or quality; one of the twenty qualities or attributes used to describe substances and determine their effects; also, one of the three universal qualities that are present in creation and that cause all phenomena. These are: sattva, the quality bringing essence, light, balance and understanding; rajas, the energy of movement and activity; and tamas, the quality bringing darkness, inertia, heaviness and materialism.

guru - Teacher; one who removes the darkness of ignorance; the channel through which understanding of the Divine comes to one; also: heavy, an attribute characterized by heaviness and bulk, it increases kapha and decreases pitta and vāta.

H

harsha - Joy, happiness, cheerfulness, all functions of healthy agni.

hrud - The heart; cardiac muscle.

I

Indra - An ancient Vedic deity; cosmic prāna.

indriya - Inner doors of perception, including sensory and motor organs and their pathways in the brain.

indriya agni - The fire component present in each of the five sense faculties, it converts sensory input into understanding, experience, and knowledge.

inorganic - being or composed of matter other than plant or animal: mineral.

J

jāthara agni - The central fire of the digestive system, responsible for digestion and assimilation of ingested food; it nourishes all bodily agni.

Jaimini - Name of the celebrated sage who founded the Mīmāmsa school of philosophy.

janma prakruti - Genetic prakruti, determined at the moment of conception by the state of the doshas in both of the parents. Once established, it does not change.

jatru agni - The fire component present in the thyroid gland; it is the bridge between bhūta agni and dhātu agni.

jihva - Tongue; one of the openings of ambu vaha srotas.

jīvātman - The individual soul.

jīva - Individual life; individual consciousness; the pure sense of "me."

jīvana - Life-giving (a special function of rakta dhātu).

ñāna - Wisdom or knowledge.

jñāna yoga - One of the main paths to liberation; the path of knowledge or wisdom to realize the Divine in oneself.

jñānamaya kosha - The sheath of knowledge, often considered to be part of vijñānamaya kosha.

jñānendriya - The five sensory faculties; the inner doors of perception, including sensory organs and their pathways in the brain.

jñānashakti - The energy of wisdom, cognition; the energy of sattva guna.

K

kālā - Time, the force that brings transformation in all matter; a measurement of movement; one of the nine causative substances of Vaisheshika.

Kāpila - The name of the sage who founded the Sānkhya school of philosophy.

kāya - Body.

kāya agni - Bodily fire; one of the synonyms for jāthara agni.

kāya chikitsā - Internal medicine; treatment of disorders relating to the entire body.

kalā - The membranous structure that holds a tissue, separating one from the other, it also lines all organs and cavities in the body.

kalala - The fertilized ovum; the first expression of creation; the primordial expression of the union between male and female.

kali - Flower bud.

Kanāda - The name of the sage who founded the Vaisheshika school of philosophy; considered to be the father of atomic theory.

kandara - One of the superior by-products of rakta dhātu; small tendons and sinews, such as hamstring muscles.

kapha - One of the three doshas, combining the water and earth elements; the psycho-physiological energy that forms the body's structure and holds the cells together.

karaja tejas - The fire component of foods; enzymes.

karma - Action; the law stating that for every action there is an equal and opposite reaction; specific action of a substance or herb; along with guna (attribute), karma makes up the inherent nature of a substance, according to Vaisheshika.

karma yoga - One of the main paths to liberation; the path of taking positive action and surrendering the fruits of all actions to the Divine.

karmendriya - The five motor faculties; the faculties of action, including motor organs and their pathways in the brain.

kashāya - Astringent taste; made up of air and earth, it increases vāta dosha and pacifies pitta and kapha.

kashāya avasthā pāka - The astringent stage of digestion, which takes place in the colon during the sixth hour or so after eating.

kathīna - Hard quality; hardness; increases vata and kapha and decreases pitta; associated with strength, rigidity, selfishness, callousness, and insensitivity. Also associated with things like pneumonia, callouses, and hardening of the arteries.

kati - Pelvic girdle, waist, lumbo-sacral area, lumbar spine.

katu - Pungent taste; made up of air and fire, it increases pitta and vāta doshas, and pacifies kapha dosha.

katu avasthā pāka - The pungent stage of digestion that occurs in the jejunum during the fourth hour after eating.

kedāra kulya nyāya - Irrigation; the first law of tissue nutrition; the process by which the end product of digested food, called āhāra rasa, is carried throughout the body via the circulatory system.

kesha - Hair; the inferior by-product of asthi dhātu.

khā - Space.

khāra - Rough quality; roughness, which is connected with dryness, absorption, constipation, and which aggravates vata and decreases pitta and kapha.

khadita - Food that must be masticated in order to become soft.

khale kapota nyāya - Selectivity; the second law of tissue nutrition; the process by which every cell and tissue selects the elemental components of ingested food that nourish that particular tissue.

khamala - The inferior by-products of māmsa dhātu, including nasal crust, earwax, sebaceous secretions, tartar, and smegma.

khavaigunya - Any weak or defective space in the body that exists because of past trauma, chronic disease, or hereditary influence and becomes a place where aggravated doshas can easily lodge and create disorder.

kitta - Waste product or inferior by-product; feces; the non-essential component of ingested food that is excreted from the body.

kleda - Liquefaction, hydration, water; sebaceous secretions, mucus, and other liquid secretions associated with kapha dosha.

kledaka - One of the kapha subtypes; its function is to liquefy ingested food in the stomach; it also protects the stomach wall from the digestive enzymes and acids; the gastric mucous membrane.

kloma - Pancreas; the root of the water carrying channels; kloma also refers to the choroid plexus in the brain.

kloma agni - The digestive energy of the pancreas. It works in conjunction with bhūta agni from the liver and assists in the digestion of proteins, carbohydrates, and fats.

kosha - Sheath. There are five sheaths that make up a human being: the sheath of bliss, the sheath of knowledge, the sheath of mind, the sheath of prāna, and the sheath of food.

koshta agni - Internal fire; one of the synonyms for jāthara agni.

kriyāshakti - Kinetic energy; a characteristic of rajo guna (rajas), energy of action and movement.

kshaya - Decreased, diminished; wasted. Signs of impaired agni include decay, weakness; and emaciation.

kshipta - Hyperactive mind; one of the five states of mind.

kshira dadhi nyāya - Transformation, coagulation; the third law of dhatu nutrition; the process by which the tissue precursors are transformed into the tissues themselves. This is the conversion of asthāyi (immature, unprocessed) dhatu into sthāyi (mature, processed) dhatu, governed by the dhatu agni.

kundalinī - The coiled, serpentine, spiritual energy, which, for most people, lies dormant at the base of the spine.

kundalinī shakti - The power of pure energy; the term used in describing the awakening of spiritual energy.

L

lāja - Roasted rice; apara ojas is described as possessing the smell of roasted rice.

laghu - Light; an attribute characterized by radiance and/or lightness, it aids in digestion, cleansing, and promotes freshness and alertness. In excess it may cause insomnia and ungroundedness; an attribute of both vāta and pitta doshas.

laukika - Ordinary; ordinary perception as opposed to extraordinary perception, relative reality.

lavana - Salty taste; made up of fire and water elements, it increases pitta and kapha dosha but pacifies vāta dosha

lavana avasthā pāka - The salty stage of digestion, which occurs in the duodenum during the third hour after eating.

lehya - Food that is licked, like ice cream. It is also one of the methods of ingesting medicines, especially bhasmas.

lekhana - "Scraping" action, the action of cleansing and removing fat and toxins from the body

lepana - Plastering; holding; one of the main important functions of māmsa dhātu

M

māmsa dhātu - One of the seven bodily tissues, māmsa consists of all types of muscle. Its functions include movement, coordination, "plastering," protection, maintenance of body temperature and body shape, ambition, confidence, and strength.

māmsa vaha srotas - The channel carrying nutrients for māmsa dhātu, or muscle tissue. The roots or governors of this channel are the fascia and small tendons. The passageway of the channel is the entire musculature system, and the opening of the channel is the pores of the skin.

mārga - Passageway; a synonym for the word srotas

mātroshna - Regulation of body temperature, one of the signs of healthy agni.

māyā - Universal illusion; the perceivable form of the Divine Mother

madhura - Sweet taste; made up of earth and water, it increases kapha dosha and pacifies pitta and vāta dosha

madhura avasthā pāka - The sweet stage of digestion, which occurs in the first hour after eating.

maha srotas - The largest channel in the body, the digestive tract

Mahad - The great principle; cosmic intelligence; the cosmic aspect of the intellect, it contains buddhi, the individual intellect, ego, and mind.

majjā dhātu - One of the seven bodily tissues, majjā consists of bone marrow, connective tissue, and nerve tissue, and associated with the endocrine system and erythrogenesis. Its main functions are

communication and filling space in the body, especially the spaces within the bones.

majjā vaha srotas - The channel carrying nutrients for majjā dhātu, or bone marrow and nervous tissue. The roots or governors for this channel are the brain, spinal cord, and joints. The pathway is the central, sympathetic, and parasympathetic nervous system. The opening is the synaptic space.

mala agnis - The fire located in the membranous structure of the organs of elimination, governing the elimination of waste products related to those organs.

mala vaha srotas - Another name for the channel carrying feces, or the purisha vaha srotas.

manas - Mind; one of the causative substances according to the Vaisheshika philosophy; the faculty arising from sattva guna according to the Sankhya school of thought; the sensory-feeling part of the mind that manifests thoughts and emotions, as contrasted with buddhi, the intellectual faculty of mind. Manas can be anu (individual) and vibhu (universal).

manas prakruti - Mental constitution, which is manifested at the time of fertilization and described in terms of the three gunas—sattva, rajas, and tamas. In the cosmic mind, equilibrium of the gunas is maintained; in an individual mind, these three are in unequal proportion, according to the karmas expressing in that individual's consciousness.

manda - Slow quality; an attribute that increases kapha and decreases vata and pitta, creates sluggishness, slow action, relaxation and dullness, as well as calm, quiet, and silence.

manda agni - Slow digestion; one of the three categories of disturbed agni; digestion affected by the heavy, slow, and cool qualities of kapha dosha, causing slow metabolism.

mano vaha srotas - The channel that carries the mind. The roots or governors of this channel are the heart and the sensory pathways. Its pathway is the entire body, and the opening or mouth of this channel is the sense organs and the marmāni.

manomaya kosha - The sheath made of mind; related to manas, the sensory and emotional mind.

mantra - A form of vocal or silent suggestion, usually repetitive; a syllable, word, or group of words that illuminate consciousness, bringing clarity, understanding, stillness, peace, prolonged concentration, and eventually samādhi; words uttered from the heart of a wise being. Mantra must be spoken, heard, or felt.

marmāni - The plural form of marma; vital energy points, similar to acupuncture points, where consciousness is most expressive.

marma - A vital point on the body that is used therapeutically and diagnostically.

maya - "Made of" as in prāna maya kosha, the sheath made of prāna.

meda dhātu - One of the seven bodily tissues, meda is a loose connective tissue that includes fat, steroids such as cholesterol, and other types of lipids. Its functions include storing energy, giving shape, beauty, and insulation to the body, sweet tone to the voice, and lubrication and protection of all bodily systems.

medhā - Mental and physical intelligence.

medhāhāra - Loss of intelligence, both mental and cellular; one of the signs of impaired agni.

medhākāra - The creation of intelligence and clear cellular communication; one of the functions of healthy agni.

medo vaha srotas - The bodily channel carrying nutrients for the fat tissue. The roots or governors of this channel are the omentum and the adrenals. The passageway is the subcutaneous fat tissue, and the opening is the sweat glands.

Mīmāmsa - One of the major philosophies that Ayurveda utilizes; Purva Mīmāmsa, founded by Jaimini, is based on the initial teachings of the Vedas, expounding liberation through performance of ritual, celebration, and duty; Uttara Mīmāmsa, also known as Vedanta, is based on the later, higher teachings of the Vedas, the Upanishads.

mithuna - Male and female energy merging together; sex.

moksha - Freedom, liberation; the final aim of all knowledge, work, and activity; the ultimate aim of life; the ending of involuntary and unconscious participation in the relative world

mrudu - Soft quality; softness, delicacy; promotes mucus, adipose tissue, relaxation, tenderness, love, care, promotes kapha and pitta and decreases vata.

mudrā - A gesture or positioning of the fingers practiced in devotional worship or yogic practice that allows for communication between the individual and the deity or the mind and body

mukta - The free or liberated mind that is completely aware, clear, attentive, and blissful; one of the five states of mind

mūdha - Deluded mind; hallucinating mind; one of the five states of mind.

mūlādhāra - The first chakra located in the root area of the trunk of the body; related to the gonads; associated with survival, groundedness, stability, security, and instincts.

mūrdhni - The head, the primary site of prāna vāyu.

mūtra agni - The fire component of the membranous structure surrounding the kidneys and bladder, it governs the functions of the urinary system. It maintains the glomeruli threshold, acid-alkali balance of urine, and specific gravity of urine.

mūtra vaha srotas - The channel that carries urine; the root or governor of this channel is the kidneys. The pathway of this channel is the ureters, urethra, and bladder. The opening or mouth of this channel is the opening of the urethra.

N

nādī - Literally, a river; a channel or passageway; the pulse; there are innumerable nādis in the human body, from the very subtle to the very gross, all carrying substances into, out of, or throughout the body

nabhasa agni - The fire component inherent in Ether element.

nakha - Nails; the inferior by-products of asthi dhātu.

nava karna dravya - The nine causative factors of the universe in the Vaisheshika school of philosophy, they are: the five elements, soul, mind, time, and direction.

nirvāna - State of pure existence; no-mind state.

nitya - Eternal; one of the characteristics of tejas, the eternal flame of life.

niyama - The five habits or codes of ethical/moral conduct expounded as the second limb in the eight-limbed Yoga system of Patañjali; the means of putting oneself into harmony with nature and establishing harmony in all relationships, niyama consists of: physical and mental purity, contentment, self-discipline/austerity, self-study, and surrender to God.

Nyāya - A major philosophy applied in Ayurveda; founded by Gautama; a system of obtaining valid knowledge of the material universe through reasoning and proper perception.

O

ojas - The subtle, positive energy of kapha dosha, it maintains immunity, strength, integrity, and vitality and has a functionally integrated relationship with tejas and prāna.

ojaskāra - Creation of ojas, the end product of tissue nutrition; one of the functions of healthy agni.

ojas kshaya - Quantitatively decreased ojas

ojodushti - Qualitative disturbance of ojas

ojohāra - Depletion of ojas; weakened immunity; one of the signs of impaired agni

ojo visramsa - Displaced ojas; impairment of the distribution of ojas, due to leakage and escape through one or more of the srotamsi (channels)

ojo vruddhi - Quantitatively increased ojas

ojo vyāpad - Ojas that is disturbed by one or more of the doshas

organic - Of, relating to, or derived from living organisms.

oshtha yoni - The labia, or lips of the vagina.

P

pāchaka - One of the five subtypes of pitta, located in the stomach and small intestine. It includes hydrochloric acid, digestive enzymes, pepsin, and intestinal juices secreted from the villi of the small intestine.

pāchana - Digestion; that which promotes digestion.

pāka - Digestion.

pārthiva agni - The fire component inherent in Earth element.

pakti - Digestion, absorption, and assimilation of food and sensory experience; one of the functions of agni.

pakvāshaya - The large intestine, colon.

pakvāshaya agni - The fire component in the large intestine or colon.

pancha rasa alavana - Five tastes except for salty; a name for triphala, which contains all the tastes except for salty taste.

panchakarma - The five methods for eliminating excess dosha and/or āma from the body for internal purification: vomiting, (vamana), purgation (virechana), decoction or oil enema (basti), bloodletting (rakta moksha), and nasal administration (nasya). In the panchakarma process, excessive dosha and/or āma is brought back to its main site in the body and

then eliminated through one or more of the five measures.

para - Beyond; superior; one of the two types of ojas, para ojas is the eight drops of superfine that stays in the heart.

Para Brahman - The highest self, beyond the body and the mind.

paramātman - The higher self; cosmic soul.

paratva - Beyond; priority, a quality of tejas that allows the cells to prioritize their functions in order to heal a trauma or disorder.

parināma - Transformation; change; growth; dimension or expansion, one of the qualities or functions of tejas —as in expansion due to heat.

Patanjali - Name of the celebrated sage who created The Yoga Sutras.

patha - Path; a synonym for the word srotas.

peyam - Food that can be drunk, like water, juice or gruel.

pīlu agni - The digestive fire present in the membrane of every cell, it maintains semi-permeability of the cell membrane and governs the selection of cellular nutrients.

pīlu pāka - The process of cellular digestion and nutrition which takes place in the cell membrane and in the cytoplasm outside the cell nucleus.

pithara agni - The fire component in the nuclear membrane inside the cell, it nourishes the RNA and DNA. Pithara agni maintains the genetic code, which is prakruti, and transforms cellular food into consciousness, yielding sattvic, rajasic, and tamasic qualities.

pithara pāka - The fire component in the nucleus of the cell; the purest manifestation of tejas in the body; it governs the transformation of cellular food into consciousness.

pitta - One of the three doshas, made up of the fire and water elements; governs digestion, absorption, assimilation, nutrition, metabolism, and body temperature.

poshaka - The essential component of ingested food, separated from the non-essential component to nourish bodily tissues. Literally, one who nourishes and supports; a name for asthāyi (unstable) dhātu, which nourishes the sthāyi (stable) dhātu; also a name for the precursors of each dosha.

poshaka kapha - The physical precursor or nourisher of kapha dosha, produced by rasa dhātu.

poshaka pitta - The physical precursor or nourisher of pitta dosha, produced by rakta dhātu; bile.

prāna - The vital life force without which life cannot exist and which is primarily taken in through the breath; the flow of cellular intelligence that governs cellular communication, sensory perception, motor responses, and all subtle electrical impulses of the body; the subtle essence of vāta dosha. Prāna has a functionally integrated relationship with ojas and tejas.

prāna vāyu - One of the five subtypes of vāta dosha, prāna moves inward and downward and is associated with the nervous system, where it governs all sensory functions and maintains attention, and with the lungs, where it governs inhalation.

prāna vaha srotas - The bodily channels that take in and carry prāna, or life force. The roots or governors of this channel are the left chamber of the heart and the entire gastrointestinal tract. The channel continues along the respiratory tract and bronchial tree, including the alveoli, and opens at the nose.

prānahāra - Depletion of prāna; one of the signs of impaired agni.

prānakāra - Creation of prāna, one of the functions of healthy agni.

prānamaya kosha - The sheath made of electromagnetic energy or vital essence. The etheric body.

prānāyāma - The control of life-energy by various techniques that regulate and restrain breath, helping one to control the mind and improve the quality of awareness and perception; this assists meditation.

prārabdha karma - That portion of previously accumulated karma that is manifesting at the present time or the present life.

prabhā - Luster, glow; one of the functions of healthy agni.

prabhāva - The dynamic, electro-magnetic action of a substance that cannot be explained by the logic of its taste, energy, and post-digestive effects (rasa, vīrya, and vipāka).

prajanana - Producing, creating; function of shukra and ārtava dhātus.

prakruti - Primordial matter, the Cosmic Mother or cosmic womb, the root cause of the creation of the universe; on an individual level, prakruti is the psychosomatic, biological constitution of an individual, the unique combination of the three doshas that forms the person's constitution at the time of conception and creates the inborn tendencies that influence how one experiences life.

prakruti varna - Maintenance of normal color complexion, one of the functions of healthy agni.

pralaya - Disintegration or destruction; the period of dissolution of the universe at the end of its cycle of creation.

pramāna - Proof.

prasāda - Clarity, purity; an offering of holy food to a deity; the essence of food.

praspandanam - Pulsation, throbbing, a function of vyāna vayu.

pratyāhāra - Withdrawal of the senses; the fifth limb in Patañjali's eight-limbed system of Yoga; the act of bringing consciousness deeper inside the body, drawing the psychic energy from peripheral sense organs to the inner movements of the mind.

pratyaksha - Direct perception; what one sees or perceives; one of the means of acquiring valid knowledge according to Nyāya philosophy.

prīnana - Nutrition, the main function of rasa dhātu.

pruthaktva - Separation; one of the functions of tejas.

pruthivī - Earth element.

purisha agni - The fire component of the membranous structure surrounding the organs of the excretory system, it governs the elimination of feces. It also helps to absorb liquids and minerals, forms the stools, and maintains the temperature and color of the feces.

purisha vaha srotas - The bodily channel that carries feces; the root or governor of this channel is the cecum, rectum, and sigmoid colon. The pathway of the channel is the large intestine, and the opening or mouth of this channel is the anal orifice.

Purusha - Pure, undifferentiated, infinite consciousness; choiceless, passive awareness; consciousness that dwells in the "city of senses," which is the human being.

pūrana - Filling up, completing; a major function of majjā dhātu and vāta dosha, especially prāna vāyu.

Pūrva Mīmāmsa - The school of thought founded by Jaimini, based on the initial teachings of the Vedas and emphasizing rituals and actions as a path to God-consciousness. See also Mīmāmsa.

R

rāga - Affection; enthusiasm; coloration; one of the functions of healthy agni.

rajah - Menstruation; one of the superior by-products of rasa dhātu.

rajas - One of the three universal gunas or qualities of consciousness; the principle of kinetic energy; active, mobile, and responsible for all movements.

rakta dhātu - Blood; one of the seven bodily tissues, rakta consists of red blood cells, and in Āyurveda is a separate tissue from the plasma (rasa dhātu). Its main functions include maintenance of life, oxygenation, and transportation of nutrients. Rakta is said by Sushruta to be the fourth dosha because ultimately all untreated disorders will affect the blood, and because unhealthy blood causes systemic problems in the same way that an aggravated dosha does.

rakta agni - The fire component present in the blood, it is responsible for the digestion and assimilation of nutrients that nourish blood tissue.

rakta moksha - Bloodletting or blood cleansing, one of the five cleansing actions of pañchakarma; a specific treatment for removing excess pitta and purification of the blood.

rakta vaha srotas - The bodily channel that maintains the functions of rakta dhātu, or red blood cells. The root or governor of this channel is the liver and spleen. It extends throughout the arteriole circulatory system, and opens at the arterial-venous junction.

rañjaka - One of the subtypes of pitta dosha located in the liver and spleen, it gives color to the blood and is responsible for the formation of blood.

rasa - Taste; the tanmātrā relating to water element; the subtle quality of the water element that exists in objects, allowing them to be sensed by taste; the first experience of food in the mouth; there are six tastes in our diet: sweet, sour, salty, pungent, bitter, and astringent.

rasa dhātu - Plasma, the first of the seven dhātus, it includes lymph fluid, white blood cells, and the plasma component of blood. Rasa is the first tissue to be nourished from ingested food and provides nutrition to every cell and tissue of the body.

rasa vaha srotas - The bodily channel that maintains the functions of rasa dhātu, the lymph and plasma tissue. The roots or governors of this channel are the right chamber of the heart and the ten great vessels of the heart, the passage is the venous and lymphatic systems, and it opens at the juncture between the arteries and veins.

rasāyana chikitsā - Rejuvenation therapy which brings about renewal, regeneration, and restoration of all bodily cells, tissues, and organs; enhances immunity and stamina and gives longevity.

Rigveda - The oldest of the four Vedas, the ancient scriptures of India, the rig veda is said to have been produced from fire.

rishi - A seer or sage; the beings who perceived and/or recorded the Vedic hymns; the enlightened sages who shared their knowledge, medicine, philosophy, and spiritual teachings.

roma kūpa - Sweat glands; one of the openings of ambu vaha srotas.

rūksha - Dry quality; creates dehydration and causes choking, constriction, spasm, pain, and dryness of the skin, as well as isolation, separation, fear, nervousness and loneliness.

rūpa - Form; the tanmātrā relating to fire element; the subtle quality of the fire element that exists in objects, making objects visible; color.

S

sādhaka - One of the five subtypes of pitta; responsible for intelligence, memory, mental digestion, enthusiasm, and other functions of the higher mental faculties.

Sāmaveda - The third of the four Vedas.

sānkhya - Number; a particular quality or function of tejas by which cellular division takes place and the proper number of chromosomes, tissues, doshas, and malas are maintained.

Sānkhya - A major school of Indian philosophy founded by the sage Kāpila. It gives Āyurveda a systematic account of cosmic evolution according to 25 categories: purusha, cosmic spirit; prakruti, creative energy; mahad, cosmic intelligence; ahamkara, the individuating principle or "I-maker"; manas, the individual mind; indriyāni, the 10 sense and motor facilities; tanmātrās, the five subtle elements; and pañcha mahā bhūtas, the five gross elements.

sāra - The pure, stabilized tissue (as opposed to the unstable or unprocessed tissue or the wastes or by-products of a tissue; the perfect superior essence of a tissue; healthy tissue.

sahasrāra - The seventh or crown chakra, located at the topmost part of the skull, and related to the pineal gland; the "thousand petaled lotus"; "Sa" means soma, lunar, female energy; "Ha" means solar, male energy. This chakra is where male and female energies merge into one and all definitions dissolve into the undefined.

sakthi - The thigh or thigh bone; one of the sites of vāta dosha.

sama agni - Balanced agni; the state of optimal, balanced metabolism that arises when all three doshas are in balance according to the individual's constitution.

samādhi - Cosmic consciousness; an expansive state of choiceless, passive awareness that is all-inclusive equilibrium; a balanced state of body, mind, and consciousness.

samāna vāyu - One of the five subtypes of vāta, its movement is linear and outward horizontally. It is mainly present in the small intestine and navel area, and stimulates appetite and the secretion of digestive juices, so is closely connected with agni (digestive fire). It is responsible for peristalsis and the opening and closing of the pyloric and ileocecal valves during the process of digestion.

samshaya - Doubt; one of the sources for non-valid knowledge according to Nyāya philosophy.

samyoga - Combination; conjunction; union; as a quality of the intelligence of tejas, the principle that allows things that have affinity to collect together.

sandra - Dense; density; associated with substances like meat and cheese; increases kapha and decreases vata and pitta; brings compactness to the body and makes a person more grounded; promotes solidity, density, and strength.

sanga - Accumulation, stagnation; physiologically it can manifest as constipation, blood clots, lymphatic congestion, growths, or blockages.

sattva - One of the three universal gunas or qualities of consciousness; the principle of equilibrium, intelligence, essence, consciousness, and clarity of perception; potential energy; jñānshakti, the energy of wisdom, understanding, and cognition; it gives rise to the mind and senses in Sānkhya Philosophy.

shākhā - Limbs; extremities.

shāstra - Scripture or scriptural knowledge.

shabda - Sound; the tanmātrā relating to ether element; the subtle quality of the ether element that exists in objects, allowing them to be sensed by hearing; speech; one of the four valid sources of knowledge according to Nyāya philosophy: testimony that is authentic and truthful. Sacred texts and realized masters have verbal authority; their words are shabda.

shabdendriya - The auditory pathways of hearing, including the ears as the related sense organs.

Shad Darshan - The six major schools of Indian thought, consisting of Sānkhya, Nyāya, Vaisheshika, Mīmāmsa, Vedānta, and Yoga; these philosophies are incorporated and applied in Āyurveda.

shad rasa - Six tastes: sweet, sour, salty, butter, pungent, astringent are the six tastes present in substances. Each of these tastes is made up of two main elements.

shakti - Energy; the divine creative will; power, strength.

shakti apāna - The subtle form of apāna vāyu, it is present in the nervous system and governs outward moving impulses such as motor responses.

shauryam - Bravery, courage, fearlessness, all functions of healthy agni.

shilājit - A naturally occurring mineral resin used in Āyurvedic treatment.

shīta - Cold quality; associated with numbness, unconsciousness, contraction, fear, and insensitivity in the body. Slows digestion and reduces immunity.

shīta vīrya - Cooling energy of a substance.

Shiva - The third in the Hindu trinity of gods: the destroyer; Infinite Consciousness; who transforms ego into bliss.

shiva granthi - The pineal gland.

shiva randhra - A small opening located at the posterior fontanel of the cranium bone and connected to sushumna nādī; it is said that the consciousness of a yogi leaves the body at death through this opening.

shlakshna - Smooth quality; brings lubrication, flexibility, and ease of movement to the body.

shleshaka - One of the five subtypes of kapha dosha present in all joints which provides lubrication of the joints and gives freedom of movement; also protects the bone from deterioration.

shleshma - Another name for kapha; the root of shleshma means "to hug." It is the nature of kapha molecules to hug together and create a compact mass.

shukra dhātu - Male reproductive tissue, one of the seven bodily tissues; the word shukra also refers to the orgasmic fluid secreted by a woman.

shukra vaha srotas - The channel carrying nutrients for shukra dhātu, or male reproductive tissue. The roots or governors of this channel are the testicles and the nipples, the pathway includes the vas deferens, epididymis, prostate, urethra, and urino-genital tract, and the mouth is the urethral opening.

siddhi - The result or benefit of any yogāsana, meditation or endeavor; success; skill; supernatural power.

sirā - Blood vessels, veins; any tubular structure.

sirā granthi - Dilation, growth, swelling; one of the three general categories of sroto dushti.

smruti - Memory; one of the faculties of buddhi, or intellect.

snāyu - Tendons, sinews, ligaments, flat muscles.

snehana - The process of internal and external oil application that precedes and accompanies pañcha-karma; snehana softens the tissues, helping them to let go of deep-seated toxins, doshas, and emotional stresses.

snigdha - Oily quality; oiliness; unctuous; associated with nourishment, relaxation, smoothness, moisture, lubrication, love, compassion, and vigor; increases pitta and kapha and decreases vata.

soma - The subtlest essence of ojas; cosmic plasma; lunar energy; the most subtle form of matter; the food of cells and RNA/DNA molecules, which becomes consciousness.

spanda dhamanī - Pulsating arteries; associated with rakta dhātu.

spandanam - Pulsation; one of the functions of vyāna vāyu in the body; the throbbing sensation that is palpable in the movement of the pulse, or the pulsation of circulation governed by the heart.

sparsha - Touch; the tanmātrā relating to air element; the subtle quality of the air element that exists in objects, allowing them to be sensed by touch; one of the causes of suffering according to Buddhism - in this sense it means contact of objects with the senses.

sparshendriya - The faculty of tactile perception, including the skin as the related sense organ.

srotāmsi - The plural form of the word srotas, bodily channel.

srotas - Pathway; a subtle or gross channel made up of dhātus (tissues) that carries substances or energies from place to place in the body; one of the innumerable special systems in the body. Each channel has a root, which is a governing organ or area of the body, a pathway, and an opening or outlet. Examples of srotamsi (the plural form of sro-tas) are the gastrointestinal tract and the veins and arteries.

sroto agni - The fire component of a specific bodily srotas (channel). Located in the root of the srotas, it maintains the function of that channel.

sroto mārga - That portion of a specific srotas that is between the opening and the root, the entire tract of the srotas.

sroto mukha - The opening, end, or "mouth" of a particular srotas.

sroto mūla - The root, origin, or governor of a particular srotas.

stanya - Lactation; the superior by-product of rasa dhātu.

sthāyi - Stable, mature, fully formed; especially the stable, fully formed dhātu.

sthāyi dhātu dushti - Qualitative disturbance of stable, fully formed dhātu; often causes chronic disorders.

sthira - Static or stable quality; stability, promotes stability and support, associated with all supportive structures in the body, also with fixity, obstructiveness, constipation, stubbornness, and lack of flexibility; increases kapha and decreases vata and pitta.

sthūla - Gross quality, grossness; associated with obstruction, obesity, and substances like meat and cheese. The gross quality increases kapha and decreases vata and pitta.

sūkshma - Subtle quality; associated with any subtle thing, including cells, thoughts, emotions, etc.

sūkshma apāna - The subtle form of apāna vāyu which is present in the nervous system and governs outward moving impulses such as motor responses. (See also apāna vāyu and shakti apāna.)

sūrya - The sun; solar energy that maintains life along with soma (lunar energy) and anila (cosmic prāna).

sūtra - A small, easily memorized phrase or aphorism that contains a great deal of knowledge and awakens the intuition. A sutra is analogous to the seed of a tree, which contains within itself all the forms of the tree in its stages of growth.

svādhishthāna - The second chakra, located in the pelvic cavity; the seat of self-esteem, courage, and self-confidence; where vital energy meets the vital organs; associated with prāna maya kosha, or the body of life-force.

sveda - Sweat.

sveda agni - The fire component of the organs and structures related to the excretion of sweat. It regulates body temperature, maintains the moisture, softness, oiliness, and acid-alkali balance of the skin, and helps govern the water-electrolyte balance in the body.

svedana - Sudation; the use of heat to loosen toxins, doshas, and emotional stress from the deep tissues and encourage them to move into the gastro-intestinal tract where they can be removed by cleansing procedures.

sveda vaha srotas - The bodily channels that carry sweat; this channel is governed by the sweat glands, it continues through the sweat ducts, and opens at the pores of the skin.

T

tālu - The soft palate; one of the roots of ambu vaha srotas.

tamas - One of the three universal gunas or qualities of consciousness (along with sattva and rajas), tamas gives rise to the five elements and the tanmātrā (subtle qualities of the elements) in Sānkhya Philosophy. It is the principle of inertia and is responsible for sleep, heaviness, slowness, unconsciousness, and decay. When it predominates in the mind, it brings ignorance, laziness, violence, and inertness.

tanmātrā - Sound, touch, form, taste, and smell; the objects of perception; the subtlest energy of the five elements, through which the gross elements are evolved.

tantra - A spiritual path utilizing a set of demanding practices that require great discipline, strength, and understanding.

tapas - Austerity, discipline, that which heats up and burns one's karmas.

tarka - Hypothetical argument; one of the three sources of non-valid knowledge according to Nyāya philosophy.

tarpaka - One of the five kapha subtypes. Associated with the white matter of the brain and the cerebrospinal fluid, it forms the protective and nourishing membranes and fluids of the nervous system. Tarpaka kapha is the film on which all experience, emotions, and knowledge are recorded in the form of memory.

tarpana - That which nourishes; that which records and retains the memories.

taruna asthi - Cartilage.

tejas - The subtle essence of fire (agni) and pitta dosha, tejas governs digestion on both subtle and gross levels; the energy of intelligence, discrimination, and of all bodily fire; gives luminosity, brightness, brilliance, enthusiasm, passion; solar energy.

tejaskāra - Creation of tejas, one of the functions of healthy agni.

tejo agni - The fire component inherent in Fire element.

tejo hāra - Depletion of tejas; one of the signs of impaired agni.

tīkshna - Sharp quality; associated with concentration, understanding, discrimination, appreciation, and comprehension.

tīkshna agni - Sharp digestion; one of the three categories of disturbed agni; digestion that is affected by the hot, sharp, and penetrating attributes of pitta dosha, causing excessively strong appetite and hyperactive metabolism.

tikta - Bitter taste; made up of air and ether, it increases vāta dosha, and pacifies pitta and kapha.

tikta avasthā pāka - The bitter stage of digestion, which takes place in the ileum, (the last and longest portion of the small intestine) during the fifth hour or so after eating.

tikta ghrita - Bitter ghee (clarified butter with bitter herbs).

tridoshic - A word to describe something that affects or involves all three doshas, either in a beneficial or detrimental way.

trikatu chūrna - An herbal compound of dry ginger, black pepper, and piper longum (pippali) that kindles agni, burns āma, detoxifies the body, and improves digestion.

trushna - Thirst. As the thirst for enjoyment, it is one of the causes of suffering according to Buddhism.

tvacha - Skin; one of the superior by-products of māmsa dhātu.

U

udāna vāyu - One of the five subtypes of vāta dosha; the upward moving energy, it mainly moves through the diaphragm, lungs, bronchi, trachea, and throat. It governs exhalation and is responsible for speech, expression, and any action that requires effort. It also stimulates memory and helps a person rise from confusion, attachment, depression, and other daunting experiences.

udaraka tejas - The subtle fire of the stomach.

udvāhana - Upward movement; a function of udāna vāyu.

upachaya - Improvement; nutrition, good muscle tone; cheerfulness; one of the qualities of healthy ojas and a function of normal tejas.

upadhātu - The superior by-product that results from the formation of a dhātu.

upamāna - Comparison, one of the four sources of valid knowledge according to Nyāya.

Upanishad - The later, higher teachings of the Vedas; implies sitting in the vicinity of an enlightened one and listening to him or her without any doubt, delusion, or comparison. The entire teaching of vedānta is upanishad.

Upa-vedas - Secondary or subordinate Vedas. Ayurveda is an upa-veda.

ushna - Hot quality; stimulates gastric fire, improving circulation, digestion, absorption, and assimilation. Promotes cleansing, expansion, anger, and irritability.

ushna vīrya - Heating energy of a substance.

Uttara Mīmāmsa - School of thought founded by the celebrated sage, Jaimini; the later, higher teachings of Vedānta found in the Upanishads. *See also* Mīmāmsa.

ūrdhva gamitva - Upward movement; a quality of tejas; psychologically, the ability to move upward or forward, going beyond depression, sadness, etc.; transcendence.

ūrdhva jatru granthi - The thyroid gland.

V

vāta dosha - One of the three doshas, vāta is associated with ether and air elements. It governs all movements and activities in the body.

vāyavya agni - The fire component inherent in the air element.

vāyu - Air element, the second of the five basic elements; wind; another name for vāta.

vāyu tejas - The subtle fire component present in air element.

vadavanala - The fire component inherent in water.

vaigunya - Literally: lack of good qualities; defective; impairment.

Vaisheshika - School of thought founded by Kanada. Seeking to understand the physical universe.

vaishvānala - The fire component inherent in the Earth.

vardhati - To grow to maturity. Vardhamāna is a noun of the same root meaning growing or increasing.

varna - Color complexion, one of the qualities of healthy agni and tejas.

vasā - Subcutaneous fat; one of the superior by-products of māmsa dhātu.

vastu - Object.

Vedānta - Literally "the ending of knowledge;" the ultimate aim and scope of the Vedas; the last of the six philosophies, which expounds that duality is artificial and all creation is nothing but Brahman.

veda - Knowledge; teaching; also the name of the ancient scriptures of India.

vega - Velocity; random movement, relating to functions of vāta such as the creation of natural urges.

vibhāga - Distinction; categorization; one of the qualities or functions of tejas whereby the proper forms of all cells and organs are maintained

vibhu - Universal.

vichitra pratyaya arabdha - Substances having similar rasa, vīrya, and vipāka, but different atomic structures. The basis of prabhāva, otherwise unexplained actions.

vīrya - The energy or potency of a substance; the secondary action of an ingested substance, experienced after taste; two primary kinds: hot or cold.

vijñānamaya kosha - The sheath made of intellect or discernment.

vikruti - Unnatural, imbalanced, or modified state; the current state of the individual, as opposed to prakruti, the original state of the constitution; a state of the body and mind in which the individual is more prone to disease.

vikruti varna - Abnormal color complexion, one of the signs of impaired agni.

vikshipta - Changeable mind; sometimes active, sometimes slow and dull; one of the five states of mind.

vimārga gamanam - False passage; something passing through the wrong channel; one of the three general categories of sroto dushti

vipāka - The final post-digestive effect of food that occurs in the colon and has an action on the excreta: urine, feces, and sweat. Vipāka is described as sweet, sour, or pungent.

virāga - Revulsion; depression; withdrawal; lack of enthusiasm; one of the signs of impaired agni.

vishada - Clear quality, associated with clarity, understanding, communication, cleansing.

vishāda - Confusion or deep grief.

vishama - Imbalanced; irregular.

vishama agni - Irregular digestion; one of the three categories of disturbed agni; digestion that is affected by vāta dosha, which can quickly enkindle agni but also quickly slow it down.

Vishnu - The supreme all-pervading lord; the second in the Hindu trinity of gods: the preserver, whose qualities are knowledge, strength, power, virility, and splendor; cosmic prāna, which is present in the atmosphere and protects global life.

vishuddha - The fifth chakra, located at the throat; related to the thyroid and parathyroid glands; associated with communication, will, and the vijñāna maya kosha.

vit sneha - Epithelial and mucous secretions that help discharge the bowel.

viveka - One of the important functions of vāta especially associated with samāna vāyu; discrimination; splitting apart or isolating; physiologically it manifests as the function of separating essential components of ingested food from inessential ones during digestion; mentally it manifests as discernment.

vruddhi - Increase (of a dosha or substance); one of the nine types of dosha gati.

vrukka - Kidney; one of the openings of ambu vaha srotas. (*Vrukkau is the plural of vrukka.*)

vyāna - The subtype of vāta dosha that is primarily located in the heart and circulates all over the body. It is responsible for pulsation and circulation of venous blood and lymph fluid, and it maintains cardiac activity and oxygenation of cells, tissues, and organ systems, through the circulation of nutrients. Also responsible for all reflex actions, and the movement of the joints and skeletal muscles through the reflex arc.

vyāna dushti - Qualitative disturbance of vyāna vāyu, the subtype of vāta related to circulation.

vyakta - Manifestation; the manifested universe; also, the 5th stage of pathogenesis during which the cardinal signs and symptoms of a disease manifest.

Y

Yajurveda - One of the four main Vedas, this is a collection of sacred ceremonies and rituals.

yakrut - The liver.

yama - The first limb of Patañjali's eight limbed yoga system; restraints or abstentions including nonviolence, non-lying, non-misuse of sex energy, nonpossessiveness; these restraints have the purpose of bringing the Yogi into a harmonious relationship with Nature and with all beings.

yantra - A mystical or astronomical diagram used for the worship of a deity; the āsana, or seat of the deity into which that deity can be invited and established for worship.

Yoga - One of the six philosophies; the science expounded by celebrated sage Patañjali including the practical means of uniting the higher and lower self and merging with cosmic consciousness through a gradual unfolding of inner strength and wisdom.

Yoga Sūtras (of Patañjali) - The garland of sūtras expounding the science of yoga.

yogāsana - The third limb of Patañjali's eight limbed Yoga system; the means of bringing awareness, stability, and ease to the body through the use of physical postures and mūdrās for the purpose of supporting meditation.

yogi - One who practices yoga; a blissful or enlightened one.

yoni - Vagina.

Bibliography and Selected Readings

REFERENCES

Bhishagratna, Kaviraj Kunjalal, editor-translator. *Sushruta Samhita*. 4th ed., 2 vols. Chowkhamba Sanskrit Series Office: Varanasi, India, 1991

Lad, Vasant. *Ayurveda: The Science of Self-Healing*, Santa Fe: Lotus Press, 1985.

Lad, Dr. Vasant and Usha. *Ayurvedic Cooking for Self-Healing*, 2nd ed., Albuquerque: The Ayurvedic Press, 1997.

Lad, Vasant. *The Complete Book of Ayurvedic Home Remedies*. New York: Harmony Books 1998.

——. *Secrets of the Pulse: The Ancient Art of Ayurvedic Pulse Diagnosis*, 2nd ed., Albuquerque: The Ayurvedic Press, 2006.

Lad, Vasant and Frawley, David. *The Yoga of Herbs: An Ayurvedic Guide to Herbal Medicine*, Santa Fe: Lotus Press, 1986.

Murthy, K. R. Srikantha, translator. *Sharngadhara Samhita: A Treatise on Ayurveda*. Chaukhambha Orientalia: Varanasi, India, 1984.

Sharma, Priyavrat V. editor-translator. *Caraka Samhita*. 4 vols. Chowkhamba Sanskrit Series Office: Varanasi, India, 1981-1994.

Sharma, Ram Karan, and Vaidya Bhagwan Dash, editors-translators. *Caraka Samhita*. 3rd ed., 3 vols. Chowkhamba Sanskrit Series Office: Varanasi, India, 1992.

Tigunait, Pandit Rajmani, Ph.D. *Seven Systems of Indian Philosophy*, Honesdale: Himalayan Institute Press, 1984.

Vagbhata. *Ashtanga Hridayam*, translated by K. R. Srikantha Murthy. 2 vols. Krishnadas Academy: Varanasi, India, 1991-1992.

READING LIST

Lad, Vasant. *Strands of Eternity*, Albuquerque: The Ayurvedic Press, 2004.

Morrison, Judith H. *The Book of Ayurveda: A Holistic Approach to Health and Longevity*. New York: Simon & Schuster Inc., 1995, A Fireside Book.

Shankaracharaya, H.H. Adi., author. Chinmayananda, H.H. Swami, commentary. *Atma Bodha*. Bombay: Central Cinmaya Mission Trust 1999.

Svoboda, Robert E. *Ayurveda: Life, Health and Longevity*. Penguin: London, 1992; reprint, The Ayurvedic Press: Albuquerque, 2004.

——. *Prakriti: Your Ayurvedic Constitution*. 2nd ed., Lotus Press: Twin Lakes, 1998.

——. *The Hidden Secret of Ayurveda*. Pune, India, 1980; reprint, The Ayurvedic Press: Albuquerque, 1994.

Acknowledgements

आयुर्वेद

The author would like to acknowledge those whose dedication and insight brought the knowledge of Āyurveda to the world, especially my teachers who lovingly showed the way and shared their knowledge and experience, and all the friends and staff at the Ayurvedic Institute without whose contributions this book would not exist. I deeply acknowledge the work of Margaret Smith Peet, Laura Humphreys, Glen Crowther, and Barbara Cook who made profound efforts to put together the vast amount of material for this book.

Index

A

āhāra rasa 57, 105, 107, 251
ākāsha. *See* Ether element
ālochaka agni 86
ālochaka pitta 59, **63-64**
āma **90**
ānandamaya kosha 195
āpo agni 95
āpas. *See* Water element
āpo agni 59, 94, 100
āpya tejas 220, 221
ārtava agni 97
ārtava dhātu 168, **172-174**
    by-products of 169
    conception and 263
    disorders of 174
    formation of 169
    qualities of 172
ārtava vaha srotas 178, **188**
āsana 20
    See also Yoga philosophy
ātman (soul) **15**
Ātreya (sage) 4
āvila (cloudy) guna 35, 44
    See also picchila (sticky) guna
Āyurveda **1-5**
    definition of health according to 275
    factors affecting health 278-280
    history of 2-4
    individualized treatments with 2, 83, 167
    philosophies of. *See* Shad Darshan
    See also agni; digestion; dhātus; doshas;
        five elements; gunas; srotāmsi
abdominal distention 91
abhrak bhasma 166
abhyanga massage 272
acid indigestion 240
acne 65, 112, 119, 241
actions (karmas) 25
actuality, compared to reality 61
adarshanam 86
addiction 221
adhīrata 89

adipose tissue 132
adrenals 135, 187
aerobic breathing 265
aging 67
    agni affecting 81-82
    anaerobic breathing and 265
    doshas affecting 67
    ojas, prāna, tejas affecting 228
    rasa dhātu and 113
    See also longevity
agni **81-85**
    acronym for 84
    balanced 276
    bhūta agni 58, 59, 94-96
    dhātu agni 97, 104-105
    digestion and 84-85, 86, 92-101
    of doshas 100
    doshas affecting 89-90
    five elements and 83-84
    functions of 86-89
    indriya agni 99
    jāthara agni 84, 92-94
    jatru agni 96-97
    kloma agni 94
    of malas 101
    ojas and 210
    pīlu agni 98-99, 266
    pithara agni 99
    pitta and 276
    qualities of 89
    smell and 83
    subtypes of 92-101
    vīrya and 247
    varieties of 90-92
    See also Fire element; specific types of
        agni
agni nārāyana 83
agni tejas 220
Agnideva (deity) 82
Agnivesa (sage) 4
ahamkāra. *See* ego
aharsha 87
AIDS 119, 165, 214, 215

Air element (vāyu) **13**
    bhūta agni corresponding to 94
    at cellular level 267
    creation of 25
    disorders of 15
    dosha corresponding to 30
    foods corresponding to 236
    gunas associated with 9
    in human body 26
    senses related to 28
    tanmātrās related to 28
alcohol 136, 192
allergies 92, 94
amātroshna 87
ambu vaha srotas 178, **184-185**
amino acids, related to gunas 98
amla. See sour taste
anabolic diseases 180
anabolism 276
anaerobic breathing 265
anemia 59, 221
anesthesia 65
anger
    blood vessels and 120
    fever and 111
    Fire element and 15
    muscle rigidity and 130
    pitta dosha and 30, 109, 163
    prāna vāyu and 50
    rakta dhātu and 118
    sweat and 192
    tīkshna agni and 91
    ushna (hot) guna and 33
anila (cosmic prāna) 82-83
anna vaha srotas 178, **181-183**
annamaya kosha 194
anorexia 57
antara agni. See jāthara agni
antibiotics 151, 244
anumāna (inference) **12**
anxiety
    agni and 87
    Alr element and 15
    awareness and 143
    fever and 111
    kledaka kapha and 70

    laghu (light) guna and 32
    meda dhātu and 138
    muscle rigidity and 130
    ovulation and 172
    prāna vāyu and 50
    REM and 164
    srotāmsi and 181
    vāta dosha and 30, 109, 163
    vishama agni and 91
apāna vāyu 46, 47, 52
apakti 86
aparatva, quality of tejas 219
appendicitis 119
appendix 190
appetite
    excessive 237
    irregular 91
    kledaka kapha and 70
    loss of 52, 92, 111, 239
    pitta dosha and 55
    samāna vāyu and 51
    See also food
arrangement. See vastu shilpa shāstra
arteriosclerosis 142, 150, 180
arthritis
    asthi dhātu and 149
    catabolism and 67
    cholesterol and 132
    meda dhātu and 135, 139
    obesity and 141
    ojas and 215
    shlakshna (smooth) guna and 33
    shleshaka kapha and 77
    tonsillitis and 127
ashauryam 87
ashita type of food 252
Ashtānga Hridayam text 4
Ashtānga Sangraha text 4
ashthavidhā vīrya 246
Ashvin twins (sages) 4
asthāyi dhātu 105, 262
asthāyi rakta 105, 107
asthi agni 97, 146, 147
asthi dhātu **144-151**
    by-products of 145-147
    disorders of 147-151

five elements in 144, 146
    formation of 144
    functions of 144
asthi sāra 147
asthi vaha srotas 178, 179, **187**
asthma 50, 71, 215
astringent stage of digestion 256, 257
astringent taste **244-245**
    elements corresponding to 237
    excessive intake of 238, 245
    organs related to 237
atheroma 142
atipravrutti 180
atom, discovery of 266
attachment 30, 35, 41, 50, 92, 109
attention, double-arrowed 232
attributes. *See* gunas
auditory neuritis 66
Aum (soundless sound) 25
aura 217, 228
autoimmune disorders 88, 118, 214
autonomic nervous system 159
avalambaka kapha 68, **70-71**
avyakta 6
awareness 168, 197-198, **231-233**
    as behavioral medicine 280
    five elements and 227
    majjā dhātu and 157, 158
    meda dhātu and 142-143
    prāna vāyu and 49
    soma and 231
    states of 202-205
    in a substance 250
    suspension of breath during 266
    witnessing 204-205

B

Bādarāyana (established Vedānta) 20, 21
backache 91, 141, 172
bala 89
behavioral medicine 280
Bell's palsy 128, 245, 253
bhāsvara, quality of tejas 220
Bhagavad Gītā 269
Bhakti Yoga 19
bhakti yoga 271
bhaumī tejas 220

bhrājaka agni 94, 64
bhrājaka pitta 64-65
bhrama (faulty cognition) 11
bhūta agni 58, 59, **94-96**
    cellular digestion and 98
    tejas and 220
bilateral symmetry of the body 225
biological clock of doshas 279
birth 152-155
    apāna vāyu and 52
    desire as cause of 36, 269
    dharma associated with 37
    doshas present at 37
    existence before 169
    reincarnation and 147
    See also fetus; pregnancy
bitter ghee 139
bitter stage of digestion 255, 257
bitter taste **243-244**
    elements corresponding to 237
    excessive intake of 238, 244
    organs related to 237
bladder, agni of 101
bleeding disorders 242
bliss 280
    absent of form 157
    ambu vaha srotas and 185
    as transcendental state 273
    awareness and 158
    chakras associated with 196
    love and 204
    in a loving relationship 174
    meda dhātu and 135, 143
    mother's womb as state of 153-155
    mukta mind and 193
    ojas and 210
    samādhi as 176
    soma and 212, 231
    tarpaka kapha and 140
    as ultimate fate of food 274
bloating 86
blood
    channel for. *See* rakta vaha srotas
    components of 113
    movement of 123
    pitta dosha and 54

purification of 122
ranjaka pitta and 57, 58
blood clots 180
blood pressure
　high. See hypertension
　meditation affecting 121
　salt affecting 73, 241
　sweating affecting 192
blood types, doshas corresponding to 120
blood vessels 114, 120-122
bloodletting treatment 119
blue light, treating jaundice using 221
bodhaka agni 94, 237
bodhaka kapha 68, **71-74**
bodily channels. See srotāmsi
body temperature
　Fire element and 13, 27, 83
　mātroshna and 87
　meda dhātu and 133
　normal, mātroshna 87
　pitta dosha and 30, 54
　rising before death 267
　sveda agni and 101
　sveda vaha srotas and 192
　vīrya and 247
body type. See prakruti
boils 119, 139, 241
bone marrow 151
　channel for. See majjā vaha srotas
　dhātu for. See majjā dhātu
　rakta agni in 116
　rakta dhātu and 114
　ranjaka pitta and 57, 58
bones
　channel for. See asthi vaha srotas
　cholesterol and 132
　dhātu for. See asthi dhātu
　fractures of, healing time for 145
　fractures of, spontaneous 146
　kapha dosha and 67
bowel movements, time of 190
Brāhma (deity) 6, 21, 82
　See also God
brāhmanda 21
brahmī, treatment using 165
Brahmā, Lord (sage) 4

brain 152, 188
　emotional part of 163
　gray matter of 155
　kapha dosha and 67
　left and right side of 175, 225
　sādhaka pitta and 59-62
　tarpaka kapha and 74
　udāna vāyu and 50
　use of 160
　See also intelligence; mind
brain tumors 77
breasts
　fibrocystic changes in 136, 139
　size of 111
　tenderness 172
breath
　left and right nostrils 175
　as offering to God 222
　See also lungs; respiration
breathlessness 49, 118, 214
bronchiectasis 71
bronchitis 50, 71
bruising 119
Buddha, Lord 21
buddhi (intellect) 8, **197**, 198, 267
buddhihāra 88
buddhikāra 88
Buddhism 5, **21-22**, 23

C

calcium 146-147, 150
callouses 34
calmness 30
cancer 89, 129, 215, 243
canker sores 117
cardiac muscles 124
cardiac spasm 245
cartilage 132, 145
catabolic diseases 180
catabolism 276
cataracts 167
causative substances. See nava karna dravya
cavities 148
cecum 190, 256
celibacy 171, 172
cells, agni for 98, 99
cellular consciousness 83, 268

cellular intelligence 6, 89
    buddhi as 267
    healthy cravings and 246
    meditation and 270
    nervousness and anger affecting 215
    tejas as 217, 219
    toxins affecting 246
cellular metabolism 88, 265-273
cerebral embolism 166
cerebral hemorrhage 165
cerebrospinal fluid 159, 185
cerebrovascular accident 165
cervix, apāna vāyu and 52
chāyā 89
chakra system
    koshas and 196
    majjā dhātu and 160
    mind and 195-196, 200-202
    srotāmsi and 178
chala (mobile) guna **34**, 42, 43
channels of movement. See srotāmsi
chaos and order 229
Charaka (Āyurvedic physician) 30
Charaka Samhitā text 3
chemical energy 14
chest pain 214
cholesterol
    functions of 132
    ghee and 139
    high 70, 215, 239
    recommended amount of 132
    types of 132
choroid plexus 137
chronic ascites 215
chronic fatigue syndrome
    herpes and 165
    ojas and 214, 215
    rakta dhātu and 119
    rañjaka pitta and 59
    rasa dhātu and 111
circulation
    rakta dhātu and 114
    vyāna vāyu and 53
cirrhosis 128, 136, 141
city of senses. See Purusha
clarity 37, 87

clear (vishada) guna **35**, 42
cleft palate 37
clotting 245
cloudy (āvila) guna 35, 44
    See also sticky (picchila) guna
coffee 243
cold (shīta) guna **33**, 42, 44
cold, exposure to 277
colds 239
colicky pain 91
colitis 91, 243
colon 184, 238
    apāna vāyu and 52
    cleansing 116, 184
    lungs and 184
    mineral absorption and 145
    post-digestive effect on 248
    vāta dosha and 47
color
    associated with kapha individuals 44
    associated with pitta individuals 43
    associated with vāta individuals 42
    of complexion, prakruti varna and 87
    of complexion, rasa dhātu and 109
    quality of tejas 217
    of tissues, rañjaka pitta and 57
coma 214
comparison (upamāna) **12**
compassion
    agni and 87
    drava (liquid) guna and 34
    kapha dosha and 41
    māmsa dhātu and 126
    meda dhātu and 134
    rasa dhātu and 109
    sattva guna and 37
    snigdha (oily) guna and 33
    sweet taste and 240
complexion 87, 109
comprehension 33, 87
concentration 168
conception 173
    apāna and 52
    difficulty in 148
    nutrition beginning at 263-265
    See also pregnancy

confidence 126
confusion
    āma and 90
    apakti agni and 86
    majjā dhātu and 157
    tarpaka kapha and 76
    udāna vāyu and 50
    vishāda and 87
congestive disorders 30, 180, 239, 241
conjunctivitis 15, 64, 117
connective tissue 125, 143
consciousness 267
    agni and 82, 83
    beginning of 152, 153, 156
    at birth 154
    center of, ego 8, 60
    cosmic, five elements originating from 26
    evolving, in Sānkhya philosophy 5
    expanding to universal, Yoga system for
        19
    first expression of, Ether 13, 83
    flow of. See prāna
    food transformed into 55, 99
    heaven as a quality of 77
    journey into matter 6
    movement of, Air 13
    pure. See Brahman; Purusha
    as reality 61
    soul and 15
    universal qualities of. See gunas (three)
    unmanifested, avyakta 25
    Vedānta philosophy and 21
constipation
    āma and 90, 190
    apāna vāyu and 52
    apakti agni and 86
    astringent taste and 238, 245
    fever and 111
    khāra (rough) guna and 33
    meda dhātu and 139
    ovulation and 172
    pungent vipāka and 249
    srotāmsi and 180
    vishama agni and 91
convulsions 128, 245
cooling vīrya 247

coordination of muscle groups 163
cosmic prāna 8, 228
cosmic representatives of life 82-83
cosmic soma 160
cough 239
courage 87
craniosacral therapy 147, 272
cravings 139, 143, 172, **246**, 269
    See also food
creation
    ātman as causative factor of 16
    cosmic representatives of 82-83
    five elements manifested in 25
    Mahad as first expression of 6
    principles of, in Sānkhya 6
    as union of atoms, in Vaisheshika 10
creative intelligence. See Mahad
creativity
    lack of 50, 242
    vāta and 30, 39, 278
    See also Prakruti
criticism 163
crown chakra 181, 196, 202
crystals 250

D

dairy products 269
dark versus light 199
darshan 4
    See also Shad Darshan
darshanam 86
dates, treating rasa dhātu using 112
death 81, 147, 169, 267, 269
decision-making capacity 88
defective space 180
degenerative diseases 180
deha prakruti **37**, 38
dehydration 110, 111, 214
deities 82
delusion 157
demyelinating disorders 66, 166
dense (sandra) guna **34**, 44
depression
    aharsha and 87
    astringent taste and 245
    Earth element and 15
    meda dhātu and 140

rasa dhātu and 109
resistance and 211
tamas guna and 37
udāna vāyu and 50
virāga and 88
dermatitis 65, 118, 241
desire 268-270
choice and 160
sexual 175
soma and 230
dhārana 47
dhātu agni **97**, 104-105
dhātu disorders affecting 107
functions of 82, 88
kshira dadhi nyāya and 262
medications and 94
pīlu agni and 98
dhātu dhara kalā 97, 105
dhātu dushti 106
dhātu kārshyana 88
dhātu poshanam 88
dhātu sāra 106
dhātu srotāmsi 179, 185-189
dhātus **103-107**
Agnideva's extremeties representing 82
balanced 276
by-products of 106
development in fetus 264
disorders of 106-107
nourished by srotāmsi 180
nutrition of 88, 96, 104-106
processed and unprocessed 105
pure essence of. See ojas
sweet taste and 239
See also specific dhātus
dhairyam 89
Dhanvantari, Lord (deity) 119, 274
dharma 18
diabetes 215
boils and 139
excess salivation and 253
kledaka kapha and 70
manda agni and 92
meda dhātu and 136-137
ojas and 215
polyneuritis and 164

rakta dhātu and 120
sweet taste and 239
diagnosis 64
doshas used in 166
gunas used in 35
perception used in 11
tongue, observing for 73
diaphragm
prāna vāyu and 48
udāna vāyu and 50
diarrhea
āma and 90
apāna vāyu and 52
apakti agni and 86
astringent taste and 244
fever and 111
pungent taste and 243
pungent vipāka and 249
rañjaka pitta and 59
sour taste and 241
sour vipāka and 249
srotāmsi and 180
tīkshna agni and 91
vishama agni and 91
diet. *See* nutrition
dig (direction) **17**
digestion **251-257**, 273-274
agni and 81, 84-85, 86, 92-101
astringent stage 256, 257
bitter stage 255, 257
bodhaka kapha and 74
channel for. *See* anna vaha srotas
dhātu nutrition and 104-105
kledaka kapha and 69
of medicines 93-94
ojas and 208, 209
pāchaka pitta and 56
pitta dosha and 54
poor 52, 57
post-digestive effect. *See* vipāka
pungent stage 255, 257
rañjaka pitta and 58
salty stage 254, 257
samāna vāyu and 51
sour stage 254, 257
stages of **252-256**, 257

sweet stage 253, 257
tejas and 216-217, 220
time required for 182
See also metabolism
dīrgham 89
dimension, quality of tejas 218
direction (dig) **17**
disease
āma causing 90
awareness and 122
classifications of 209-210
See also specific diseases and disorders
distinction, quality of tejas 218
Divine Mother. See Prakruti
divya tejas 221
dizziness 163
dosha gati 17
dosha prakruti **37**
doshas **29-30**
agni affected by 89-90
agni of 100
Agnideva's tongues as 82
balanced 276
biological clock of 279
blood types corresponding to 120
channels they move along. See srotāmsi
determining a person's constitution. See
prakruti (body type)
diagnosis using 166
elements associated with 15
exercise appropriate for 279
food qualities related to 259
interaction of 276-278
present state of. See vikruti
pure essences of. See ojas; prāna; tejas
seasons corresponding to 32
srotāmsi associated with 181
stages of digestion associated with 256
subtypes of. See subdoshas
tastes affecting 238-245
times of day associated with 16
twenty attributes (gunas) and 31-35
water requirements for 137
See also kapha dosha; pitta dosha; vāta
dosha
double-arrowed attention 232

doubt (samshaya) 11
drava (liquid) guna **34**, 43, 44
dravatva, quality of tejas 219
dravyamaya tejas 221
dreams
majjā dhātu creating 161
REM and 164
drugs
medicines, digestion of 93-94
recreational 121-122
dry (rūksha) guna **33**, 42
dull guna. See slow (manda) guna
dullness 37
dysentery 91, 111, 241, 244
dyspepsia 57
dyspnea 49

E
ear wax 129
ears
element corresponding to 27
vāta dosha and 47
Earth element (pruthivī) **14**
agni in 83
bhūta agni corresponding to 94
at cellular level 267
creation of 26
disorders of 15
dosha corresponding to 30
foods corresponding to 236
gunas associated with 9
in human body 27
muscles derived from 122
senses related to 28
tanmātrās related to 28
eczema 65, 118, 241
edema
ambu vaha srotas and 185
manda agni and 92
rakta dhātu and 118
rasa dhātu and 112
salt taste and 242
sour taste and 241
srotāmsi and 180
sweet taste and 239
vyāna vāyu and 53
Water element and 15

ego **8**
    at cellular level 267
    as "I" memory 60
    majjā dhātu and 156
    sādhaka pitta and 60
ekagra mind 193
electrical energy 14
emaciation 110, 112, 127, 245
emotions 270-273
    accumulation of 147
    awareness of 280
    biochemical responses of 280
    bone marrow and 151
    honesty about 232
    in lungs 227
    māmsa dhātu and 129-130
    muscles expressing 123
    prāna and 227
    prāna vāyu and 49
    rañjaka pitta and 58
    rasa dhātu and 109
    repression of 86, 97
    sādhaka pitta and 60
    tears and 161
emphysema 50, 71
Empty Bowl Meditation 266
endocrine system
    dhātu for. See majjā dhātu
    ojas and 208
endometriosis 112, 148
endometrium 173
endurance 135, 147
enema 35, 184
energy
    directions associated with 17
    doshas corresponding to 29
    potent. See vīrya
    types of, from five elements 14
enlightenment 280
    birth and death cycle and 169
    glimpses of 199
    individual and universal 271
    opposite of 223
    postponement of 221
    sex and 175
enthusiasm

loss of 118
    rāga and 88
epididymis 171
Epstein Barr virus 165, 214
erysipelas 117
esophagus 182
estrogen 148, 173, 175
eternal quality of tejas 220
Ether element (ākāsha) **13**
    awareness and 226
    bhūta agni corresponding to 94
    at cellular level 267
    creation of 25
    dosha corresponding to 30
    foods corresponding to 236
    gunas associated with 9
    in human body 26
    motor organ related to 28
    tanmātrās related to 28
    See also prāna; vāta dosha
exercise
    asthi vaha srotas and 187
    blood flow to muscles during 122
    bowel movements requiring 190
    excessive 215
    guidelines according to doshas 279
    māmsa dhātu and 128
    recommended forms of 78
    role of fat and cholesterol in 132
exhalation 50, 183
extrasensory perception 60, 160
eyes
    ālochaka pitta and 63-64
    color of, rañjaka pitta and 57
    darshanam and 86
    desire and 170
    directly looking into 164
    element corresponding to 27
    movement of, while talking 164
    pitta dosha and 54, 55
    secretions of 161

F

fainting 242
faith 109, 110
fallopian tubes 173
fanaticism 269

farsightedness 64
fascia 125
fat
    amount of, measuring 133
    channel for. See meda vaha srotas
    characteristics of 132, 133
    dhātu for. See meda dhātu
    excess 133
    functions of 132, 133, 135
    ideal amount of 134, 138, 139
    locations of 133
    metabolism of 133, 136, 187
    See also obesity; weight
fatigue 90, 112
faulty cognition (bhrama) 11
fear
    Air element and 15
    ashauryam and 87
    awareness and 143
    blood vessels and 120
    laghu (light) guna and 32
    majjā dhātu and 163
    meda dhātu and 138
    muscle rigidity and 130
    observing 271
    ojas and 214
    ovulation and 172
    prāna vāyu and 50
    rūksha (dry) guna and 33
    rasa dhātu and 109
    relationship to 272
    srotāmsi and 181
    suppressing 272
    vāta dosha and 30, 39, 163
    vishama agni and 91
feces
    channel for. See purisha vaha srotas
    purisha agni for 101
feelings 270-273
    See also emotions
feet, temperature of 110, 118, 163
female energy. See Prakruti
female reproductive tissue
    channel for. See ārtava vaha srotas
    dhātu for. See ārtava dhātu
fetus

consciousness of 152, 153, 156
dhātu development in 264
gender of, determined during pregnancy
    264
kundalinī in 152
majjā dhātu and 152-155
mind and heart development of 38
ojas in 263-264
prāna in 153, 224, 263-264
prakruti of 37
samādhi experienced by 152
shukra dhātu in 263
tejas in 263-264
See also birth; pregnancy
fever 15, 111, 112
Fire element (agni) **13**
    bhūta agni corresponding to 94
    at cellular level 267
    creation of 26
    disorders of 15
    dosha corresponding to 30
    foods corresponding to 236
    gunas associated with 9
    in human body 26
    senses related to 28
    tanmātrās related to 28
    See also agni; pitta dosha; tejas
five elements 9, **12-15**
    agni and 83-84
    and tanmātrā 98
    bhūta agni associated with 59, 94
    at cellular level 267
    creation manifesting 25
    directions associated with 17
    doshas associated with 15
    energy associated with 14
    house arrangements based on 17
    in human body 26-27
    of individuals, required for health 15
    in rasa dhātu 107
    senses corresponding to 27-29
    taste made up of 236
    tridosha and 29
    See also Air element; Earth element;
        Ether element; Fire element;
        Water element

fluidity, quality of tejas 219
food
    balanced diet 258-260, 278-279
    channel for. See anna vaha srotas
    combining 260-261
    four types of 252
    gunas and 267
    intake of 143
    nutritional disorders 259
    qualities of, related to doshas 259
    See also appetite; cravings; digestion;
        rasa (taste)
forgiveness 30
form. See rūpa
Four Noble Truths 21

G
gallstones 59, 136, 137, 139, 146
gandha (smell) 9, 27
    agni and 83
    pitta dosha and 43
    srotāmsi for 178
Ganga 159
gastritis 57, 69, 91, 238, 240
gati, quality of tejas 220
Gautama (seer) 10
gemstones 250
gender determined during pregnancy 264
genetic disorders 142
genetic prakruti. See janma prakruti
genitals, element corresponding to 27
ghee
    and honey 261
    cholesterol and 132, 139
    during pregnancy 264
    prabhāva effects of 250
gingivitis 150
glaucoma 215
global majjā 160
God
    as Brāhma 21
    meditation and 212, 222
    nature of, Buddhism and 22
    nature of, Mīmāmsa philosophy and 18
    union with, Yoga philosophy and 19
golden mean 269
grand mal epilepsy 50

gravity, resisting 124
greed 30, 163
grief 130, 141, 161, 181
gross (sthūla) guna **35**, 44
guduchi, treatment using 165
gulwel sattva 165
gums
    bleeding 118, 181
    infection of 148
    receding 149
    strengthening 149
gunas (three universal) **8**
    Agnideva's tongues as 82
    food having qualities of 99, 267
    manas prakruti and 37
    in rasa dhātu 108
    See also rajas; sattva; tamas
gunas (twenty) **30-35**
    amino acids related to 98
    bhūta agnis and 95
    eight types of vīrya among 246
    See also specific gunas
guru (heavy) guna **32**, 44

H
hair
    asthi dhātu and 145
    asthi vaha srotas and 187
    color of, rañjaka pitta and 57
    heavy metals in 144
    pitta dosha and 54, 55
    pubic hair 145
    rasa dhātu and 109
    sweat glands near 192
hair loss 54, 138, 148, 242
hallucinations 157, 164
hands
    element corresponding to 27
    temperature of 110, 118, 163
hard (kathina) guna **34**, 44
harsha 87
head, prāna vāyu and 48
headache 111
health
    defined 275
    factors affecting 278-280
    individualized treatments for 2, 83, 167

hearing
    asthi dhātu and 144
    sādhaka pitta and 60
    srotāmsi for 178
heart 183, 238
    avalambaka kapha and 71
    cardiac muscles of 124
    prāna and 224
    prāna vāyu and 48
    sādhaka pitta and 59, 62
    vyāna vāyu and 53
heart attack 120, 150, 215
heart chakra 196, **200-201**
heartburn 15, 240, 243
heating vīrya 247
heavy (guru) guna **32**, 44
heavy metals, retained in asthi dhātu 144
hematoma 181, 213
hematopoietic system, ojas and 208
hemorrhoids 117, 249
hepatitis
    mūtra vaha srotas and 191
    meda dhātu and 141
    ojas kshaya and 214
    ojo visramsa and 213
    rakta dhātu and 115, 119
    rañjaka pitta and 59
hepatomegaly 117
herniation 127
herpes 119, 129, 165
high cholesterol 59
higher self (paramātman) 19
HIV 214
hives 112, 119
holiness 87
hot (ushna) guna **33**, 43
hot flashes 172
house, arranging according to elements 17
Hubble, Edwin Powell (astronomer) 21
hunger. See appetite
hyperacidity 57, 91, 242
hyperactivity 164
hyperglycemia 70
hypertension
    majjā dhātu and 165
    manda agni and 92

meda dhātu and 134, 136
obesity and 139
ojo vruddhi and 215
rakta dhātu and 117, 120
hyperthyroidism 134
hypoglycemia 57, 70, 91
hypothalamus 152, 155, 226
hypothermia 87
hypothetical argument (tarka) 11

I

identification 158
identity 156
    See also ego
ileocecal valve 190
illumination, quality of tejas 220
immune system 88
    agni and 81
    majjā dhātu and 165
    ojas and 88, 154, 208-210, 214
    rakta dhātu and 118
    tonsils and 127
impatience 89
indigestion 90, 91
individual mind 193, 198-200, 271
Indra (deity) 82
Indra (sage) 4
indriya agni **99**
indriya. See sensation; senses
infections 117
infectious diseases 180
inference (anumāna) **12**
inflammation 117
inflammatory diseases 180
inhalation 48, 183
injections, digestion of 93-94
inner reality, darshan associated with 5
insecurity
    asthi dhātu and 149
    chala (mobile) guna and 35
    food used to satisfy 143
    meda dhātu and 138
    ovulation and 172
    REM and 164
    srotāmsi and 181
insensitivity 34
insight 156

insomnia
    fever and 111
    majjā dhātu and 163
    meda dhātu and 138
    ovulation and 172
    pungent taste and 243
    vishama agni and 91
intelligence
    cellular. *See* cellular intelligence
    cosmic 229
    creative. *See* Mahad
    during crisis 218
    intellect and reasoning. *See* buddhi
    medhākāra and 89
    of the body 229
    pitta dosha and 30, 55
    pure. *See* tejas
    soma and 230
    See also knowledge; mind
intuition 193, 230
iritis 64
irrigation, first law of nutrition 262
ischemia 53

J

jāthara agni 84, **92-94**
    bhūta agni and 58
    pāchaka pitta and 56
    tastes stimulating 253
    tejas and 221
Jaimini (philosopher) 18
janma prakruti **36**, 38
jatru agni **96-97**
jaundice 115, 140, 191
jīvātman (lower self) 19
jñānamaya kosha 194
jñānashakti 9
jñānendriya 9
Jñana Yoga 19
joints
    cracking and popping 132, 138
    majjā vaha srotas and 188
    shleshaka kapha and 77
judgment 163

K

kāma dudha 165

Kāpila (seer) 5
kālā. *See* time
kāya agni. *See* jāthara agni
kāya chikitsā (internal medicine) 83
kalā 105
Kanāda (seer) 10, 230, 266-267
kapha dosha **29-30**, 276
    agni affected by 89, 90, 91
    agni of 100
    balanced 278
    biological clock of 279
    characteristics of 40, 44
    color associated with 87
    disorders of 66, 166-168, 180, 278
    elements associated with 15
    exercise guidelines for 279
    in fat 133
    interaction with other doshas 277
    locations of 65-67
    majjā dhātu and 166-168
    pure essence of. *See* ojas
    qualities of 65
    soma represented by 83
    subtypes of 65-78
    times of day associated with 16
    water requirements for 138
karma prakruti. *See* janma prakruti
Karma Yoga 19
karma, tejas and 221-223
karmas (actions) 25
karmendriya 9
kashāya. *See* astringent taste
kathina (hard) guna **34**, 44
katu. *See* pungent taste
khāmala 126
khavaigunya 180, 268
khāra (rough) guna **33**, 42
khadita type of food 252
kidney stones 146
kidneys
    agni of 101
    ambu vaha srotas and 184
    apāna vāyu and 52
    meda vaha srotas and 187
    salt taste and 237, 238
    water intake and 138

kitta. See mala by-product
kledaka kapha 68-70
    digestion and 84
    disorders of 69
    in jāthara agni 56
kloma agni **94**
knowledge 62
    ending of. See Vedānta philosophy
    experience as food of 197
    sādhaka pitta and 59, 62
    sources of 11-12
    See also intelligence
koshas 194-196
koshta agni. See jāthara agni
kriyāshakti 9
kshaya 89
kshipta mind 193
kundalinī shakti 176, 201
    fetus and 152
    tejas and 223-224

L

lactation
    channel for. See stanya vaha srotas
    rasa dhātu and 109
laghu (light) guna **32**, 42, 43
Lakshmi (deity) 184
lavana. See salty taste
laziness 37, 89, 239
leeches 119
legs, element corresponding to 27
lehya type of food 252
leprosy 166
lethargy 92
libido, low 132, 249
life force. See prāna
life span. See aging; longevity
life, definition and purpose of 1
lifestyle, balanced 279
light (laghu) guna **32**, 42, 43
light versus dark 199
lipomas 136, 139, 215
liquid (drava) guna **34**, 43, 44
liver
    agni in 94-96
    bitter taste and 238
    cirrhosis 136, 141

cleansing 140
enlarged 117, 141
fats processed by 140
māmsa dhātu and 128
pitta dosha and 54
rakta agni in 116
rakta dhātu and 114
rañjaka pitta and 57, 58
samāna vāyu and 51
testosterone and 139
loneliness 33, 70, 109, 149
longevity 41, 126, 135
    asthi dhātu and 147
    dīrgham and 89
    mercury and 108
    rakta dhātu and 117
    respiration and 17
    sweet taste and 239
    See also aging
love
    agni and 87
    awareness and 204, 211
    food's relationship to 134
    kapha dosha and 30, 41
    māmsa dhātu and 126
    meda dhātu and 134
    meditation and 132
    mrudu (soft) guna and 34
    rasa dhātu and 109
    sattva guna and 37
    sex and 175
    snigdha (oily) guna and 33
    soma and 270
    sweet taste and 239, 240
    transformation and 223
    See also sex
lower self (jīvātman) 19
lungs 183, 238
    avalambaka kapha and 71
    colon and 184
    emotions in 227
    grief and sadness in 141
    kapha dosha and 65
    prāna vāyu and 48
    udāna vāyu and 50
lupus 118

lymph fluids, movement of 123
lymphatic congestion 112
lymphatic system 184, 186
lymphomas 215

M
māmsa agni 97, 126, 129
māmsa dhātu **122-132**
    by-products of 125-127
    disorders of 127-129
    emotions and 129-130
    five elements in 122
    formation of 122
    functions of 123-125
    meda dhātu and 133
    meditation and 130-132
    qualities of 123
māmsa dhara kalā 125
māmsa kshaya 127
māmsa sāra 126
māmsa vaha srotas 178, 179, **186**
māmsa vruddhi 127
mātroshna 87
madhura. *See* sweet taste
maha agni. *See* jāthara agni
maha srotas 177
Mahad **6**, 200
majjā agni 97, 155
majjā dhātu **151-168**, 268
    awareness and 157, 158
    by-products of 161
    chakra system and 160
    disorders of 162-168
    dreams and 161
    ego and 156
    formation of 152, 155
    functions of 155-159
    kapha dosha and 166-168
    pitta dosha and 164-166
    prenatal development and 152-155
    senses and 155, 157
    vāta dosha and 163-164
majjā sāra 157
majjā vaha srotas 178, **188**
mala by-product 106
mala srotāmsi 179
mala vaha srotas. *See* purisha vaha srotas

malabsorption syndrome 52
malas, agni of **101**
male energy. *See* Purusha
male reproductive tissue
    channel for. *See* shukra vaha srotas
    dhātu for. *See* shukra dhātu
manas (sensory mind) 197, 198
    See also mind
manas prakruti **37-38**
manda (slow) guna **32**, 44
manda agni 90, **91**
mano sāra 203
mano vaha srotas 178, 179, **193-205**
manomaya kosha 194
mantras
    division removed by 199
    oral versus written 3
    prabhāva and 250
    sex and 176
    so'ham 222, 231
marijuana 121
marmāni 130, 193
marma point therapy 272
massage 130, 186, 271, 272
masturbation 175
material world. *See* physical world
mechanical energy 14
meda agni 97
meda dhātu 126, **132-143**
    awareness and 142-143
    by-products of 134-135
    disorders of 135-142
    five elements in 133
    formation of 134
    functions of 132-135
    māmsa dhātu and 133
meda sāra 135
meda vaha srotas 178, 179, **186-187**
medhāhāra 89
medhākāra 89
medicines, digestion of 93-94
meditation 211-213, 270-273, 280
    anaerobic breathing during 265
    awareness and 158, 168, 203, **204-205**
    Empty Bowl 266
    eye movements during 164

māmsa dhātu and 130-132
muscle stress and 130
physical consciousness and 159
postponement of 221
rakta dhātu and 121
respiration and 226
sex and 176
sound and 201
subconscious revealed by 16
tejas and 223
memory 198
day-to-day 268
genetic **268**, 270
lack of 50
of past lives 155
sādhaka pitta and 60
subconscious 268
tarpaka kapha and 75-76
thought as response of 271
udāna vāyu and 50
menopause 148, 187
menstrual irregularities 138
menstruation 173
apāna vāyu and 52
channel for. See rajah vaha srotas
profuse 119
rasa dhātu and 109, 111
mercury, as semen of Shiva 108, 171
metabolism 276
agni and 134
cellular 265-273
hyperactive 128
types of 90-92
typhoid affecting 135
vīrya and 247
See also digestion
Mīmāmsa philosophy 4, **18-19**, 22
mind **16**, 270-273
awareness and 197-198
chakra system and 195-196, 200-202
channel for. See mano vaha srotas
components of 197
five states of 193-194
layers of 194-195
perception and 197-198
prāna vāyu and 48-49

universal and individual 193, 198-200, 271
See also brain; intelligence
minerals
absorption of 145
deposits of 147
how much to take 150
metabolism of 147
mithuna 175
mobile (chala) guna **34**, 42, 43
mononucleosis 59, 119, 140, 165, 213, 214
moon (soma) 82-83, 228, 235
morphology 230
motor organs, elements corresponding to 28-29
motor pathways. See karmendriya
mouth 71-74
mrudu (soft) guna **34**, 44
mudrā 176
mukta mind 193
multiple sclerosis 66, 128, 166, 214
muscle hypertrophy 127
muscle pain 243
muscle wasting 214
muscles
channel for. See māmsa vaha srotas
coordination of 163
dhātu for. See māmsa dhātu
disorders of 128
kapha dosha and 67
ojas and 208
relaxation of 130
rigid 163
types of 124-125
mūdha mind 193
mūtra agni 101
mūtra vaha srotas 178, 185, **191-192**
myasthenia 127
myocarditis 127
myofibrosis 151
myomas 127
mysticism 168

N
nabhasa agni 59, 94, 95, 100
Nagarjuna (sage) 3
nails

asthi dhātu and 145
asthi vaha srotas and 187
condition of 145
disorders of 147
nasal crust 129
nausea 91, 92, 110, 111, 243
nava karna dravya (nine causative
substances) 10, **12-17**
navel 51, 152
neem toothpaste 149
nerve tissue
channel for. *See* majjā vaha srotas
dhātu for. *See* majjā dhātu
nervous system
majjā dhātu and 152
muscles controlled by 124
ojas and 208
sādhaka pitta and 62
tarpaka kapha and 74
nervousness
asthi dhātu and 149
majjā dhātu and 163
ovulation and 172
REM and 164
srotāmsi and 181
vāta dosha and 163
neuralgia 165
neuromuscular junction 125, 130, 165
neurotransmitters 159
nightmares 164
nine causative substances. *See* nava karna
dravya
nine gates of the body 5
nirvāna 22
nitya, quality of tejas 220
nose, element corresponding to 27
nuclear energy 14
number, quality of tejas 217
nutrition
guidelines for 258-260, 278-279
ojas, tejas, prāna related to 263-265
three laws of 261-262
See also food
nutritional disorders 259
Nyāya philosophy 4, **10-12**, 22

O
obesity
agni and 133
alcohol and 136
arthritis and 141
awareness and 143
backache and 141
body location of 140
depression and 140
early signs of 136
Earth element and 15
hypertension and 139
kledaka kapha and 70
lack of love and 135
manda agni and 92
meda dhātu and 136
meda vaha srotas and 187
ojas and 215
sadness and 141
steroids and 135
sthūla (gross) guna and 35
sweet taste and 237, 239
typhoid and 135
See also fat; weight
objective experience 158
odor. *See* gandha (smell)
oil
anemia treatment using 221
massage using 130, 271
vāta diseases and 47
oily (snigdha) guna **33**, 43, 44
ojah kāra 88
ojas 207, **208-215**
apara ojas 210, 214
balanced 276
beginning of, in fetus 263-264
depleted 214-215, 264
disorders of 213-215
displaced 213
disturbed 213-214
in egg cells 172
formation of 169, 208, 262
functional integrity with tejas and prāna
228-229
and the heart 171
in the newborn 154

increased 215
para ojas 210-213, 214
prāna governing 224
production of 88
protecting through awareness 232
repressed emotion and 270
shukra dhātu and 171
sweet taste and 239
types of 210-212
ojaskshaya 214-215
ojohāra 88
ojovisramsa 213
ojovruddhi 215
ojovyāpat 213-214
oleation treatment 219
omentum 134, 187
optic neuritis 66
order and chaos 229
original face 157
osteomas 151
osteoporosis
apāna vāyu and 52
asthi agni and 148
bitter taste and 244
meda dhātu and 135, 138
ojaskshaya and 214
shlakshna (slimy) guna and 33
outer reality. See physical world
ova 169, 242
ovaries 173
ovulation 52, 111, 173
oxygen, as food of prāna 229

P

pīlu pāka. See cellular metabolism
pāchaka pitta 55, 56-57, 69
pāchana. See digestion
pākvāshaya agni 95
pārthiva agni 94, 95, 100
Patañjali (pioneer of Yoga) 19
pakti 86
pallor 118
palpitations 49, 118, 214
pañchakarma 107, 119, 128, 130, 271
pancreas 94, 137, 184, 238
pancreatic cancer 129
Para Brahman 82

paralysis from stroke. See stroke paralysis
paralysis of muscles 128
paramātman (higher self) 19
paraplegia 128
parasites 73, 151, 244
parathyroid gland 146-147, 149
paratva, quality of tejas 218
parināma, quality of tejas 218
Parkinson's disease 50, 73, 77, 253
Patañjali 19
patience, dhairyam and 89
pelvis, apāna vāyu and 52
peptic ulcers 57, 243
perception **11**, 168, 197-198
diagnosis using 11
majjā dhātu and 157
past images affecting 156
prāna vāyu and 49
See also senses
periosteum 145, 147
peristalsis, increased or decreased 52
personality 227
petit mal epilepsy 50
peyam type of food 252
photophobia 64, 111
physical world, darshan associated with 4
picchila (sticky) guna **35**, 44
pīlu agni **98-99**, 266
pineal gland 210
pithara agni **99**
pithara pāka 266-268
pitta dosha **29-30**, 276
agni affected by 89, 90, 91
agni of 100
balanced 278
biological clock of 279
characteristics of 39, 43
color associated with 87
disorders of 164-166, 180, 278
elements associated with 15
exercise guidelines for 279
functions of 54
interaction with other doshas 277
locations of 53
majjā dhātu and 164-166
meditation and 131

pure essence of. See tejas
qualities of 53
sūrya represented by 83
subtypes of 53-65
water requirements for 137
pituitary gland 161, 175
plasma
ambu vaha srotas and 184
body wastes from 192
channel for. See rasa vaha srotas
dhātu for. See rasa dhātu
impurities of 192
kapha dosha and 65
pneumonia 50, 71
polarity therapy 272
polycythemia 118
possessiveness 30, 163
postponement, quality of tejas 219
potent energy. See vīrya
prāna 8, 13, 207, **224-227**
balanced 276
channel carrying. See prāna vaha srotas
cosmic 8, 82-83
in fetus 153, 224, 263-264
functional integrity with ojas and tejas
228-229
location of 226
ojas and 210
oxygen and 229
protecting through awareness 232
respiration and 224-226
soma and 229
time measured in 17
prāna vāyu 46, 47, 48-50
in brain function 60
disorders of 49
in jāthara agni 56
prāna vaha srotas 178, **183-184**, 227
prānāyāma 49, 265
prānakāra 88
prānamaya kosha 194
prabhā 89
prabhāva **249-250**
prajanana 168
prakruti (body type) **35-38**
categories of 36-38

development of 277
kapha characteristics 40, 44
pitta characteristics 39, 43
vāta characteristics 39, 42
Prakruti (Divine Mother) **6**
prāna bridging to Purusha 225
tanmātrās in womb of 28
unmanifested. See Brahman
prakruti sound 231
prakruti varna 87
prasāda 87
praspandanam 47
pratyaksha. See perception
pregnancy 263-265
apāna vāyu and 52
ghee during 264
ojas disorders during 215
rañjaka agni and 115
woman having two hearts during 153
See also birth; conception; fetus
premenopausal syndrome 112
premenstrual syndrome 112
priority, quality of tejas 218
procreation 168
progesterone 173
prostate, apāna vāyu and 52
pruthaktva, quality of tejas 218
pruthivī. See Earth element
psoriasis 118, 119, 241
psychology 272-273
pulse, indicating amount of fat 139
pungent stage of digestion 255, 257
pungent taste **242-243**
elements corresponding to 237
excessive intake of 237, 242
organs related to 237
pungent vipāka 249
pure Consciousness. See Brahman; Purusha
purgatives 35
purisha agni 97, 101
purisha vaha srotas 97, 178, **189-191**
Purusha **5**, 10
insight and 156
prāna bridging to Prakruti 225
unmanifested. See Brahman
pūrana 47

Pūrva Mīmāmsa philosophy 18
pyrexia 87

Q

quadriplegia 128
qualities. See gunas
quantum physics 230

R

rāga 88
radiant energy 14
radiation 151
rajah vaha srotas 178, **189**
rajas guna **8-10**
 foods associated with 99
 foods corresponding to 99
 manas prakruti and 37, 38
rakta agni 58, 59, 95, 97, 114, 116
rakta dhātu **113-122**
 by-products of 116-117
 disorders of 117-120
 formation of 105, 113, 114
 tastes in 116
rakta kshaya 118
rakta moksha (bloodletting) 119
rakta sāra 117
rakta vaha srotas 178, **186**
rakta vruddhi 117
rañjaka agni 59, 95
rañjaka pitta 57-59, 116
rapid eye movement 164
rasāyana chikitsā (rejuvenation therapy) 82
rasa (taste) 9, 27, **235-238**
 actions of 250
 astringent taste 244-245
 balancing 238
 bitter taste 243-244
 cravings for 246
 disorders of 110
 excessive use of 237
 five elements and 236
 kapha dosha and 44
 organs related to 237
 pitta dosha and 43, 54
 pungent taste 242-243
 rakta dhātu and 116
 rasa dhātu and 107

salty taste 241-242
 similar, but with different actions. See
  prabhāva
 sour taste 240-241
 srotāmsi for 178
 stages of digestion associated with 182,
  251, 252
 sweet taste 238-240
 tongue and 236
 tongue areas related to 237
 vīrya associated with 248
 vāta dosha and 42
 water and 235-236
 See also food
rasa agni 97, 107, 112
rasa dhātu **107-113**
 by-products of 112
 disorders of 110-112
 emotions and 109
 five elements in 107
 formation of 105
 function of 108
 gunas in 108
 kapha dosha in 111
 qualities of 108
 tastes in 107
 vāta dosha in 107, 111
rasa kshaya 111
rasa sāra 108, 109
rasa vaha srotas 178, **185-186**
rasa vruddhi 112
rashes 112, 117, 119, 241
reality, compared to truth 61
reasoning capacity, buddhikāra and 88
rectum, apāna vāyu and 52
red blood cells 114-116
 dhātu for. See rakta dhātu
reflexes, vyāna vāyu and 53
reincarnation
 asthi dhātu and 147
 desire and 269
 past life, babys experiencing 154
rejuvenation therapy. See rasāyana chikitsā
relationships
 agni and 88
 balanced 279

clarity in 203
judgment and 160
ojas and 210
purpose of 77
sex and 176, 279
as a srotas 181
tarpaka kapha and 77
relaxation 32, 33, 131
reproductive tissue
channels for. *See* ārtava vaha srotas;
shukra vaha srotas
dhātus for. *See* ārtava dhātu; shukra
dhātu
See also pregnancy; sex
respiration 183
meditation and 226
prāna and 224-226
prānakāra and 88
rate of 265
undue awareness of 49
respiratory tract
avalambaka kapha and 71
kapha dosha and 65
restlessness 34
rheumatic fever 214
rheumatism 127
rishis (seers) 3
root chakra 175, 196, 200
rough (khāra) guna **33**, 42
rūksha (dry) guna **33**, 42
rūpa (form) 9, 27
rūpa, quality of tejas 217

S

sādhaka agni 87
sādhaka pitta 59-63
sunlight and 140
tarpaka kapha and 74
sānkhya, quality of tejas 217
Sānkhya philosophy 4, **5-10**, 22, 220
sāra by-product 106
SAD (Seasonal Affective Disorder) 140
sadness
aharsha and 87
kledaka kapha and 70
majjā dhātu and 161
muscle rigidity and 130

obesity and 141
rasa dhātu and 111
srotāmsi and 181
saliva, excess 253
salty stage of digestion 254, 257
salty taste **241-242**
elements corresponding to 237
excessive intake of 237, 241
organs related to 237
samādhi 20, 158
agni and 81
fetus experiencing 152
sex and 176
soma and 210
sweet taste and 239
samāna vāyu 84
sama agni **90**
samāna vāyu 46, 51-52
disorders of 52
in jāthara agni 56
viveka and 47
samshaya (doubt) 11
samyoga, quality of tejas 218
sandra (dense) guna **34**, 44
sanga 180
sattva guna **8-10**
foods associated with 99
indicating health 276
manas prakruti and 37, 38
schizophrenia 164
sciatic nerve, apāna vāyu and 52
sciatica 91, 165
scoliotic changes 151
Seasonal Affective Disorder (SAD) 140
seasons, doshas corresponding to 32
seers (rishis) 3
selectivity, second law of nutrition 262
selfishness 34
sensation
prāna vāyu and 49
sādhaka pitta and 60
senses
as agents of the mind 198
agnis of 99
city of. *See* Purusha
five elements corresponding to 27-29

impaired perception of 100
majjā dhātu and 155, 157
mano vaha srotas and 193
objects of. See tanmātrās
pathways of. See jñānendriya
srotāmsi associated with 178
See also gandha (smell); hearing;
    perception; rasa (taste); sparsha
    (touch); vision
separation, quality of tejas 218
septicemia 213
sex 171, 175-176
apāna vāyu and 52
excessive 215
frequency of 174
low libido 132, 249
role of, in life 279
timing of 279
See also love; reproductive tissue
sexual debility 110, 242
shabda (sound) 9, 27
sādhaka pitta and 60
soma and 231
shabda (testimony) **12**
Shad Darshan 2, **4-5**
Mīmāmsa philosophy 4, 18-19, 22
Nyāya philosophy 4, 10-12, 22
Sānkhya philosophy 4, 5-10, 22, 220
Vaisheshika philosophy 4, 10, 12-17, 22,
    221, 266
Vedānta philosophy 4, 20-21, 22
Yoga philosophy 4, 19-20, 23
Shakti 10
sharp (tīkshna) guna **32**, 43
shatāvarī, treatment using 165
shauryam 87
shīta (cold) guna **33**, 42, 44
shilājit, treatment using 146
shingles 165
Shiva (deity) 82
mercury as semen of 108, 171
soma as 274
shlakshna (smooth) guna **33**, 44
shleshaka kapha 68, 77-78
shleshma 65
See also kapha dosha

shortsightedness 64
shukra agni 97
shukra dhātu 168, **169-172**
by-products of 169
disorders of 174
in fetus 263
formation of 169
shukra vaha srotas 178, **188**
sickle cell anemia 119, 166, 214
sirā granthi 180
Six Philosophies. See Shad Darshan
skeletal muscles 124, 125
skeletal system, ojas and 208
skin
bhrājaka pitta and 64-65
bleeding 118
color of, rañjaka pitta and 57
desire and 170
discoloration of 119
dry 33, 91, 118, 138, 249
element corresponding to 27
layers of 186
māmsa dhātu and 125
majjā dhātu in 159
oily 136
pitta dosha and 55
pungent taste and 243
rakta dhātu and 125
rasa dhātu and 109, 125
salty taste and 242
sour taste and 241
sweat glands in 192
vāta dosha and 47
wrinkling 110
sleep 34
deep 158
disorders of, meda dhātu and 141
excessive 239
insufficient 128
kledaka kapha and 70
mrudu (soft) guna and 34
sleep apnea 50
slimy guna. See smooth (shlakshna) guna
slow (manda) guna **32**, 44
small intestine
agni and 84, 93

pāchaka pitta and 56
pitta dosha and 54
samāna vāyu and 51
smegma 129
smell. *See* gandha
smooth (shlakshna) guna **33**, 44
smooth muscles 124
snāyu (tendons) 134
snigdha (oily) guna **33**, 43, 44
so'ham mantra 222, 231
soft (mrudu) guna **34**, 44
soma **82-83**, **229-231**
cellular 266
global life and 160, 228
ojas and 210, 212
unprocessed and desire 269
sore throat 33
soul (ātman) **15**
in egg 172
in sperm 170
sound. *See* shabda
soundless sound (Aum) 25
sour stage of digestion 254, 257
sour taste **240-241**
elements corresponding to 237
excessive intake of 237, 240
organs related to 237
sour vipāka 249
Space element. *See* Ether element
spandanam 47
sparsha (touch) 9, 27
quality of tejas 217
srotāmsi for 178
speech difficulties 50
speech, udāna vāyu and 50
sperm 170
apāna vāyu and 52
bitter taste and 244
kapha dosha and 68
pungent taste and 242
pungent vipāka and 249
as subtle atomic cell 169
spina bifida 37
spinal cord
majjā dhātu in 152
majjā vaha srotas and 188

sexual energy and 175
spine
alignment of 151
avalambaka kapha and 71
tarpaka kapha and 74
spleen 238
enlarged 117, 141
pitta dosha and 54
rakta agni in 116
rakta dhātu and 114
rañjaka pitta and 57
splenitis 119
splenomegaly 117
srotāmsi 97, **177-180**
disorders of 180-181
roles of 178
senses associated with 178
srotas. *See* srotāmsi
sroto agni 97
sroto mūla **178**
sroto mārga **178**
sroto mukha **178**
stamina 134, 147
stanya vaha srotas 178, 189
static (sthira) guna **34**, 44
steatorrhea 137
sterility, male 170
steroids 135
sthāyi dhātu 105, 262
sthāyi rasa 107
sthira (static) guna **34**, 44
sthūla (gross) guna **35**, 44
sticky (picchila) guna **35**, 44
stomach 182
agni in 84, 93
capacity of, three parts in 143
kledaka kapha and 68, 69-70
pāchaka pitta and 56
pitta dosha and 54
pungent taste and 238
rañjaka pitta and 57, 58
stools, quality of 191
strength 34
asthi dhātu and 147
bala and 89
kapha dosha and 41

rasa dhātu and 109
    sandra (dense) guna and 34
    stamina 126
stress 130, 164, 270
stroke paralysis 166
    astringent taste and 245
    majjā dhātu and 166
    prāna vāyu and 50
    rakta dhātu and 120
    sweet taste and 239
    tarpaka kapha and 77
styes 64
subconscious mind 270
subcutaneous fat 125
subdoshas 45
subjective experience 158
subtle (sūkshma) guna **35**, 42
suffering 21, 22, 223-224
sun **82-83**, 228
    as father of water 235
    tejas and 216, 217, 221
Sushruta Samhitā text 3
sūkshma (subtle) guna **35**, 42
sūrya. See sun
sūtras 3
sveda agni 101
sveda vaha srotas 178, 185, **192-193**
swallowing, difficulty 129
sweat
    channel for. See sveda vaha srotas
    movement of 123
    pitta dosha and 54
    sveda agni for 101
    as treatment 271
    urine and 192
sweat glands 184
sweet stage of digestion 253, 257
sweet taste 184, **238-240**
    digestion of 94
    elements corresponding to 237
    excessive intake of 237, 239
    organs related to 237
sweet vipāka 248
synaptic cleft 125, 130
synaptic space 159, 188, 267

T

tamas guna **8-10**
    foods associated with 99
    manas prakruti and 37, 38
tanmātrā 9, **27-29**, 98, 100
tantra 176
tarka (hypothetical argument) 11
tarpaka kapha 60, 68, **74-77**, 140
taste. See rasa
tea tree oil 149
tears 161, 188
teeth 182
    asthi dhātu and 145
    cavities in 148
    grinding of 151
    organs connected to 149
    sensitivity of 148, 240
    tartar on 136
teething 148
tejah kāra 88
tejas 207, **216-224**
    āpya tejas 220, 221
    agni tejas 220
    balanced 276
    beginning of, in fetus 263-264
    bhaumī tejas 220
    color quality of 217
    dimension quality of 218
    distinction quality of 218
    divya tejas 221
    dravyamaya tejas 221
    eternal quality of 220
    fluidity quality of 219
    formation of 88
    functional integrity with ojas and prāna 228-229
    illumination quality of 220
    karma and 221-223
    kundalinī shakti and 223-224
    manifestations of 220-221
    number quality of 217
    ojas disturbed by 215
    ojas quality maintained by 213, 216
    postponement quality of 219
    prāna governing 224
    priority quality of 218

protecting through awareness 232
qualities of 217-220
role in formation of ojas 208, 210
separation quality of 218
touch quality of 217
udaraka tejas 221
union quality of 218
upward quality of 220
vāyu tejas 220
velocity quality of 220
tejo agni 59, 94, 95, 100
tendons 125
testicles 52, 169, 170
testimony (shabda) **12**
testosterone 139, 175
third eye 196, 201
thirst
excessive 136, 137, 240
sweet taste and 239
thoughts 270-273
throat 33
prāna vāyu and 48
udāna vāyu and 50
throat chakra 196, 201
thymus gland 96, 127
thyroid gland
agni in 96
asthi dhātu and 146-147, 149
majjā dhātu and 161
meda dhātu and 135
sweet taste and 238
tīkshna (sharp) guna **32**, 43
tīkshna agni 90, **91**
tikta ghrita 166
tikta. See bitter taste
time **16**
doshas and 279
perception and 227
tarpaka kapha and 76
thought and 156
tissues. See dhatus
tongue 182
bodhaka kapha and 72-73
dark coating of 182
element corresponding to 27
enlarged 127

taste areas on 237
tonsillitis 127
tonsils
bodhaka kapha and 73
māmsa dhātu and 127
toothpaste 149
touch. See sparsha
transformation, third law of nutrition 262
trauma
asthi dhātu affected by 147
asthi vaha srotas affected by 187
to head 63, 77
incorrect eating resulting from 143
māmsa dhātu affected by 128
ojas affected by 215
personality changes resulting from 75
treatment, individualized 2, 83, 167
tremors 243
tridosha. See doshas
trigeminal neuralgia 166
triphala 238
triphala tea 73, 149
truth 160
Four Noble Truths 21
Mīmāmsa philosophy and 18
Nyāya philosophy and 10
perceiving through your eyes 64
sādhaka pitta and 61-62
Sānkhya philosophy and 5
shabda as 12
Vaisheshika philosophy and 10
tuberculosis 128, 214, 215
tumors 180, 239
24 principles of Sānkhya 5
typhoid 128, 135, 215

U
udāna vāyu 46, 47, 50
udaka vaha srotas. See ambu vaha srotas
udaraka tejas 221
udvahana 47
ulcerative colitis 215, 240
ulcers 15
kapha dosha and 68
kledaka kapha and 69, 70
salt taste and 242
sour taste and 241

srotāmsi and 181
tīkshna (sharp) guna and 33
unconsciousness 214
unctuous guna. See oily (snigdha) guna
understanding 30, 33
union, quality of tejas 218
universal attributes. See gunas (three
  universal)
universal mind 193, 198-200, 271
universe. See brāhmanda
upadhātus by-product 106
upamāna (comparison) **12**
upanishad 18, 21
     See also Vedānta philosophy
Upa-Vedas 3
upward movement, quality of tejas 220
urethra, apāna vāyu and 52
urinary disorders 52
urinary tract
     agni of 101
     apāna vāyu and 52
urine
     channel for. See mūtra vaha srotas
     color of 191
     mūtra agni for 101
     movement of 123
     nighttime passing of 129, 181
     passing infrequently 181
     spasm during passing of 136
     sweat and 192
urticaria 112, 119
ushna (hot) guna **33**, 43
uterus 173
Uttara Mīmāmsa philosophy 18
ūrdhva gamitva, quality of tejas 220

V

Vāgbhata (physician) 4
vāta dosha **29-30**, 276
     elements associated with 15
     agni affected by 89, 90, 91
     agni of 100
     anila represented by 83
     balanced 278
     biological clock of 279
     characteristics of 39, 42
     color associated with 87

disorders of 47, 67, 163-164, 180, 278
entering rasa dhātu 107
exercise guidelines for 279
functions of 47
interaction with other doshas 277
locations of 45, 47
majjā dhātu and 163-164
pure essence of. See prāna
qualities of 45
subtypes of 45-53
times of day associated with 16
water requirements for 138
vāyavya agni 59, 94, 95, 100
vāyu. See Air element
vāyu tejas 220
vadavanala 83
vagina, apāna vāyu and 52
Vaisheshika philosophy 4, **10**, **12-17**, 22,
  221, 266
vaishvānala 83
varicose veins 150, 180
vastu shilpa shāstra 17
Vedānta philosophy 4, **20-21**, 22
Vedas (scriptures) 2
vegetarianism 269
velocity, quality of tejas 220
vibhāga, quality of tejas 218
vīrya (potent energy) **246-248**, 250
vijñānamaya kosha 195
vikruti **36**
vikruti varna 87
vikshipta mind 193
vimārga gamanam 180
vipāka (post-digestive effect) **248-249**, 250
virāga 88
vishāda 87
vishada (clear) guna **35**, 42
vishama agni 90, **91**
vishnu 228
Vishnu (deity) 82
vision 27, 28, 178
visramsa 207
visualization 143
vitamin C 240
vitamins, how much to take 150
viveka 47

vocal cords, element corresponding to 27
void, the 226
vomiting 91, 92, 242
vyāna vāyu 46, 47, 53
vyakta 6

W
water
    amount needed 137
    channel for. *See* ambu vaha srotas
    digestion of 185
Water element (āpas) **14**
    agni in 83
    bhūta agni corresponding to 94
    at cellular level 267
    creation of 26
    disorders of 15
    doshas corresponding to 30
    foods corresponding to 236
    gunas associated with 9
    in human body 27
    moon as mother of 235
    muscles derived from 122
    senses related to 28
    sun as father of 235
    tanmātrās related to 28
    taste and 235-236
    See also kapha dosha; ojas
water retention 34, 41, 110, 127, 172
weight
    difficulty gaining 141
    gaining 128
    ideal 142
    loss of 214
    See also fat; obesity
Western medicine 2
worms 73, 151, 244
wrinkles 242

Y
yantra 176
Yoga philosophy 4, **19-20**, 23
Yoga Sūtras of Patañjali 19

Established to promote the traditional knowledge of Ayurveda, **The Ayurvedic Institute** also offers programs in the sister disciplines of Ayurveda—Sanskrit, Yoga and Jyotisha. The knowledge is taught with the body, mind and spiritual components intact, along with practical examples, ceremonies and stories.

The **Education Department** presents the nine-month residential Ayurvedic Studies Programs, Levels I and II, as well as advanced study in India. Our Ayurvedic Online Learning Program continuing education and professional development courses. Also available are the Ayurvedic correspondence course *Lessons & Lectures on Ayurveda* by Robert E. Svoboda, BAMS, and various weekend and intensive seminars with Vasant Lad, BAM&S, MASc and others.

The Herb Department has Ayurvedic and Western herbs, audio and video tapes from our programs, books, incense, and a variety of Ayurvedic and other products.

The Panchakarma Department provides traditional Ayurvedic procedures for purification and rejuvenation that include oil massage, herbal steam treatment, shirodhara, cleansing diet, herbal therapy, and other treatments.

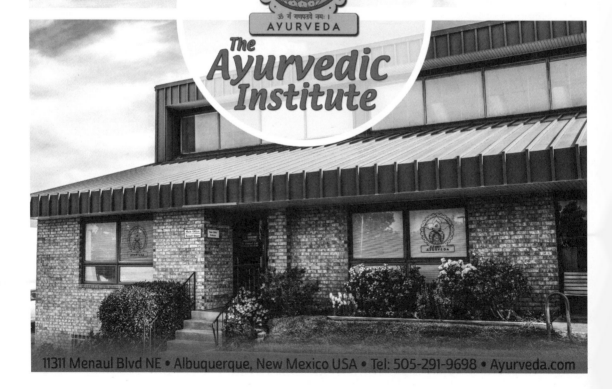

11311 Menaul Blvd NE • Albuquerque, New Mexico USA • Tel: 505-291-9698 • Ayurveda.com

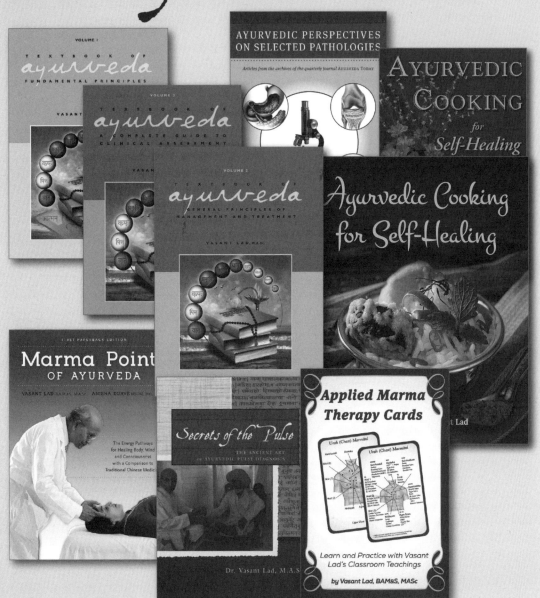

The Ayurvedic Press

VOLUME 1

TEXTBOOK OF *ayurveda*
FUNDAMENTAL PRINCIPLES

VOLUME 2

TEXTBOOK OF *ayurveda*
A COMPLETE GUIDE TO CLINICAL ASSESSMENT

VOLUME 3

TEXTBOOK OF *ayurveda*
GENERAL PRINCIPLES OF MANAGEMENT AND TREATMENT
VASANT LAD, M.A.Sc.

AYURVEDIC PERSPECTIVES ON SELECTED PATHOLOGIES
Articles from the archives of the quarterly journal AYURVEDA TODAY

AYURVEDIC COOKING for Self-Healing

Ayurvedic Cooking for Self-Healing

FIRST PAPERBACK EDITION

Marma Points OF AYURVEDA
VASANT LAD BAM&S, MASc   ANISHA DURVE MSOM, DiplAc

The Energy Pathways for Healing Body, Mind and Consciousness with a Comparison to Traditional Chinese Medicine

Secrets of the Pulse
THE ANCIENT ART OF AYURVEDIC PULSE DIAGNOSIS

Dr. Vasant Lad, M.A.S

Applied Marma Therapy Cards

Learn and Practice with Vasant Lad's Classroom Teachings

by Vasant Lad, BAM&S, MASc

To Place an Order Call 800-863-7721 or Visit Ayurveda.com

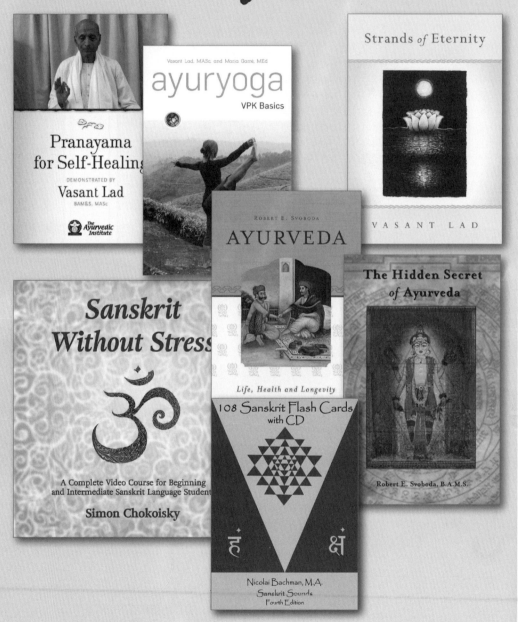